γ-Linolenic Acid

Metabolism and Its Roles
in Nutrition and Medicine

γ-Linolenic Acid

Metabolism and Its Roles in Nutrition and Medicine

Editors

Yung-Sheng Huang
Abbott Laboratories
Columbus, Ohio

David E. Mills
University of New Mexico
New Mexico Department of Health
Albuquerque, New Mexico

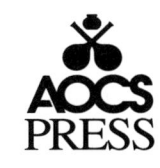

Champaign, Illinois

AOCS Mission Statement

To be a forum for the exchange of ideas, information, and experience among those with a professional interest in the science and technology of fats, oils, and related substances in ways that promote personal excellence and provide high standards of quality.

AOCS Books and Special Publications Committee

E. Perkins, chairperson, University of Illinois, Urbana, Illinois
J. Bauer, Texas A&M University, College Station, Texas
N.A.M. Eskin, University of Manitoba, Winnipeg, Manitoba
W. Farr, Owensboro Grain Co., Owensboro, Kentucky
T. Foglia, USDA—ERRC, Philadelphia, Pennsylvania
L. Johnson, Iowa State University, Ames, IA
Y.-S. Huang, Ross Laboratories, Columbus, Ohio
J. Lynn, Lever Brothers Co., Edgewater, New Jersey
G. Maerker, Oreland, Pennsylvania
M. Mossoba, Food and Drug Administration, Washington, D.C.
G. Nelson, Western Regional Research Center, San Francisco, California
F. Orthoefer, Stuttgart, Arkansas
J. Rattray, University of Guelph, Guelph, Ontario
A. Sinclair, Deakin University, Geelong, Victoria, Australia
G. Szajer, Akzo Chemicals, Dobbs Ferry, New York
B. Szuhaj, Central Soya Co., Inc., Fort Wayne, Indiana
L. Witting, State College, Pennsylvania

Copyright © 1996 by AOCS Press. All rights reserved. No part of this book may be reproduced or transmitted in any form or by any means without written permission of the publisher.

The paper used in this book is acid-free and falls within the guidelines established to ensure permanence and durability.

Library of Congress Cataloging-in-Publication Data

International Symposium of GLA (1st : 1995 : San Antonio, Tex.)
    Gamma-linolenic acid/Yung-Sheng Huang and David E. Mills, editors.
        p. cm.
    "Proceedings of the First International Symposium of GLA, held in conjunction with the annual meeting of the AOCS in San Antonio, Texas during May 7–11. 1995"--Pref.
    Includes bibliographical references and index.
    ISBN 0–935315–68–3 (alk. paper)
    1. Linolenic acids—Physiological effects—Congresses.
2. Linolenic acids—Therapeutic use—Testing—Congresses.
I. Huang, Yung-Sheng, Dr. II. Mills, David E. III. Title.
QP752.L515I58 1995
612'.01577—dc20   96-15494
                                                                                   CIP

Printed in the United States of America with vegetable oil-based inks.

00 99 98 97 96 5 4 3 2 1

Acknowledgments

The AOCS Health and Nutrition Division and the Organizing Committee would like to thank the following organizations for their generous contribution: Abbott Laboratories, Ross Products Division, Medical Nutritional Research and Development, Columbus, Ohio; Bioriginal Food and Science Corporation, Saskatoon, Saskatchewan, Canada; Hoffman-La Roche Ltd., Mississauga, Ontario, Canada; Nestlé Ltd., Lausanne, Switzerland; Nippon Gohsei, Osaka, Japan; Rokin bv, Zaandam, The Netherlands; and Scotia Pharmaceuticals Ltd., Guilford, England.

The editor (YSH) is greatly indebted to Mr. Kulow, president of Bioriginal Food and Science Corp., Saskatchewan, Canada, for his help in soliciting funds, inviting speakers, and co-chairing the three lengthy meeting sessions. He is also very grateful to Ms. Mary Lane, Director of the AOCS Press, for her invaluable advice and - constant encouragement.

We wish to acknowledge the great assistance provided by members of the AOCS Books and Special Publication Committee, and the AOCS staff in Champaign, Illinois. Finally, we wish to express our deep appreciation to all of the authors. Through scientific evidence, these authors have demonstrated comprehensively the dynamic relationship between dietary γ-linolenic acid and the biological system.

Yung-Shung Huang
David E. Mills

Preface

The essentiality of long-chain n-6 fatty acids is well recognized. In humans, linoleic acid (LA) is metabolized to n-6 polyunsaturated fatty acids (PUFAs) and other 20-carbon eicosanoids, which play vital roles in normal physiological functions. Because of an abundance of LA in the diet, one tends to assume that the formation of long-chain n-6 PUFAs is adequate. This is far from the truth because the process of converting LA to long-chain metabolites is rate-limited by the activity of Δ6-desaturase, whose activity is further modulated by many nutritional and physiological factors. Under these circumstances, even if the intake of LA is adequate, the depressed Δ6-desaturase activity may substantially reduce the formation of long-chain n-6 PUFAs, and subsequently, result in a state of functional n-6 essential fatty acid deficiency. Clinical evidence has associated this deficiency with many pathological conditions. Fortunately, this inadequacy may be alleviated by dietary supplementation of γ-linolenic acid (GLA), the Δ6-desaturation product of LA.

GLA was first isolated from the evening primrose. This herbal plant was traditionally used by the Native Americans to treat various diseases, and later discovered by the European settlers. In the 17th century, this plant was transplanted to Europe and became a popular folk remedy. Its wide range of use as a general vulnerary and treatment earned it the name of "king's cureall". When the oil was first extracted from the evening primrose in 1919, Heiduschka and Lueft reported the presence of an unusual linolenic acid which yielded a hexabromide derivative of linolenic acid with very different physical characteristics from the other two common forms (α- and β-isomers) found in linseed oil. Thus, they named it γ-isomer, or gamma-linolenic acid (GLA). The exact chemical structure of GLA was later characterized by Eibner et al. (1927) and verified by Riley in 1949. Since then, GLA has been found in many other plants, fungi, algae, and microorganisms.

During the past 20 years, interest in the potential of GLA for medical use has grown rapidly, but not without great skeptism. Even the nutritional value of GLA was frequently criticized by some nutritionists. Nonetheless, the number of researchers engaged in GLA research has significantly increased, and, in many parts of the world, GLA has been accepted as a health food or a prescription drug.

It was this continued growing interest in GLA that convinced the Health and Nutrition Division of the American Oil Chemists' Society that it would be most timely and informative to the public to convene an international conference to examine the biological value of GLA. Yung-Sheng Huang of Ross Products Division, Abbott Laboratories, and Mr. Frederick of Bioriginal Food and Science Corporation were given the responsibility of organizing this meeting. Subsequently, the First International Symposium of GLA was held in conjunction with the annual meeting of the AOCS in San Antonio, Texas, May 7–11, 1995. This meeting brought together many world-renowned experts who explored in depth the biochemistry, metabolism, nutritional, and clinical uses of GLA. This monograph represents the record of that symposium. The book is divided into seven major areas, Source and Biosynthesis, Absorption and Metabolism, Inflammation and Immune Response, Cardiovascular Disease and Hypertensions, Development, Diabetes and Cancer, and Regulatory Status. Each area includes several relevant chapters.

Yung-Sheng Huang and David E. Mills
Editors

Contents

Preface vii

Source and Biosynthesis

Chapter 1 Natural Source and Biosynthesis of γ-Linolenic Acid:
An Overview. 1
James C. Phillips and Yung-Sheng Huang

Chapter 2 Pathways for the Biosynthesis of Polyunsaturated Fatty Acids. . . 14
*Howard Sprecher, Devanand Luthria, Svetla P. Baykousheva,
and B. Selma Mohammed*

Chapter 3 Biosynthesis of γ-Linolenic Acid in the Cyanobacterium
Spirulina platensis. 22
Norio Murata, Patcharaporn Deshnium, and Yasushi Tasaka

Chapter 4 Enzymatic Enrichment of γ-Linolenic Acid from Black Currant
Seed Oil 33
H.-J. Wille and J. Wang

Absorption and Metabolism

Chapter 5 Transport of Long-Chain Polyunsaturated Fatty Acids Across
the Human Placenta: Role of Fatty Acid-Binding Proteins 42
*Assim K. Dutta-Roy, Fiona M. Campbell, Samson Taffesse,
and Margaret J. Gordon*

Chapter 6 Absorption of γ-Linolenic Acid from Borage, Evening Primrose,
and Black Currant Seed Oils. Fatty Acid Profiles, Triacylglycerol
Structures, and Clearance Rates of Chylomicrons in the Rat 54
Carl-Erik Høy and Michael S. Christensen

Chapter 7 Metabolism of [3-^{13}C]γ-Linolenic Acid in the Suckling Piglet
and Rat. 66
*Stephen C. Cunnane, J. Vogt, S.S. Likhodii, G. Moine,
R. Muggli, K.-H. Tovar, G. Kohn, and G. Sawatzki*

Chapter 8 *In Vivo* and *In Vitro* Metabolism of Linoleic and
γ-Linolenic Acids 84
*Yung-Sheng Huang, David E. Mills, Richard C. Cantrill,
and Jean-Pierre Poisson*

Inflammation and Immune Response

Chapter 9 γ-Linolenic Acid and Immune Function 106
Dayong Wu and Simin N. Meydani

Chapter 10 The Biological/Nutritional Significance of γ-Linolenic Acid in the Epidermis: Metabolism and Generation of Potent Biological Modulators 118
V.A. Ziboh

Chapter 11 γ-Linolenic Acid, Inflammation, Immune Responses, and Rheumatoid Arthritis 129
Robert B. Zurier, Pamela DeLuca, and Deborah Rothman

Chapter 12 The Anti-Inflammatory Role of γ-Linolenic and Eicosapentaenoic Acids in Acute Lung Injury 137
Michael D. Karlstad, John D. Palombo, Michael J. Murray, and Stephen J. DeMichele

Cardiovascular Disease and Hypertension

Chapter 13 Effects of Feeding a Supplement of γ-Linolenic Acid Containing Oils with Fish Oil on the Fatty Acid Composition of Serum Phospholipids in Healthy Volunteers. 168
Armand Christophe

Chapter 14 Comparative Evaluation of the Hypocholesterolemic Effect of Octadecatrienoic Acids 175
Michihiro Sugano and Ikuo Ikeda

Chapter 15 γ-Linolenic Acid Attenuates Blood Pressure Responses to Environmental Stimuli: Implications for Human Essential Hypertension. 189
David E. Mills, Yung-Sheng Huang, and Jean-Pierre Poisson

Chapter 16 γ-Linolenic Acid: A Potent Blood Pressure Lowering Nutrient . . 200
Marguerite M. Engler

Chapter 17 Impact of Dietary γ-Linolenic Acid on Macrophage-Smooth Muscle Cell Interaction: Down-Regulation of Vascular Smooth Muscle Cell DNA Synthesis 218
Robert S. Chapkin, Yang-Yi Fan, and Kenneth S. Ramos

Development

Chapter 18 Effects of γ-Linolenic Acid on Brain Fatty Acid Composition and Behavior in Mice 227
Patricia E. Wainwright and Yung-Sheng Huang

Chapter 19 γ-Linolenic Acid in Infant Formula 246
G.L. Crozier, M. Fleith, and M.-C. Secretin

Diabetes and Cancer

Chapter 20 γ-Linolenic Acid Biosynthesis and Chain Elongation
in Fasting and Diabetes Mellitus. 252
*Jean-Pierre Poisson, Michel Narce, Yung-Sheng Huang,
and David E. Mills*

Chapter 21 Essential Fatty Acids in the Management
of Diabetic Neuropathy 273
David F. Horrobin

Chapter 22 Anti-Cancer Actions of γ-Linolenic Acid with Particular
Reference to Human Brain Malignant Glioma 282
U.N. Das

Chapter 23 Metabolism of Li-γ-Linolenate (LiGLA) in Human Prostate,
Ovarian, and Pancreatic Carcinomas Grown in Nude Mice 293
*R.J. de Antueno, M. Elliot, K. Jenkins, G.W. Ells,
and D.F. Horrobin*

Regulatory Status

Chapter 24 Global Regulatory Status of γ-Linolenic Acid 304
F.C. Kulow

Index 311

Chapter 1

Natural Sources and Biosynthesis of γ-Linolenic Acid: An Overview

James C. Phillips[a] and Yung-Sheng Huang[b]

[a]Pediatric Nutritional Research and Development and
[b]Medical Nutritional Research and Development,
Ross Products Division, Abbott Laboratories,
Columbus, OH

Introduction

The chemical formula of γ-linolenic acid is shown in Figure 1.1.

```
Δ        18  17  16  15  14  13  12  11  10   9   8   7   6   5   4   3   2   1
         CH₃·CH₂·CH₂·CH₂·CH₂·CH=CH·CH₂·CH=CH·CH₂·CH=CH·CH₂·CH₂·CH₂·CH₂·COOH
n- or ω   1   2   3   4   5   6   7   8   9  10  11  12  13  14  15  16  17  18
```

Fig. 1.1. Chemical structure of γ-linolenic acid

Like other natural polyunsaturated fatty acids, the three double bonds in γ-linolenic acid are arranged in a methylene-interrupted fashion and are of *cis* configuration. According to the delta (Δ) nomenclature system, this fatty acid can be expressed as all-*cis*-6,9,12-octadecatrienoic acid or *c*6,*c*9,*c*12-octadecatrienoic acid where *c* indicates the *cis*-configuration, and the numbers (6, 9, and 12) indicate the positions of double bonds related to the carboxyl carbon of the acyl chain (-COOH). This systematic name can also be simplified to 18:3 (Δ6,9,12), 18:3 (Δ6,9,12), 18:3 (6,9,12), or 6,9,12-18:3, where 18 indicates the number of total carbon atoms, and 3 represents the number of double bonds in the molecule. However, γ-linolenic acid is conveniently abbreviated to GLA, or represented by its shorthand name, 18:3n-6 (or 18:3ω-6), where n-6 (or ω-6) indicates the position of the first double bond beginning from the methyl end (CH_3_).

In mammals, GLA is formed from linoleic acid (LA, 18:2n-6) by Δ6-desaturase. Once formed, GLA is rapidly elongated (by elongase) to dihomo-γ-linolenic acid (DGLA, 20:3n-6), which is then metabolized to arachidonic acid (AA, 20:4n-6) by Δ5-desaturase (Fig. 1.2) (1). The endogenous conversion of LA to GLA is considered to be the rate-limiting step for the formation of DGLA, AA, and their important metabolites, e.g., 1- and 2-series of prostaglandins (PG) and thromboxanes (TX) (2,3).

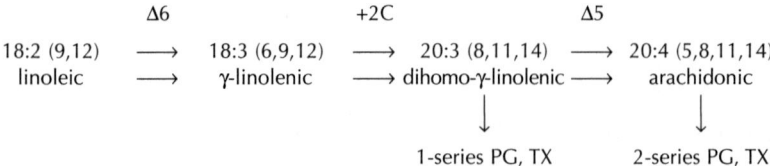

Fig. 1.2. Metabolism of n-6 fatty acids

There are many pathological conditions which are known to suppress the conversion of LA to GLA (6). A decrease in formation of long-chain n-6 polyunsaturated fatty acids has been related to many chronic degenerative diseases such as rheumatoid arthritis, high blood pressure, hyperlipidemia and diabetic neuropathy. Because many clinical symptoms can be alleviated by dietary supplementation of GLA by-passing the suppressed D6-desaturation (4), the potential nutritional and medical use of GLA has generated a great deal of interest in recent years in the discovery of more potential sources of GLA. This chapter examines the sources and biosynthesis of GLA in nature.

Distribution of γ-Linolenic Acid in Natural Sources

Animal Tissues

In animals, GLA is rapidly metabolized to DGLA, and hence, a very small amount of GLA is accumulated in animal tissues (5–9) (Table 1.1). However, noticeable amounts of GLA can be found in human breast milk, ranging from 0.35 to 1.0% by weight of milk fat (10,11).

TABLE 1.1 GLA Content (% fatty acids) in Animal Tissues

Tissue	Animal	PL	TG	Others	Reference
Adenoma	Human	0.4	0.1	0.5**	5
Adrenal	Rat	tr	tr	0.2*	5
	Human	0.1	0.1	0.3**	5
Adrenal mitochondria	Pig	1.5	2.6	—	6
Bile (PC)	Cow	0.6	—	—	7
	Pig	0.3	—	—	7
Testes	Pig	tr	tr	1.7++	8
Ovarian	Pig	0.5	tr	0.6+,0.8**	8
	Beef	0.5	1.9	0.8+,1.0**	8
Graafin follicles	Pig	0.7	0.1	0.4+,0.2**	8
	Beef	0.8	0.4	0.4+,0.3**	8
Gray matter (PC)	Human	0.1	—	0.1§	9
White matter (PC)	Human	0.1	—	0.1§	9
Milk	Human	—	0.35	—	10
		0–0.13	0.36–1.0	—	11

Abbreviations: PC, phosphatidylcholine; PL, total phospholipids; TG, triacylglycerol.
*, Ether glycerolipids; **, Cholesteryl esters; +, Free fatty acids; ++, Diacylglycerol; §, Phosphatidylethanolamine.

Higher Plants

In higher plants, GLA is distributed mainly among species of the Onagraceae, Boraginaceae, Scrophulariaceae and Saxifragaceae families (12–29) (Table 1.2).

Onagraceae Family. Evening primrose (*Oenothera biennis* L.) is a biennial crop with yellow flowers that bloom in the evening. This plant grows widely in North America. It is also being cultivated in countries such as Australia, China, France, Holland, Hungary, New Zealand, the United Kingdom, and Yugoslavia. The evening primrose seed contains approximately 15% protein, 43% cellulose and lignin and 24% oil (12). The oil contains 65–80% linoleic acid, 7–14% γ-linolenic acid, but no significant amounts of n-3 fatty acids (13,14). The highest amount of GLA was found in *O. acerviphilla* and *O. paradoxa* with 16 and 14%, respectively (15). The evening primrose seed oil was the first seed oil to become available commercially and is the most used source of GLA for clinical and pharmaceutical applications (4). It is currently available in over 30 countries as a nutritional supplement or as a constituent of specialty foods.

Boraginaceae Family. Borage, an herbaceous hardy annual, has starlike bright blue flowers. Its native habitats include regions of the Mediterranean, Asia Minor and North Africa. Traditionally, this plant has been used as a refreshing tea and as a folk remedy for some diseases. However, this plant is of greatest interest today for the rich content of GLA in its seed. The seed oils of *Borago officinalis*, L. and *Symphytum officinale*, L. contain high levels of GLA (20–27% of total fatty acids), but only 35–40% of LA (16,17). In comparison with evening primrose oil, borage oil contains significant higher amounts (8%) of long-chain monounsaturated fatty acids, gadoleic acid (20:1), erucic acid (22:1), and 24:1. It may also contain the toxic unsaturated pyrrolidizine alkaloids (UPA), particularly in oil from *S. officinale* (30,31). Some other species in this family such as *Echium vulgare* (17), *Onosmodium occidentale* (18), *O. hipidissimum* (19), and *E. plantagineum* (20) and even the leaf lipids of borage (21) contain high levels of α-linolenic acid (ALA, 18:3n-3) and stearidonic acid (SDA, 18:4n-3).

Saxifragaceae Family. Another attractive source of GLA-containing oils is seeds of the *Ribes*. Among them, blackcurrant (*Ribes nigrum*) is the richest source of GLA (19%) (22,23). This shrub is grown mainly in Europe. The seed is a by-product of blackcurrant juice production and is available in large quantities as a pomace (residue) from the production of jams, jellies, and juice liquors. The seeds are washed with alcohol to eliminate waxes and coloring agents; the oil (about 30%) is recovered by pressing or by hexane extraction. The extracted oil contains up to 15–19% GLA, and 92% of the mixed fatty acids are unsaturated (15). Blackcurrant seed oil also contains substantial amounts of n-3 fatty acids, i.e., ALA (12–14%) and SDA (2–4%) (24,25).

Others. In Scrophularaceae family, *Scrophularia marilandica* contains 10% GLA and only traces of ALA (13). In the Aceraceae family, the seed oil of *Acer negundo*,

L. contains 7% GLA and 1% ALA (26). In Liliaceae, the seed oil of *Astelia trinerva* contains 25% GLA and only trace amounts of ALA (27). The seed oil of English hops (*Humulus lupulus*) in the Moraceae family contains 5% GLA (28). In the Ranunculaceae family, the oil from *Anenome cylindrica* contains 19% GLA (29).

Microorganisms

Many species of microorganisms are rich in GLA (30–43). Oils obtained from the fermentation of these microorganisms are called microbial oils. The term single-celled oils was referred primarily to the triacylglycerol fraction (Table 1.3).

Fungus. Nakajima and Izu (32) have isolated and characterized 300 strains of fungi from soil and identified 10 strains with high GLA content ranging from 10–25.2%. Bernhard and Albrecht (33) and Shaw (34) have shown that the mycelial fat of the Phycomycete molds, such as *P. blakesleeanus* contained GLA in amounts up to 16% of the total fatty acids. Shimitzu et al. (35) have shown that *Mortierella alpina* produced large amounts of 20-carbon n-6 fatty acids (i.e., DGLA and AA) and also small amounts of 18-carbon n-6 fatty acids (mainly GLA). Hiruta et al. (36)

TABLE 1.2 Fatty Acid Composition and Seeds in Higher Plants

Organism	Fatty acid composition (% of total)							
	18:1 n-9	18:2 n-6	18:3 n-6	18:3 n-3	18:4 n-3	20:1/ 22:1	20:3/ 20:4	Ref.
Onagraceae								
Oenothera biennis	9.0	72.0	10.0	—	—	—	—	13
O. lamarckiana Ser.	12.3	62.2	8.2	0.2	—	—	—	14
Boraginaceae								
Borago officinalis	16.3	38.1	22.8	0.2	—	7.7	—	14
Symphytum officinale	15	43	27	1	0.5	3.0	—	16
Onosmodium occidentale	15.5	17.0	18.3	30.4	8.2	1.6	—	18
O. hipidissimum	13.5	18.2	20.1	26.8	8.1	2.0	—	19
Echium vulgare	16	18	11	37	10	0.8	—	17
E. plantagineum	17.1	14.9	9.7	33.6	13.1	—	—	20
Saxifragaceae								
Ribes alpinum	18.1	39.0	22.0	8.9	—	0.1	—	13
R. rubrum	15	42	5	30	3	—	—	13
R. uva crispa	10	48	17	13	4	—	—	22
R. nigrum	10.3	46.5	18.2	13.6	3.7	0.6	—	23
Scrophulariaceae								
Scrophularia lanceolata	16.6	66.0	0.5	8.0	—	—	—	13
S. marilandica	14.9	62.6	0.6	9.6	—	—	—	13
Aceraleae								
Acer negundo	21.0	34.0	7.0	1.0	—	28.8	—	26
A. tataricum	18.0	35.0	6.0	0.8	—	32.9	—	26
A. ginnala	23.9	37.4	3.5	1.0	—	25.8	—	26
Humulus lupulus	10	60	5	15	—	—	—	28

have reported that *Mortierella ramanniana* var. *angulispora* contains about 7% of GLA in the wild type, and up to 13.9% in the mutant, MM 15-1 strain. Ratledge (37) screened a number of molds of the order *Mucorales*, and noted that strains which produced the larger amounts of oil tended to have a lower content of GLA, and vice versa. Oil extracted from *Mucor javanicus* contains about 15–18% GLA along with 9% linoleic and 40% oleic acid (36).

Algae. Spirulina, a cyanobacterium, is a blue-green aquatic vegetable plankton (alga) found in highly alkaline waters in many parts of the world. For centuries, this microorganism has been used by many cultures. It serves as food to people in Africa and Central America: the ancient Egyptians had found all of the nutrients in spirulina, and the Aztec population of Mexico used it for making bread and preparing health-giving soups. Even today, spirulina is widely available in nutrition stores throughout Europe and North America. Spirulina contains 65–71% protein in dry weight, 10% carbohydrate, 7% fiber, 9% minerals and less than 5% nucleic acids.

TABLE 1.3 Fatty Acid Composition of Microorganisms

Organism	Fatty acid composition (% of total)							
	18:1 n-9	18:2 n-6	18:3 n-6	18:3 n-3	18:4 n-3	20:1/ 22:1	20:3/ 20:4	Ref.
Fungi								
Mortierella alpina	12.1	5.1	3.4	—	—	3.0/—	3.2/56.2	35
M. isabelina	43.9	12.0	8.3	—	—	0.4/0.2	—	35
M. ramanniana var. angulispora	51.0	10.8	7.0	—	—	—	—	36
Mucor javanicus	39.9	8.9	17.9	—	—	—	—	38
Rhizopus arrhizus	40.6	15.8	9.8	—	—	—	—	34
Phycomyces blakesleeanus	32.1	20.8	5.4	—	—	—	—	34
Algae								
Anacystis nidulans	—	0	0	0	0	—	—	41
Anabaena variabilis	—	17	16	0	0	—	—	41
Synechocystis 6714	—	17	0	31	0	—	—	41
Tolypothrix tenuis	—	15	6	13	11	—	—	41
Spirulina maxima	4	9	12	—	—	—	—	39
S. platensis	6	22	18	<1	—	—	—	39
Protozoa								
Tetrahymena pyriformis	8.7	17.9	37.7	—	—	<1.0	—	43
T. corlissi	11.6	26.1	30.6	—	—	4.4	—	43
T. selifera	4.2	13.2	47.2	—	—	0.7	—	43
T. paravorax	1.0	15.5	33.3	—	—	—	—	43
Crithidia fasciculata	26.0	10.3	17.2	—	—	1.0/10.5	—	44
C. oncopelti	26.8	9.8	17.9	—	—	1.4/10.3	—	44
C. lucilae	17.2	12.6	16.7	—	—	1.8/10.8	—	44
C. acanthocephali	22.8	20.6	13.0	—	—	0/4.8	—	44
Blastocrithidia culicis	23.1	17.7	29.3	—	—	0/7.7	—	44
Leishmania tarentolae	25.0	5.7	11.4	—	—	9.2/0	—	44
Ochromonas danica	8	16	10	2	—	—	5/11	45

Although low in total fat, this microorganism can synthesize polyunsaturated fatty acids. Nichols and Wood (39) have examined six blue-green algae and found that *Spirulina platensis* differs from all other photosynthetic tissues in containing a high proportion of GLA, ranging from 12 to 21% of total fatty acids. Cieferri and Tiboni (40) have also found that lipids in this microorganism contain 20–25% GLA. Based on the type of fatty acid synthesized, Murata and Nishida (41) have grouped cyanobacteria into four groups. Group 1 synthesizes saturated and monounsaturated but not polyunsaturated fatty acids. The other three can synthesize LA and in addition, ALA, GLA and SDA, respectively. In the latter three groups, GLA is located primarily in the photosynthesizing lamellae structures and has a function analogous to that fulfilled by ALA in many other algae and in the leaves of higher plants.

Protozoa. Many species of ciliated protozoa in the familiy Tetrahymenidae, e.g., *Tetrahymena pyriformis*, are rich (≥30%) in GLA (43). The lipids in these microorganisms consist of 68% phospholipids (54% phosphatidyl ethanolamine and 30% phosphatidyl choline) and 28% of neutral lipids (90% triglycerides). Saturated (52.2%) and monounsaturated (9%) fatty acids are the principal fatty acids in the neutral lipids, whereas GLA (29.5%) and LA (22.8) are the two major fatty acids in the phospholipids (44). In four genera of zooflagellates belonging to the order of Kinetoplastida, three genera (*Crithidia*, *Blastocrithidia*, and *Leishmania*) synthesize GLA (42,44). The phytoflagellates, *Ochromonas danica*, when cultivated in light and defined medium contain significant amounts of GLA (10%) (45).

Biosynthesis of γ-Linolenic Acid

Animals

In the animal body, both 18:2n-6 and 18:3n-3 are essential to normal physiological functions. However, animals cannot synthesize these acids and have to obtain them from the diet. During the course of evolution, animals lost the ability to insert double bonds into fatty acids beyond the $\Delta 9$ position, e.g., into the $\Delta 12$ and $\Delta 15$ positions, and cannot convert 18:1n-9 to 18:2n-6 and 18:2n-6 to 18:3n-3. Nonetheless, animals have retained the ability to insert double bonds between the existing bond and the carboxyl end of the acyl chain. For example, animals can metabolize dietary 18:2n-6 and 18:3n-3 through $\Delta 6$-desaturation, elongation and $\Delta 5$-desaturation to form long-chain n-6 and n-3 metabolites, respectively (Fig. 1.2). The activity of $\Delta 6$-desaturase in animal tissues requires the CoA derivatives of LA as the substrate (1,46).

Higher Plants

In most of the higher plants, double bonds can be inserted at the $\Delta 9$, $\Delta 12$, and $\Delta 15$ positions (Fig. 1.3). The activities of the first two enzymes result in formation of oleic acid and linoleic acid, respectively. The presence of $\Delta 15$-desaturase results in the occurrence of ALA in plant tissues and seeds. In several higher plants such as

```
           Δ9              Δ12                Δ15
18:0    →    18:1 (9)   →   18:2 (9,12)   →   18:3 (9,12,15)
stearic       oleic          Linoleic          α-linolenic
                                ↓ Δ6              ↓ Δ6
                             18:3(6,9,12)     18:4(6,9,12,15)
                             γ-linolenic       Stearidonic
```

Fig. 1.3. Biosynthesis of γ-linolenic acid in plants and microorganisms

Oenothera and *Boraginaceae* the activity of Δ15-desaturase is absent, hence they can synthesize LA but not ALA. The presence of Δ6-desaturase enables the plant tissues to insert the double bond into the Δ6 position of LA. As a result, these plants are rich in GLA. In *Ribe*, both Δ15-desaturase and Δ6-desaturase are active, hence both GLA and SDA are synthesized in this plant. The level of GLA in the plant is modulated by the balance of activities of the desaturation enzymes (Δ12, Δ15, and Δ6). This balance varies during different developmental stages. For example, at the early stage of seed maturation in the evening primrose, LA is either Δ6-desaturated to form GLA or Δ15-desaturated to form ALA. With progressive seed maturation, the activity of Δ6-desaturase predominates. As a result, ALA disappears from the seed lipids whereas GLA is accumulated (47). Dissimilar to its synthesis in the animal system, the synthesis of GLA in plants such as evening primrose, borage and blackcurrant uses the linoleoyl moiety linked to phospholipids as the substrate for the Δ6-desaturase enzyme. The enzyme converts PC-linked linoleic acid (*sn*-2) to PC-linked GLA (48,49).

Lower plants

As in the higher plants, the enzyme Δ12-desaturase in lower plants such as yeast, *Torulopsis utilis* (50), alga, *Candida lipolytica* (51), chloroplast of *Chorella vulgaris* (52), and microsomes of *Neurospora crassa* (53), uses the phosphatidylcholine-linked oleoyl (at both *sn*-1 and *sn*-2) to form linoleoyl-phosphatidylcholine (54). The linoleic acid thus formed is then desaturated by Δ15-desaturase to form α-linolenic acid (55). However, in GLA-rich microorganisms, the linoleoyl-phosphatidylcholine is desaturated by Δ6-desaturase to form GLA. In cyanobacteria, however, Δ6-desaturation takes place with LA bound to glycerolipids as a mono- and di-galactosyl diacylglycerol derivative (56).

Bioavailability of γ-Linolenic Acid

As shown above, GLA can be obtained from various sources, having its origin in a plant or a microorganism. However, the bioavailability of GLA may differ significantly among these oil sources (57). In addition to a difference in total GLA content (58), GLA in different GLA-rich oils may not be equally absorbed. Evidence has shown that absorption of any given fatty acid is a function of stereospecific distribution and the nature of the adjacent fatty acids (59,60).

Association of γ-Linolenic Acid and Other Fatty Acids

To assess the effect of adjacent fatty acids on the biological activity of GLA in the oil, the composition of the individual GLA-containing triacylglycerol (TG) molecules in the oil source has to be determined. Several reports using reverse-phase HPLC have distinguished the distribution of GLA-containing triacylglycerol molecular species in evening primrose seed, borage seed and blackcurrant seed oils (61–63). Data in Table 1.4 highlight the distribution patterns of GLA in these oils. Briefly, in evening primrose oil, the TG species containing two or more GLA molecules represent less than 1% of the total TG mass. Most of the GLA-containing species consist of only one molecule of GLA per TG molecule, accompanied primarily (80%) by two molecules of linoleic acid or, in some cases, one molecule of linoleic acid and one molecule of either palmitic or oleic acid. In borage oil, the TG species containing two or more molecules of GLA represent over 13% of the total

TABLE 1.4 Distribution (mole %) of Major GLA-containing Triacylglycerol Molecular Species (>1%) in Evening Primrose, Borage, and Blackcurrant Seed Oils

Species	Primrose[a]	Borage[a]	Blackcurrant[b]
Overall G (mol %)	9.3	24.8	15.9
GGG	—	0.24	0.55*
GGX			
18:3n-3	—	—	1.19*
18:2n-3	0.71	9.84	3.82
18:1n-9	—	0.83	1.24*
16:0	—	2.39	0.68*
GXX			
18:4n-3/18:2n-6	—	—	1.48
18:3n-3/18:3n-3	—	—	0.85*
18:3n-3/18:2n-3	—	—	7.90
18:3n-3/18:1n-9	—	—	1.77*
18:3n-3/16:0	—	—	0.97*
18:2n-6/18:2n-6	17.63	15.41	12.54
18:2n-6/18:1n-9	1.55	12.30	5.11
18:2n-6/16:0	1.19	9.53	5.26
18:2n-6/18:0	—	—	0.64*
18:2n-6/20:1	—	2.53	0.39*
18:2n-6/22:1	—	0.55	—
18:1n-9/18:1n-9	—	—	1.03
18:1n-9/16:0	—	—	1.01*
16:0/16:0	—	1.47	0.28*
16:0/20:1	—	0.78	0.06

G: Gamma-linolenic acid; X: fatty acid other than GLA.
[a]*Source:* Huang et al. (62).
[b]*Source:* Perrin et al. (61).
*Estimated value.

TG mass. Most of them are accompanied by one molecule of linoleic or palmitic acid. More than 43% of the GLA-containing TG molecular species consist of only one molecule of GLA and two molecules of LA, or one molecule of GLA, one molecule of LA, and one molecule of either oleic or palmitic acid. Substantial proportions (4%) of the GLA-containing TG species contain one molecule of long-chain monounsaturated fatty acid, i.e., 20:1, 22:1, and 24:1. In BCO, approximately 7.7% of total TG mass contains two molecules of GLA and one molecule of either ALA, LA, oleic, or palmitic acid. About 38% of the total TG mass contains only one molecule of GLA, more than one-third of these contain at least one molecule of n-3 fatty acid (i.e., ALA, SDA), and two-thirds of them contain at least one molecule of LA.

Stereospecific Positional Distribution of γ-Linolenic Acid

The stereospecific position of GLA varies among different oil sources. Lawson and Hughes (38) have examined the stereospecific distribution of GLA in triglyceride from plant oils such as evening primrose, borage, and blackcurrant and from *Mucor javanicus* fungal oil (Table 1.5). They found that GLA is concentrated in the *sn*-3 position of evening primrose and blackcurrant oils and in the *sn*-2 position of borage oil, but evenly in both the *sn*-2 and *sn*-3 positions of fungal oil.

Previously, it has been suggested that tissue levels of GLA and its metabolite DGLA in animals were modulated by the level of GLA in the diet regardless of the GLA source (58). However, Huang et al. (62) recently compared the *in vitro* hydrolysis rate of different GLA-containing TG species by pancreatic lipase, and found that the lipolytic rates were significantly slower in TG species containing two or three molecules of GLA than in those containing only one GLA in the same TG molecule. The presence of long-chain saturated or monounsaturated fatty acids in some GLA-containing oils also affects the bioavailability of GLA. Myher et al. (59) have shown that the atherogenic native peanut oil contains a significantly greater proportion of TG with LA in the *sn*-2 position, and long-chain saturated fatty acids are located at the *sn*-3 position. They suggested that the atherogenicity may arise from a relative metabolic unavailability of the LA from the natural oil, which may be due in part to the presence of long-chain saturated fatty acids in the outer position. Similarly, Huang et al. (62) have shown that the release of GLA from either the outer position (*sn*-1 or *sn*-3) or the middle position (*sn*-2) was significantly slower when two other stereospecific positions in the same TG molecule were occupied by saturated or long-chain monounsaturated fatty acids.

TABLE 1.5 Stereospecific Distribution (mole %) of GLA in Triacylglycerols in Four GLA Oils

Position	Primrose	Borage	Blackcurrant	Mucor
ALL	9.3	24.8	15.9	17.9
sn-1	3.6	4.0	4.1	13.3
sn-2	10.7	40.4	17.4	19.6
sn-3	13.5	30.1	25.8	19.6

Source: Lawson and Hughes (38)

Comments

The growing interest in GLA for human nutrition has driven the development of commercial processes for producing GLA-rich oils. Through careful seed selection, GLA levels can be increased. For example, the GLA level in evening primrose seeds has been raised from 8% many years ago to 14% in recent years. However this is a long and tedious process. In many microbial oils, the proportion of GLA is about twice that of evening primrose oil and can be increased further by screening mutants growing at low temperature (41). Under tightly controlled fermentation culture conditions, bacteria and fungi can increase the production capability of microorganisms to a large-scale production of GLA. For example, molds of the *Mucorales* and *Mortierella* species have been used for the production of GLA-rich oils (64,65). In recent years, this process has became an attractive alternative to the use of plant oils for commercial purposes in both the pharmaceutical and food industries. The major drawback is that the high production cost makes it difficult for fungal oils to compete directly with oilseeds as cost-effective sources of GLA. Another concern in the use of microbial oils is their relatively high levels of saturated and monoene acids and low levels of linoleic acid. This feature may be of limited dietary interest, but these types of oils are more suitable as oil sources of pure GLA or upgraded triacylglycerols (24).

Acknowledgments

The authors wish to express their sincere appreciation to their colleagues, Dr. Bob Miller, Mr. Dave Wynsen, Dr. Rob Miller, and Dr. Stan Keely, for their overall support of time and other resources in the preparation of this manuscript.

References

1. Mead, J.F. Synthesis and Metabolism of Polyunsaturated Acids (1961) *Fed. Proc. 20*, 952–955.
2. Sprecher, H. Biochemistry of Essential Fatty Acids (1981) *Prog. Lipid Res. 20*, 13–22.
3. Brenner, R.R. Nutritional and Hormonal Factors Influencing Desaturation of Essential Fatty Acids (1981) *Prog. Lipid Res. 20*, 41–47.
4. Horrobin, D.F. Nutritional and Medical Importance of Gamma-Linolenic Acid (1992) *Prog. Lipid Res. 31*, 163–194.
5. Takayasu, K., Okuda, K., and Yoshikawa, I. Fatty Acid Composition of Human and Rat Adrenal Lipids: Occurrence of ω-6 Docosatrienoic Acid in Human Adrenal Cholesterol Ester (1970) *Lipids 5*, 743–750.
6. Cmelik, S., and Ley, H. Distribution of Cholesteryl Esters and Other Lipids in Subcellular Fractions of the Adrenal Gland of the Pig (1975) *Lipids 10*, 707–713.
7. Christie, W.W. The Structure of Bile Phosphatidylcholine (1973) *Biochim. Biophys. Acta 316*, 204–211.
8. Holman, R.T., and Hofstetter, H.H. The Fatty Acid Composition of the Lipids from Bovine and Porcine Reproductive Tissues (1965) *J. Am. Oil Chem. Soc. 42*, 540–544.
9. Svennerholm, L. Distribution and Fatty Acid Composition of Phosphoglycerides in Normal Human Brain (1968) *J. Lipid Res. 9*, 570–579.

10. Gibson, R.A., and Kneebone, G.M. Fatty Acid Composition of Human Colostrum and Mature Breast Milk (1981) *Am. J. Clin. Nutr. 34*, 252–257.
11. Harzer, G., Haug, M., Dieterich, I., and Gentner, P.R. Changing Patterns of Human Milk Lipids in the Course of Lactation and during the Day (1993) *Am. J. Clin. Nutr. 37*, 612–621.
12. Whipkey, A., Simon, J.E., and Janick, J. In Vivo and In Vitro Lipid Accumulation in *Borago officinalis* L. (1988) *J. Am. Oil Chem. Soc. 65*, 979–984.
13. Wolf, R.B., Kleiman, R., and England, R.E. New Sources of γ-Linolenic Acid (1983) *J. Am. Oil Chem. Soc. 60*, 1858–1860.
14. Hudson, B.J.F. Evening Primrose (*Oenothera* spp.) Oil and Seed (1984) *J. Am. Oil Chem. Soc. 61*, 540–543.
15. Gunstone, F.D., Harwood, J.L., and Padley, F.B. (Eds.) (1994) *The Lipid Handbook*, 2nd edition, Chapman and Hall, London.
16. Kleiman, R., Earle, F.R., Wolff, I.A., and Jones, Q. Search for New Industrial Oils. XI. Oils of Boraginaceae (1964) *J. Am. Oil Chem. Soc. 41*, 459–460.
17. Miller, R.W., Earle, F.R., Wolf, I.A., and Barclay, A.S. Search for New Seed Oils. XV. Oils of Boraginaceae (1968) *Lipids 3*, 43–45.
18. Craig, B.M., and Bhatty, M.K. A Naturally Occurring All-*cis* 6,9,12,15-Octadecatetraenoic Acid in Plant Oils (1964) *J. Am. Oil Chem. Soc. 41(3)*, 209–211.
19. MacKenzie, S.L., Giblin, E.M., and Mazza, G. Stereospecific Analysis of *Onosmodium hispidissimum* Mack. Seed Oil Triglycerides (1993) *J. Am. Oil Chem. Soc. 70*, 629–631.
20. Smith, C.R., Jr., Hagemann, J.W., and Wolff, I.A. The Occurrence of 6,9,12,15-Octadecatetraenoic Acid in *Echium plantagineum* Seed Oil (1964) *J. Am. Oil Chem. Soc. 41*, 290–291.
21. Jamieson, G.R., and Reid, E.H. The Leaf Lipids of Some Members of the Boraginaceae Family (1969) *Phytochemistry 8*, 1489–1494.
22. Traitler, H., Winter, H., Richli, U., and Ingenbleek, Y. Characterization of γ-Linolenic Acid in Ribes Seeds (1984) *Lipids 19*, 923–928.
23. Traitler, H., Wille, H.J., and Studer, A. Fractionation of Blackcurrant Seed Oil (1988) *J. Am. Oil Chem. Soc. 65*, 755–760.
24. Gunstone, F.D. Gamma Linolenic Acid-Occurrence and Physical and Chemical Properties (1992) *Prog. Lipid Res. 31*, 145–161.
25. Muderhwa, J.M., Dhuique-Mayer, C., Pina, M., Galzy, P., Grignas, P., and Graille, J. Répartition Interne/Externe des Acides Gras des Triglycérides de Quelques Huiles Gamma Linoléniques (1987) *Oleagineux 42*, 207–211.
26. Bohannon, M.B., and Kleiman, R. γ-Linolenic Acid in *Acer* Seed Oils (1976) *Lipids 11*, 157–159.
27. Morice, I.M. Seed Fats of *Astelia* and *Collospermum*, Family Liliaceae (1969) *J. Sci. Food Agric. 20*, 343–346.
28. Roberts, J.B., and Stevens, R. The Seed Fat of Hops (*Humulus lupulus*, L.) (1963) *Chem. Ind.* 608–609.
29. Spencer, G.F., Kleiman, R., Earle, F.R., and Wolff, I.A. Unusual Olefinic Fatty Acids in Seed Oils from Two Genera in the Ranunculaceae (1970) *Lipids 5*, 277–278.
30. Awang, D.V.C. Herbal Medicine: Borage (1990) *Can. Pharm. J. 123*, 121–126.
31. de Smet, P.A.G.M. Safety of Borage Oil (1991) *Can. Pharm. J. 124*, 5 (lett.).

32. Nakajima, T., and Izu, S. (1992) Microbial Production and Purification of Omega-6 Polyunsaturated Fatty Acids. In: *Essential Fatty Acids and Eicosanoids* (Sinclair, A.J., and Gibson, R.E.), pp.57–64, American Oil Chemists' Society, Champaign, IL, pp. 57–64.
33. Bernhard, K., and Albrecht, H. Die Lipide aus *Phycomyces blakesleeanus* (1948) *Helv. Chim. Acta 31*, 977–988.
34. Shaw, R. The Occurrence of γ-Linolenic Acid in Fungi (1965) *Biochim. Biophys. Acta 98*, 230–237.
35. Shimitzu, S., Shinmen, Y., Kawashima, H., Akimoto, K., and Yamada, H. Production of C-20 Polyunsaturated Fatty Acids by Fungi. In: *Proceedings of ISF-JOCS World Congress 1988*, pp. 1000–1006, The Japan Oil Chemists' Society, 1989.
36. Hiruta, T., Takebe, H., Uotani, K., Fukatsu, S., Kamisaka, Y., Yokochi, T., Nakahara, T., and Suzuki, O. Breeding of *Mortierella ramanniana* var. *angulispora* MA26 for Gamma-Linolenic Acid Production. In: *Proceedings of ISF-JOCS World Congress 1988*, pp. 1114–1119, The Japan Oil Chemists' Society, 1989.
37. Ratledge, C. Single Cell Oils—Have They a Biotechnological Future? (1993) *Trends Biotechnol. 11*, 278–284.
38. Lawson, L.D., and Hughes, B.G. Triacylglycerol Structure of Plant and Fungal Oils Containing γ-Linolenic Acid (1988) *Lipids 23*, 313–317.
39. Nichols, B.W., and Wood, B.J.B. The Occurrence and Biosynthesis of Gamma-Linolenic Acid in Blue-Green Alga, *Spirulina platensis* (1968) *Lipids 3*, 46–50.
40. Ciferri, O., and Tiboni, O. The Biochemistry and Industrial Potential of *Spirulina* (1985) *Ann. Rev. Microbiol. 39*, 503–526.
41. Murata, N., and Nishida, I. (1987) Lipids of Blue-Green Algae (Cyanobacteria), In: *The Biochemistry of Plants* (Stumpf, P.K., and Conn, E.E.), vol. 9, Academic Press, New York, pp. 315–347.
42. Korn, E.D., Greenblatt, C.L., and Lees, A.M. Synthesis of Unsaturated Fatty Acids in the Slime Mold Physarum polycephalum and the Zooflagellates *Leishmania tarentolae, Trypanosoma lewisi,* and *Crithidia* sp.: A Comparative Study (1965) *J. Lipid. Res. 6*, 43–50.
43. Erwin, J., and Bloch, K. Lipid Metabolism of Ciliated Protozoa (1963) *J. Biol. Chem. 238*, 1618–1624.
44. Meyer, H., and Holz, G.G., Jr. Biosynthesis of Lipids by Kinetoplastid (1966) *J. Biol. Chem. 241*, 5000–5007.
45. Haines, T.H., Aaronson, S., Gellerman, J.L., and Schlenk, H. Occurrence of Arachidonic and Related Acids in the Protozoon, *Ochromonas danica* (1962) *Nature (London) 194*, 1282–1283.
46. Okayasu, T., Nagao, M., Ishibashi, T., and Imai, Y. Purification and Partial Characterization of Linoleoyl-CoA Desaturase from Rat Liver Microsomes (1981) *Arch. Biochem. Biophys. 206*, 21–28.
47. Mukherjee, K.D., and Kiewitt, I. Formation of γ-Linolenic Acid in the Higher Plant Evening Primrose (*Oenothera biennis* L.) (1987) *J. Agric. Food Chem. 35*, 1009–1012.
48. Stymne, S., and Stobart, A.K. Biosynthesis of γ-Linolenic Acid in Cotyledons and Microsomal Preparations of the Developing Seeds of Common Borage (*Borago officinalis*) (1986) *Biochem. J. 240*, 385–393.
49. Griffith, G., Stobart, A.K., and Stymne, S. Δ6- and Δ12-Desaturase Activities and Phosphatidic Acid Formation in Microsomal Preparations from the Developing Cotyledons of Common Borage (*Borago officinalis*) (1988) *Biochem. J. 252*, 641–647.

50. Talamo, B., Chang, N., and Bloch, K. Desaturation of Oleyl Phospholipid to Linoleyl Phospholipid in *Torulopsis utilis* (1973) *J. Biol. Chem. 248*, 2738–2742.
51. Pugh, E.L., and Kates, M. Desaturation of Phosphatidylcholine and Phosphatidylethanolamine by a Microsomal Enzyme System from *Candida lipolytica* (1973) *Biochim. Biophys. Acta 316*, 305–316.
52. Gurr, M.I., Robinson, M.P., and James, A.T. The Mechanism of Formation of Polyunsaturated Fatty Acids by Photosynthetic Tissue: The Tight Coupling of Oleate Desaturation with Phospholipid Synthesis in *Chlorella vulgaris* (1969) *Eur. J. Biochem. 9*, 70–78.
53. Baker, N., and Lynen, F. Factors Involved in Fatty Acyl CoA Desaturation by Fungal Microsomes. The Relative Roles of Acyl CoA and Phospholipids as Substrate (1971) *Eur. J. Biochem. 19*, 200–210.
54. Pugh, E.L., and Kates, M. Characterization of a Membrane-Bound Phospholipid Desaturase System of *Candida lipolytica* (1975) *Biochim. Biophys. Acta 380*, 442–453.
55. Bloch, K., Baronowsky, P., Goldfine, H., Lennarz, W.J., Light, R., Norris, A.T., and Scheuerbrandt, G. Biosynthesis and Metabolism of Unsaturated Fatty Acids (1961) *Fed. Proc. 20*, 921–927.
56. Sato, N., Seyama, Y., and Murata, N. Lipid-Linked Desaturation of Palmitic Acid in Monogalactosyl Diacylglycerol in the Blue-Green Alga (Cyanobacterium) *Anabaena variabilis* Studied in Vivo (1986) *Plant Cell Physiol. 27*, 819–835.
57. Jenkins, D.K., Mitchell, J., Manku, M.S., and Horrobin, D.F. Effects of Different Sources of Gamma-Linolenic Acid on the Formation of Essential Fatty Acid and Prostanoid Metabolites (1988) *Med. Sci. Res. 16*, 525–526.
58. Raederstorff, D., and Moser, U. Borage or Primrose Oil Added to Standardized Diets Are Equivalent Sources for γ-Linolenic Acid in Rats (1992) *Lipids 27*, 1018–1023.
59. Myher, J.J., Marai, A., Kuksis, A., and Kritchevsky, D. Acylglycerol Structure of Peanut Oils of Different Atherogenic Potential (1977) *Lipids 12*, 775–785.
60. Mattson, F.H., Nolen, G.A., and Webb, M.R. The Absorbability by Rats of Various Triglycerides of Stearic and Oleic Acid and the Effect of Dietary Calcium and Magnesium (1979) *J. Nutr. 109*, 1682–1687.
61. Perrin, J.-L., Prevot, A., Traitler, H., and Bracco, U. Analysis of Triglyceride Species of Blackcurrant Seed Oil by HPLC via a Laser Light Scattering Detector (1987) *Rev. Fr. Corps Gras 34*, 221–223.
62. Huang, Y.-S., Lin, X., Redden, P.R., and Horrobin, D.F. In Vitro Hydrolysis of Natural and Synthetic γ-Linolenic Acid-Containing Triacylglycerols by Pancreatic Lipase (1995) *J. Am. Oil Chem. Soc. 72*, 625–631.
63. Redden, P.R., Huang, Y.-S., Lin, X., and Horrobin, D.F. Separation and Quantification of the Triacylglycerols in Evening Primrose and Borage Oils by Reverse-Phase High-Performance Liquid Chromatography (1995) *J. Chromatogr. 694A*, 381–389.
64. Ratledge, C. (1989) Biotechnology of Oils and Fats. In: *Microbial Lipids,* Ratledge, C., and Wilkinson, E.G., vol. 2, Academic Press, London, pp. 567–668.
65. Ratledge, C. (1989) Microbial Oils and Fats: Perspectives and Prospects. In: *Fats for the Future,* Cambie, R.C., Ellis Horwood, Chichester, pp. 153–171.

Chapter 2

Pathways for the Biosynthesis of Polyunsaturated Fatty Acids

**Howard Sprecher, Devanand Luthria,
Svetla P. Baykousheva, and B. Selma Mohammed**

Department of Medical Biochemistry,
The Ohio State University,
Columbus, Ohio 43210

Arachidonic Acid Biosynthesis

It is generally accepted that linoleic acid is metabolized to arachidonic acid in the endoplasmic reticulum as follows: 9,12-18:2 → 6,9,12-18:3 → 8,11,14-20:3 → 5,8,11,14-20:4. This pathway requires the participation of position-specific acyl-CoA-dependent 6- and 5-desaturases with an intervening malonyl-CoA-dependent chain-elongation step. When the pathways of unsaturated fatty acid biosynthesis were being elucidated, Stoffel and Ach (1) presented evidence that linoleate was chain-elongated to 11,14-20:2, which was then desaturated at position 8 to yield 8,11,14-20:3. We synthesized [1-^{14}C]11,14-20:2 and [1-^{14}C]11,14,17-20:3. When they were incubated with rat liver microsomes, they were desaturated at position 5 to yield 5,11,14-20:3, and 5,11,14,17-20:4, respectively. At that time, we concluded that rat liver microsomes did not contain an 8-desaturase, and that 6,9,12-18:3 was an obligatory intermediate in the biosynthesis of arachidonate (2). Our results were corroborated by Dhopeshwarkar and Subramanian (3,4) who showed that brain also lacked an 8-desaturase. At about the same time, Albert et al. (5) incubated [1-^{14}C]11,14-20:2 with testes microsomes and isolated the radioactive trienoic acids. When they degraded them, they found radioactive 5- and 8-carbon aldehydo methyl esters, suggesting that rat testes contained an 8-desaturase. More recently, Cook et al. (6) reported that cultured C6 glioma cells metabolized deuterium-labeled fatty acids via a number of pathways, one of which could proceed via desaturation at position 8.

Acyl-CoA-dependent desaturase reactions are routinely assayed by incubating a radioactive fatty acid with microsomes in the presence of NADH, Mg^{2+}ATP, CoASH, and ATP. The introduction of a double bond, at a given position, is frequently assumed to indicate that microsomes contain a position-specific desaturase. However, relatively little is known about the proteins that catalyze position-specific desaturation reactions. The 9-desaturase that catalyzes the conversion of stearoyl-CoA to oleoyl-CoA has been purified from rat liver. It is a single polypeptide of 53,000 Da. The introduction of a double bond at position 9 is an aerobic process and it requires cytochrome b_5, cytochrome b_5 reductase and the desaturase (7). It is now known that two different 9-desaturases are expressed in tissue-specific ways in mice (8,9). A partially purified 6-desaturase from rat liver also requires cytochrome b_5 and cytochrome b_5 reductase for activity (10). There are no reported attempts to purify a hepatic acyl-CoA-dependent 5-desaturase. It is not known how many desaturases are expressed in mammalian tissue, or if any given protein can accept multiple substrates, or perhaps even introduce double bonds at different positions. For example, both 8,11,14-20:3 and 11,14-20:2 are desaturated at position 5. Does a single enzyme desaturate both substrates? In this regard, it is interesting to note that Gurr et al. (11) reported that *cis*-12-18:1 was desaturated at position 9, to yield linoleate, in a number of animal and plant species. It seems very unlikely that the synthesis of arachidonate, via 11,14-20:2, is a major pathway. If 11,14-20:2 is desaturated at position 8, it remains to be determined if liver expresses an 8-desaturase, or whether another protein is simply not absolutely position specific.

When rats are fed a chow diet, their membrane lipids generally contain large amounts of both linoleate and arachidonate but only low levels of 18:3(n-6) and 20:3(n-6). Microsomal reaction rates have frequently been used as a predictor of what types of fatty acids are made for subsequent esterification into membrane lipids. Desaturation of linoleate to 6,9,12-18:3 by a 6-desaturase is generally recognized as the rate-limiting step in the synthesis of arachidonate (12). The biosynthesis of unsaturated fatty acids and their subsequent incorporation into membrane lipids are processes that are both localized primarily in the endoplasmic reticulum. The rate of chain-elongation of 18:3(n-6) to 20:3(n-6) was 2.5 nmol/min/mg of microsomal protein (12), whereas the rate of acylation of 6,9,12-18:3 into 1-acyl-*sn*-glycero-3-phosphocholine was 28 nmol/min/mg of microsomal protein (13). If reaction rates *per se* are predictors of membrane fatty acid composition, it would be predicted that 6,9,12-18:3 should be preferentially esterified rather than being chain-elongated to 8,11,14-20:3. *In vivo*, it is possible that linoleate may be channeled to arachidonate, so that 6,9,12-18:3 and 8,11,14-20:3 are not readily made available for acylation reactions. Alternatively, a more complex type of fatty acid metabolism may take place. When we incubated [1-^{14}C]6,9,12-18;3 or [1-^{14}C]6,9,12,15-18:4 with hepatocytes, both substrates were initially incorporated into phospholipids. After about 60 min, all of the exogenous substrate had been metabolized. However, from 60 to 120 min, there was a continued increase in the amount of esterified arachidonate and 20:5(n-3). The continued synthesis of these acids was accompanied by a decrease in the amount of esterified 18:3(n-6) and 18:4(n-3). We suggested that the 18-carbon acids may have entered a very labile phospholipid pool and that they were rapidly hydrolyzed by a phospholipase A_2 for further metabolism to arachidonate (14). Many tissues, including liver (15), contain a CoASH-dependent, ATP-independent pathway for remodeling the fatty acid composition of membrane lipids. It is thus possible that when 6,9,12-18:3 is produced *in vivo*, it is initially incorporated into membrane lipids. If the CoASH-dependent pathway was highly fatty acid-specific, the esterified 6,9,12-18:3 might simply be transferred to CoASH for subsequent metabolism to 8,11,14-20:3 and then to arachidonate. If this pathway is operative, it implies that when 6,9,12-18:3 is produced, it is initially esterified, but sufficient amounts do not accumulate to detect when the fatty acid composition of membrane lipids is quantified.

It is well established that many physiological processes are modified by the types of unsaturated fatty acids found in membrane lipids. Three basic different nutritional models have been used to determine how changes in membrane fatty acid composition alter function. When animals are fed no fat or a diet devoid of essential fatty acids, their membrane lipids accumulate 5,8,11-20:3. The essential fatty acid-deficient model has been used extensively to study the role of essential fatty acids as they relate to a variety of parameters. The second dietary model may be called a fatty acid replacement strategy. In this dietary model, a fat is added to a basal diet that already contains an adequate level of essential fatty acids. The addition of fish oils to the diet is an example of this type of dietary intervention. When a typical Western diet is consumed, the membrane lipids contain only trace amounts of 20:5(n-3). When fish oil is added to the diet, some of the esterified arachidonate is replaced by 20:5(n-3). This type of dietary intervention has been most frequently used to determine how eicosanoid-mediated processes, such as platelet aggregation, and inflammation, are altered. The third dietary model has as its basic premise the addition to the diet of an oil containing a fatty acid that is beyond the rate-limiting step in a biosynthetic sequence. The addition of oils containing 6,9,12-18:3 to the diet is an example of this type of strategy, because the rate-limiting 6-desaturase step is circumvented. However, it has never been determined to what extent the addition of 6,9,12-18:3 to the diet affects the metabolism of linoleate to arachidonate. We carried out a number of feeding studies, using deuterium-labeled fatty acids, to quantify how they modified both the mass amounts of esterified arachidonate and its isotopic composition. In these studies, male weanling rats were fed a modified AIN-76 diet for 4 wk in which the fat content was 3.3% by weight, consisting of 2.1% ethyl oleate, 1% ethyl linoleate and 0.2% ethyl linolenate. After 4 wk on this diet, the rats were changed to one in which all of the linoleate was replaced by an equal amount of $17,17,18,18-d_4-18:2(n-6)$. The rats were killed 4 d later, and the molar fraction of esterified deuterium-labeled 20:4(n-6) in liver phospholipids, as determined by mass spectrometry, was found to be 33.9%. The second group of rats was preconditioned by feeding them an identical diet, except for a reduction of oleate content to 1.9%, with 0.2% ethyl 6,9,12-18:3 included in the diet. After 4 wk, all of the linoleate was again replaced by the deuterium-labeled analog. Now the molar fraction of deuterium-labeled arachidonate was reduced to 27.1%. The third group of animals was fed the same diet as group 2, but now the unlabeled 18:3(n-6) was replaced by an equal amount of $17,17,18,18-d_4-18:3(n-6)$. The molar fraction of labeled 20:4(n-6) in phospholipids was 24.6%. In these studies, the amount of 18:3(n-6) that was fed was 20% of the level of linoleate. However, the molar fraction of esterified labeled 20:4(n-6) derived from 18:3(n-6) was 70% of that produced from 18:2(n-6), i.e., 27.1/33.9 = 70%. When 18:3(n-6) was added to the diet, it depressed the amount of d_4-18:2(n-6) metabolized to esterified d_4-20:4(n-6). However, it can be calculated that the amount of esterified labeled 20:4(n-6) that was produced from the combined metabolism of 18:2(n-6) plus 18:3(n-6) was greater than what was produced from linoleate alone. When 18:2(n-6) was the only dietary (n-6) acid, 33.9% of the arachidonate was labeled. When unlabeled 18:3(n-6) was added to the diet, this value was reduced to 27.1%. However, it can be calculated that when 0.2% 18:3(n-6) was added to a diet containing 1% 18:2(n-6), the molar fraction of labeled 20:4(n-6) in liver phospholipid was 51.7%, i.e., 27.1% plus 24.6%. None of these dietary manipulations altered the actual amount of arachidonate esterified in phospholipids. It can thus be concluded that dietary supplements of 18:3(n-6) increase the production of 20:4(n-6), but they do not alter the amount of this acid esterified in phospholipids. Obviously, additional studies are required to determine if this type of phenomenon is observed when other levels of linoleate and 18:3(n-6) are fed.

Intracellular Movement in Fatty Acid Biosynthesis

It has generally been accepted that 7,10,13,16-22:4 and 7,10,13,16,19-22:5 are desaturated at position 4 in the endoplasmic reticulum to yield 4,7,10,13,16-22:5 and 4,7,10,13,16,19-22:6, respectively. When we incubated [1-^{14}C]7,10,13,16,19-22:5 with rat liver microsomes and appropriate cofactors, the substrate was not desaturated. However, when NADPH and malonyl-CoA were added to the incubation, the substrate was initially chain-elongated to yield 9,12,15,18,21-24:5, which was subsequently desaturated at position 6 to yield 6,9,12,15,18,21-24:6. When we incubated [1-^{14}C]7,10,13,16,19-22:5 and [3-^{14}C]labeled 9,12,15,18,21-24:5 or 6,9,12,15,18,21-24:6 with hepatocytes, all three substrates were metabolized to yield esterified 4,7,10,13,16,19-22:6 (16). Comparable studies have shown that 7,10,13,16-22:4 is metabolized to 4,7,10,13,16-22:5 via an analogous pathway (17).

The above studies show that 7,10,13,16-22:4 and 7,10,13,16,19-22:5 are the respective precursors of 4,7,10,13,16-22:5 and 4,7,10,13,16,19-22:6, but their synthesis is independent of an acyl-CoA-dependent 4-desaturase. Indeed, the synthesis of these two acids implies that there is intracellular communication between the endoplasmic reticulum and a site for partial β-oxidation. Both 6,9,12,15,18,21-24:6 and 6,9,12,15,18-24:5 are made in the endoplasmic reticulum. These acids must then move to a site for β-oxidation where they are chain-shortened, to 4,7,10,13,16,19-22:6 and 4,7,10,13,16-22:5, respectively, followed by their esterification into membrane lipids. It is well recognized that peroxisomes chain-shorten fatty acids, and these catabolites may then move to mitochondria where the process is completed (18). It is also possible that peroxisomes partially β-oxidize long-chain acids, and that the chain-shortened products move to the endoplasmic reticulum where they are esterified. We used 7,10,13,16-22:4 as a model substrate to study this partial β-oxidation esterification process. The rationale for using this acid as a model substrate is based on three types of studies. When 7,10,13,16-22:4 was fed to rats raised on a diet devoid of fat, it was primarily metabolized to yield esterified arachidonate (19). When [3-^{14}C]7,10,13,16-22:4 was injected into the tail vein of rats fed chow, 96% of the esterified radioactivity in liver phospholipids was arachidonate with the substrate accounting for only 4% (20). When [3-^{14}C]7,10,13,16-22:4 was incubated with fibroblasts, it was metabolized to yield esterified arachidonate. However, when it was incubated with fibroblasts from patients with Zellweger's disease, who lack peroxisomes, it was not possible to detect any esterified arachidonate (21).

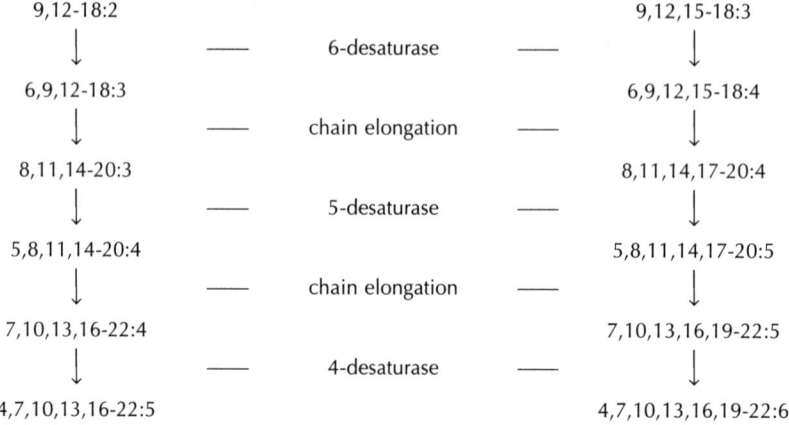

Fig. 2.1. The pathways, as commonly depicted, for showing how dietary linoleate and linolenate are metabolized to 4,7,10,13,16-docosapentaenoic acid and 4,7,10,13,16,19-docosahexaenoic acid, respectively, in the endoplasmic reticulum.

When we incubated [1-^{14}C]7,10,13,16-22:4 with rat liver peroxisomes, its rate of β-oxidation, as measured by the generation of acid-soluble radioactivity, was not depressed when microsomes and 1-acyl-*sn*-glycero-3-phosphocholine (1-acyl-GPC) were included in the incubation. Conversely, when [3-^{14}C]7,10,13,16-22:4 was incubated with peroxisomes, its rate of β-oxidation, as measured by the generation of acid-soluble radioactivity, was depressed when 1-acyl-GPC and microsomes were included in the incubation. The data show that the preferred metabolic rate of [1-^{14}C]5,8,11,14-20:4, when it was produced via β-oxidation, was to move out of peroxisomes to the endoplasmic reticulum where it was esterified into the acceptor, rather than serving as a continued substrate for β-oxidation. When [1-^{14}C]7,10,13,16-22:4 was incubated alone with peroxisomes, its rate of β-oxidation was about fourfold greater compared with [1-^{14}C]7,10,13,16-22:4. When the acyl-CoAs of 5,8,11,14-20:4 and 7,10,13,16-22:4 were incubated with 1-acyl-GPC and rat liver microsomes, their rates of acylation were 159 and 18 nmol/min/mg of microsomal protein, respectively. These studies show that there is an inverse relationship between rates of β-oxidation and acylation. Indeed, the studies suggest that competition between peroxisomal β-oxidation and microsomal acylation reactions may be an important *in vivo* control for determining what types of polyunsaturated fatty acids are incorporated into membrane lipids (22).

Figure 2.1 shows the classical pathway whereby dietary linoleate and linolenate are metabolized to 4,7,10,13,16-22:5 and 4,7,10,13,16,19-22:6, respectively. Figure 2.2 shows a revised pathway for the biosynthesis of those two acids. There are three major differences between the two reaction sequences. According to the revised pathway, both 6,9,12,15,18-24:5 and 6,9,12,15,18,21-24:6 are made in the endoplasmic reticulum. These acids must then move to peroxisomes where they are chain-shortened by two carbon atoms. The resulting products presumably must then move back to the endoplasmic reticulum where they are esterified into acceptors. It

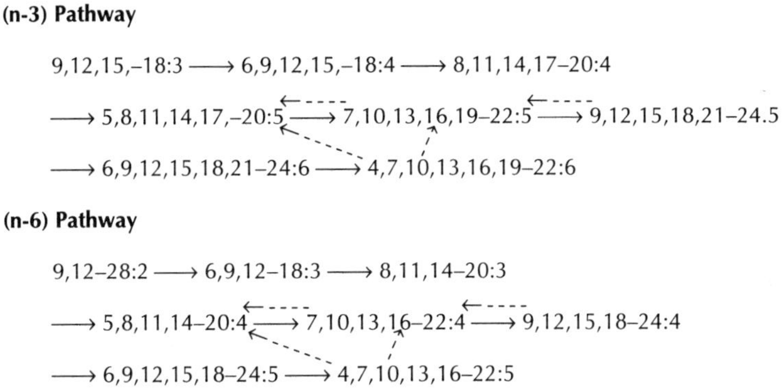

(n-3) Pathway

9,12,15,-18:3 ⟶ 6,9,12,15,-18:4 ⟶ 8,11,14,17–20:4

⟶ 5,8,11,14,17,-20:5 ⇌ 7,10,13,16,19–22:5 ⇌ 9,12,15,18,21–24.5

⟶ 6,9,12,15,18,21–24:6 ⟶ 4,7,10,13,16,19–22:6

(n-6) Pathway

9,12–28:2 ⟶ 6,9,12–18:3 ⟶ 8,11,14–20:3

⟶ 5,8,11,14–20:4 ⇌ 7,10,13,16–22:4 ⇌ 9,12,15,18–24:4

⟶ 6,9,12,15,18–24:5 ⟶ 4,7,10,13,16–22:5

Fig. 2.2. Revised pathways for the biosynthesis of 4,7,10,13,16-docosapentaenoic acid and 4,7,10,13,16,19-docosahexaenoic acid. The solid arrows denote reaction taking place in the endoplasmic reticulum. The dashed arrows show acids that are substrates for partial β-oxidation followed by esterification of chain-shortened products into membrane lipids.

remains to be determined what regulates this intracellular movement. According to Figure 2.1, two acids in each sequence are chain-elongated. According to the revised pathway, three acids in each pathway are chain-elongated and two of these reactions take place in sequence. In a recent review Cinti and his colleagues (23) summarize the evidence suggesting that separate malonyl-CoA-dependent condensing enzymes are used for saturated vs. unsaturated primers. The resulting β-ketoacyl-CoA derivatives are then channeled into a common set of enzymes to complete the chain-elongation process. It would seem unlikely that a single condensing enzyme could accept six different primers, as would be required by the revised pathway. Clearly, additional studies are required to determine what regulates microsomal fatty acid chain-elongation and how many enzymes are present. Desaturation at position 6 has generally been recognized as the rate-limiting step in the biosynthesis of arachidonate. According to the revised pathway, four different fatty acids must be desaturated at position 6. In a series of competitive substrate studies, we were unable to obtain any conclusive evidence that microsomes contain chain length-specific 6-desaturases (24). Further studies are also clearly required to determine what regulates desaturation at position 6 as it now relates to the biosynthesis of both 4,7,10,13,16-22:5 and 4,7,10,13,16,19-22:6.

Acknowledgment

The studies were supported in part by National Institutes of Health Grant DK-20387.

References

1. Stoffel, W., and Ach, K.L. Der Stoffwechsel der Ungesättigten Fettsäuren. II.

Eigenschaften des Kettenverlängernden Enzyms zur Frage der Biohydrogenierung der Ungesättigten Fettsäuren (1964) *Hoppe-Seylers Z. Physiol. Chem. 337,* 123–132.

2. Sprecher, H., and Lee, C.-J. The Absence of an 8-Desaturase in Rat Liver, a Reevaluation of Optional Pathways for the Metabolism of Linoleic and Linolenic Acids (1975) *Biochim. Biophys. Acta 388,* 113–125.

3. Dhopeshwarkar, G.A., and Subramanian, C. Intracranial Conversion of Linoleic Acid to Arachidonic Acid: Evidence for Lack of Δ^8 Desaturase in the Brain (1976) *J. Neurochem. 26,* 1175–1179.

4. Dhopeshwarkar, G.A., and Subramanian, C. Biosynthesis of Polyunsaturated Fatty Acids in the Developing Brain, II. Metabolic Transformation of Intracranially Administered [3-^{14}C]Eicosatrienoic Acid—Evidence for Lack of Δ^8 Desaturase (1976) *Lipids 11,* 689–692.

5. Albert, D.H., Rhamy, R.K., and Coniglio, J.G. Desaturation of Eicosa-11,14-Dienoic Acid in Human Testes (1979) *Lipids 14,* 498–500.

6. Cook, H.W., Byers, D.M., Palmer, F.B.S.C., Spence, M.W., Rakoff, H., Duval, S.M., and Emken, E.A. Alternate Pathways in the Desaturation and Chain Elongation of Linolenic Acid, 18:3(n-3), in Cultured Glioma Cells (1991) *J. Lipid Res. 32,* 1265–1273.

7. Strittmatter, P., Spatz, L., Corcoran, D., Rogers, M.J., Setlow, B., and Redline, R. Purification and Properties of Rat Liver Microsomal Stearyl Coenzyme A Desaturase (1974) *Proc. Natl. Acad. Sci. U.S.A. 71,* 4565–4569.

8. Kaestner, K.H., Natambi, J.M., Kelly, T.J., and Lane, M.D. Differentiation-Induced Gene Expression in 3T3-L1 Preadipocytes (1989) *J. Biol. Chem. 264,* 14755–14761.

9. Ntambi, J.M. Dietary Regulation of Stearyl-CoA Desaturnase 1 Gene Expression in Mouse Liver (1992) *J. Biol. Chem. 267,* 10925–10930.

10. Okayasu, T., Nagao, M., Ishibashi, T., and Imai, Y. Purification and Partial Characterization of Linoleoyl-CoA Desaturase from Rat Liver Microsomes (1981) *Arch. Biochem. Biophys. 206,* 21–28.

11. Gurr, M.J., Robinson, M.P., James, A.T., Morris, C.J., and Howling, D. The Substrate Specificity of Desaturase: The Conversion of *cis*-12-Octadecenoic Acid into Linoleic Acid in Different Animal and Plant Species (1972) *Biochim. Biophys. Acta 280,* 415–421.

12. Sprecher, H., Voss, A.C., Careaga, M., and Hadjiagapioú, C. (1987) in *Polyunsaturated Fatty Acids and Eicosanoids,* Lands, W.E.M., American Oil Chemists' Society, Champaign, IL, pp. 154–168.

13. Lands, W.E.M., Inoue, M., Sugiura, Y., and Okuyama, H. Selective Incorporation of Polyunsaturated Fatty Acids into Phosphadidylcholine by Rat Liver Microsomes (1983) *J. Biol. Chem. 257,* 14968–14972.

14. Voss, A.C., and Sprecher, H. Metabolism of 6,9,12-Octadecatrienic and 6,9,12,15-Octadecatetraenoic Acids by Rat Hepatocytes (1988) *Biochim. Biophys. Acta 958,* 153–162.

15. Sugiura, T., Kudo, N., Ojima, T., Mabuchi-Itoh, K., Yamashita, A., and Waku, K. Coenzyme A-Dependent Cleavage of Membrane Phospholipids in Several Rat Tissues; ATP-Independent Acyl-CoA Synthesis and the Generation of Lysophospholipids (1995) *Biochim. Biophys. Acta 1255,* 167–176.

16. Voss, A.C., Reinhart, M., Sankarappa, S., and Sprecher, H. The Metabolism of 7,10,13,16,19-Docosapentaenoic Acid to 4,7,10,13,16,19-Docosahexaenoic Acid in Rat Liver Is Independent of a 4-Desaturase (1991) *J. Biol. Chem. 266,* 1995–2000.

17. Mohammed, B.S., Sankarappa, S., Geiger, M., and Sprecher, H. Reevaluation of the Pathway for the Metabolism of 7,10,13,16-Docosatetraenoic Acid to 4,7,10,13,16-Docosapatenoic Acid in Rat Liver (1995) *Arch. Biochem. Biophys. 317,* 179–184.

18. Osmundsen, H., Bremer, J., and Pedersen, J.I. Metabolic Aspects of Peroxisomal β-Oxidation (1991) *Biochim. Biophys. Acta 1085,* 141–158.
19. Sprecher, H. The Total Synthesis and Metabolism of 7,10,13,16-Docosatetraenoate in the Rat (1967) *Biochim. Biophys. Acta 144,* 296–304.
20. Voss, A., Reinhart, M., and Sprecher, H. Differences in the Interconversion between 20- and 22-Carbon (n-3) and (n-6) Polyunsaturated Fatty Acids in Rat Liver (1992) *Biochim. Biophys. Acta 1127,* 33–40.
21. Christensen, E., Woldseth, B., Hagve, T.-A., Poll-the, B.T., Wanders, R.J.A., Sprecher, H. Stokke, O., and Christophersen, B.O. Peroxisomal β-Oxidation of Polyunsaturated Long Chain Fatty Acids in Human Fibroblasts. The Polyunsaturated and the Saturated Long Chain Fatty Acids Are Retroconverted by the Same Acyl-CoA Oxidase (1993) *Scand. J. Clin. Lab. Invest. 536 (Suppl. 215),* 61–74.
22. Baykousheva, S.P., Luthria, D.L., and Sprecher, H. Arachidonic Acid Formed by Peroxisomal β-Oxidation of 7,10,13,16-Docosatetraenoic Acid Is Esterified into 1-Acyl-*sn*-glycero-3-phosphocholine by Microsomes (1994) *J. Biol. Chem. 269,* 18340–18344.
23. Cinti, D.L., Cook, L., Nagai, M.N., and Suneja, S.K. The Fatty Acid Chain Elongation System of Mammalian Endoplasmic Reticulum (1992) *Prog. Lipid Res. 31,* 1–52.
24. Geiger, M., Mohammed, B.S., Sankarappa, S., and Sprecher, H. Studies to Determine If Rat Liver Contains Chain Length-Specific Acyl-CoA 6-Desaturases (1993) *Biochim. Biophys. Acta 1170,* 137–142.

Chapter 3

Biosynthesis of γ-Linolenic Acid in the Cyanobacterium *Spirulina platensis*

Norio Murata, Patcharaporn Deshnium, and Yasushi Tasaka

Department of Regulation Biology,
National Institute for Basic Biology,
Myodaiji, Okazaki 444, Japan

Lipids and Fatty Acids in Cyanobacteria

Cyanobacteria are autotrophic prokaryotes with the capacity for photosynthesis. Cyanobacterial cells resemble the chloroplasts of plants in terms of both membrane structure and glycerolipid composition (1). There are three types of membrane in cyanobacterial cells: the plasma membrane, the outer membrane, and the thylakoid membrane. The thylakoid membranes are closed systems and are separate from the plasma membrane (1,2). This architecture corresponds to that of the eukaryotic chloroplast, which has inner and outer envelope membranes and thylakoid membranes.

The major glycerolipids of cyanobacterial cells are monogalactosyl diacylglycerol (MGDG), digalactosyl diacylglycerol (DGDG), sulfoquinovosyl diacylglycerol (SQDG), and phosphatidylglycerol (PG) (2), and in eukaryotic chloroplasts these same glycerolipids predominate (3,4). MGDG accounts for about half of the total glycerolipids, and the other three glycerolipids contribute to the remaining half to different degrees, depending on the strain and specific growth conditions (5,6).

Cyanobacterial strains can be classified into four groups by reference to the unsaturation of fatty acids (Table 3.1). Group 1 is characterized by the presence of saturated and monounsaturated fatty acids excessively, whereas groups 2, 3 and 4 contain polyunsaturated fatty acids. The latter fatty acids are unusual in that the C_{18} and C_{16} fatty acids are esterified to the *sn*-1 and *sn*-2 positions of the glycerol moiety, respectively. Strains in group 1 [e.g., *Synechococcus* sp. PCC 7942 (*Anacystis nidulans* R2) and *Mastigocladus laminosus*] introduce a double bond only at the Δ9 position of fatty acids, either at the *sn*-1 or the *sn*-2 position (5,7). Strains in group 2 (e.g., *Synechococcus* sp. PCC 7002, *Anabaena variabilis*, *Plectonema boryanum*, and *Nostoc muscorum*) can introduce double bonds at the Δ9, Δ12 and Δ15 (ω-3) positions of C_{18} fatty acids at the *sn*-1 position, as well as at the Δ9 and Δ12 positions of C_{16} fatty acids at the *sn*-2 position (7,8). Strains in group 3 (e.g., *Synechocystis* sp. PCC 6714 and *Spirulina platensis*) can also introduce three double bonds, but these are found at the Δ6, Δ9 and Δ12 positions of C_{18} fatty acids at the *sn*-1 position (5). Strains in group 4 (e.g., *Synechocystis* sp. PCC 6803 and *Tolypothrix tenuis*) can introduce double bonds at the Δ6, Δ9, Δ12 and Δ15 (ω-3) positions of C_{18} fatty acids at the *sn*-1 position (5,9). However, desaturation at the *sn*-2 position in groups 1 and 2 and Δ6 desaturation at the *sn*-1 position in groups 3 and 4 are confined to MGDG, with both SQDG and PG being excluded. It is likely that desaturation does not occur in fatty acids that are bound to DGDG; the various molecular species of DGDG are probably synthesized by galactosylation of the corresponding molecular species of MGDG (8). Among the members of the four groups of cyanobacteria, those in group 2 are the most similar to plant chloroplasts in terms of the desaturation of fatty acids.

Biosynthesis of γ-Linolenic Acid in *Spirulina*

The cyanobacterial strains in group 3 and group 4 synthesize γ-linolenic acid, while *Spirulina platensis*, which belongs to group 3, was found to contain the highest level of γ-linolenic acid among the strains examined (Table 3.1). We analyzed the fatty acid composition of individual lipid classes of *Spirulina platensis* (Table 3.2). The level of 16:0 ranged from 50 to 60% of the total fatty acids in each lipid class. γ-Linolenic acid was confined to MGDG and DGDG, whereas 18:2(9,12) was a main contributor of fatty acids to SQDG and DGDG.

The distribution of fatty acids at the *sn*-1 and *sn*-2 positions of the glycerol moieties of lipids (data not shown) indicated that the *sn*-2 position was exclusively esterified by 16:0, and that all of the C_{18} fatty acids and 16:1(9) were located at the *sn*-1 position. These findings suggest a pathway for the biosynthesis of fatty acids (or molecular species), as shown in Fig. 3.1. In MGDG, SQDG, and PG, the major precursors of all of the molecular species are *sn*-1-18:0/*sn*-2-16:0 species. In these precursors, the

TABLE 3.1 Major Fatty Acids of the Total Lipids from Various Strains of Cyanobacteria

Organism	Growth temp. (°C)	Fatty acid (mole %)							
		16:0	16:1 (9)	16:2 (9,12)	18:0	18:1 (9)	18:2 (9,12)	α18:3 (9,12,15)	γ18:3 (6,9,12)	18:4 (6,9,12,15)
Group 1										
Mastigocladus laminosus (F)	34	34	31	0	5	29	0	0	0	0
Synechococcus PCC7942 (U)	34	49	36	0	4	10*	0	0	0	0
Synechococcus PCC6301 (U)	38	48	38	0	4	7*	0	0	0	0
Synechococcus lividus (U)	38	42	36	0	1	20	0	0	0	0
Group 2										
Plectonema boryanum (F)	28	36	22	0	1	3*	10	29	0	0
Nostoc muscorum (F)	28	41	14	0	1	2	7	35	0	0
Anabaena variabilis (F)	22	29	22	3	t	7	15	24	0	0
Synechococcus PCC7002 (U)	22	35	19	0	t	10	25	10	0	0
Group 3										
Spirulina platensis (F)	32	53	3	0	1	1	13	0	29	0
Synechocystis PCC6714 (U)	34	59	2	0	t	9	16	0	12	0
Group 4										
Tolypothrix tenuis (F)	30	55	3	0	1	2	5	6	11	17
Synechocystis PCC6803 (U)	22	51	3	0	1	2	6	8	21	8

t: Trace (less than 0.5%). *Mixture of Δ9-octadecenoic acid (oleic acid) and Δ11-octadecenoic acid (*cis*-vaccenic acid). F and U in parentheses indicate filamentous and unicellular strains, respectively.

TABLE 3.2 Major Fatty Acids of the Various Lipid Classes in *Spirulina platensis* Grown at 34°C

Lipid class	Fatty acid (mole %)				
	16:0	16:1 (9)	18:1 (9)	18:2 (9,12)	γ18:3 (6,9,12)
MGDG (47%)	52	3	1	1	42
DGDG (16%)	51	5	2	3	38
SQDG (17%)	60	2	7	26	1
PG (20%)	55	1	5	35	1

first double bond is introduced at the Δ9 position of 18:0, at the *sn*-1 position, to yield 18:1(9), and the second double bond is introduced at the Δ12 position of 18:1(9), at the *sn*-1 position, to yield 18:2(9,12). In SQDG and PG, no further desaturation occurs. In MGDG, by contrast, a third double bond is introduced at the Δ6 position of 18:2(9,12) to yield 18:3(6,9,12), in other words, γ-linolenic acid.

It is likely that the molecular species of DGDG are synthesized by galactosylation of the corresponding molecular species of MGDG and that no desaturation takes place in DGDG itself (8). The scheme in Fig. 3.1 suggests the possible existence of three different types of desaturase, namely, Δ9 desaturase, Δ12 desaturase and Δ6

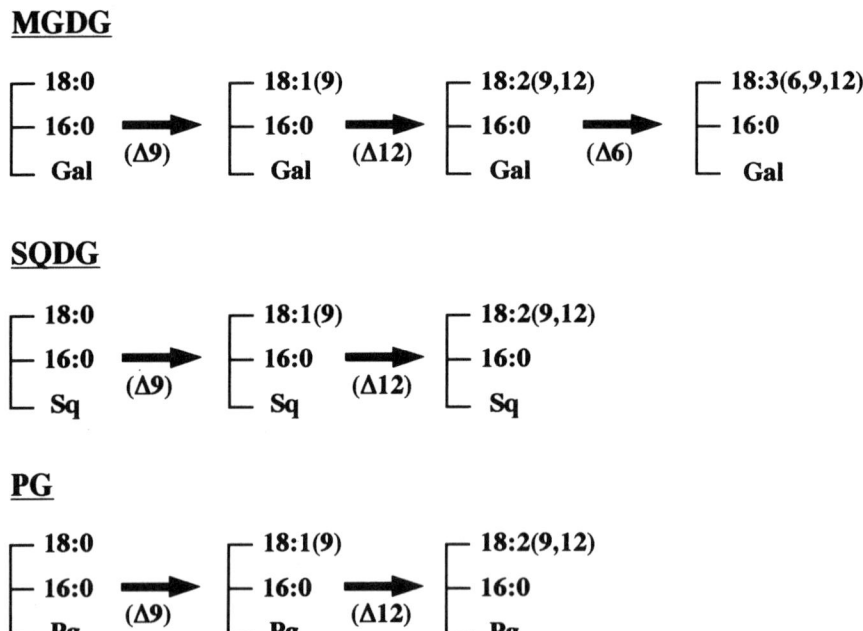

Fig. 3.1. Pathway for the desaturation of fatty acids in *Spirulina platensis*. Abbreviations: Gal, galactose; Sq, sulfoquinovose; Pg, glycerolphosphate.

desaturase. This last desaturase is specific to MGDG, whereas the former two desaturases can use SQDG and PG as their substrates, in addition to MGDG.

There are three classes of desaturases. Acyl-CoA desaturases introduce double bonds into fatty acids bound to coenzyme A; these enzymes are bound to the endoplasmic reticulum in animal, yeast and fungal cells (10). Acyl-ACP desaturases introduce double bonds into fatty acids that are bound to ACP; they are present in the stroma of plant plastids (11). Acyl-lipid desaturases introduce double bonds into fatty acids that have been esterified to glycerolipids (12–14); they are bound to the endoplasmic reticulum, the chloroplast membrane in plant cells (12), and the thylakoid membranes in cyanobacterial cells (13). This last class of desaturase is the most efficient regulator of the extent of unsaturation of membrane lipids in response to changes in temperature.

The acyl-lipid desaturases can be further classified into two subgroups by reference to their electron donors. One subgroup, present in the endoplasmic reticulum of plant cells, uses cytochrome b_5 as the electron donor (15,16). The other, present in the chloroplasts of plant cells and in cyanobacterial cells, uses ferredoxin as the electron donor (13,17,18). A unique characteristic of the acyl-lipid desaturases is that they recognize, by an unknown mechanism, exactly those positions within various carbon chains at which double bonds are to be specifically introduced.

Cyanobacterial Desaturases

All known cyanobacterial desaturases are of the acyl-lipid and membrane-bound type (19). Because purification of these enzymes by conventional methods has proved difficult, we attempted the molecular cloning of the various desaturases. A mutant that was defective in the synthesis of 18:2(9,12), 18:3(6,9,12), 18:3(9,12,15), and 18:4(6,9,12,15) was initially isolated from *Synechocystis* sp. PCC 6803 after treatment of wild-type cells with ethyl methanesulfonate (9). The mutant, designated Fad12, was defective in desaturation at the Δ12 position of C_{18} fatty acids at the *sn*-1 position of the glycerol moiety in all lipid classes. The growth rate at 22°C of the mutant was much lower than that of the wild type, whereas mutant and wild-type cells grew at about the same rate at 34°C (20).

A gene (*desA*) for the Δ12 desaturase was isolated (21) by screening of the genomic DNA library of *Synechocystis* sp. PCC 6803 for the ability to complement the Fad12 mutation with respect to both growth at low temperature and desaturation at the Δ12 position of fatty acids after *in situ* transformation. The *desA* gene contains an open reading frame of 1053 bp that corresponds to 351 amino acid residues and encodes an acyl-lipid desaturase. The enzyme can introduce a second *cis*-double bond at the Δ12 position of fatty acids bound to membrane glycerolipids. Similar *desA* genes were isolated by heterologous hybridization from *Synechococcus* sp. PCC 7002, *Synechocystis* sp. PCC 6714 and *Anabaena variabilis* with a probe derived from the *desA* gene of *Synechocystis* sp. PCC 6803 (22). The amino acid sequence deduced from the nucleotide sequence of the *desA* gene of *Synechocystis* sp. PCC 6803 is similar to that of the gene from *Synechocystis* sp. PCC 6714. The extent of sequence similarity between the amino acid sequences from *Synechocystis* sp. PCC 6803 and *Synechocystis* sp. PCC 6714 is 96%. However, the extent of conservation of the amino acid level between the sequences of polypeptides from *Synechocystis* sp. PCC 6803 and *Synechococcus* sp. PCC 7002 and that between the sequences of polypeptides from *Synechocystis* sp. PCC 6803 and *A. variabilis* are 57 and 59%, respectively (22).

The *desC* gene for a Δ9 acyl-lipid desaturase was found in the 5′-upstream region of the *desA* gene on the chromosome of *A. variabilis* (23). The *desC* gene of *Synechocystis* sp. PCC 6803 was cloned by screening a genomic library with a probe derived from the *desC* gene of *A. variabilis*. The deduced amino-acid sequences of the Δ9 acyl-lipid desaturases of *Synechocystis* sp. PCC 6803 and *A. variabilis* are similar to those of the Δ9 acyl-CoA desaturases from rat (24), mouse (25,26), and yeast (27), with homology at the amino acid level of about 25% in each case.

We have cloned the *desB* gene for the ω-3 acyl-lipid desaturase from *Synechocystis* sp. PCC 6803 by screening a genomic library with a probe derived from the *desA* gene of this strain (28). Reddy et al. (29) cloned the *desD* gene for Δ6 desaturase by the "gain-of-function" method using *Anabaena* sp. PCC 7120, which does not contain a Δ6 desaturase. Currently genes for all of the desaturases have been cloned from *Synechocystis* sp. PCC 6803.

Molecular Cloning of Desaturases of *Spirulina*

The desA *Gene for Δ12 Desaturase*

From comparisons of the sequences of the *desA* genes from *A. variabilis*, *Synechocystis* sp. PCC 6803, *Synechocystis* sp. PCC 6714 and *Synechococcus* sp. PCC 7002 (22), we selected two conserved regions, namely, amino acid positions 116–121 and 233–237, counted from the amino terminus of the *desA* gene of *Synechocystis* sp. PCC 6803. Oligonucleotides corresponding to these regions, including a synthetic *Eco RI* restriction site at each 5′ end, were synthesized. Their sequences were as follows:

5-GGGAATTCTA(TC)CC(ACGT)TT(TC)CA(TC)AG(CT)TGG-3′ and
5′-GGGAATTCAC(AG)TT(AGT)AT(AG)TC(AG)TG(AG)CA-3′.

The oligonucleotides were used as forward and reverse primers, respectively, for amplification by the polymerase chain reaction (PCR) of a partial nucleotide sequence of the *desA* gene of *Spirulina platensis*, with genomic DNA as the template. The amplified products of about 400 bp were of the size predicted for the partial sequence of the *desA* gene of *Synechocystis* sp. PCC 6803. These products of PCR were subcloned into pBluescript(SK+) (Stratagene, La Jolla, CA) and nucleotide sequences were determined. A clone with a sequence homologous to that of the *desA* gene of *Synechocystis* sp. PCC 6803 was identified. A genomic DNA library of *S. platensis*, constructed in the phage vector λ*DASHII* (Stratagene) was screened with the insert of this clone, and the *desA* gene for Δ12 desaturase was cloned (its sequence has been deposited to the EMBL Data Library with the accession number X86736). Figure 3.2 shows a comparison of the amino acid sequence deduced from the *desA* gene of *S. platensis* with those deduced from the *desA* genes of *A. variabilis*, *Synechocystis* sp. PCC 6803, *Synechocystis* sp. PCC 6714 and *Synechococcus* sp. PCC 7002. The extent of homology at the amino acid level between the *desA* gene of *S. platensis* and those of *A. variabilis*, *Synechocystis* sp. PCC 6803, *Synechocystis* sp.

```
Spirulina   MTLSIVKSEDSSSRPSAVPSDLPLEEDIINTLPSGVFVQDRYKAWMTV  48
Anabaena     MTTSTIKNQEIKNLSNPELRLKDILDTLPRSVYQQNRRKAWTQA  44
PCC 6803    MTATIPPLTPTVTPSNPDRPIADLKLQDIIKTLPKECFEKKASKAWASV  49
PCC 6714    MTATIPPLRPTETSSNPDRPIADLKLQDIIKTLPKECFEKKASKAWASV  49
PCC 7002     MTSVTVRPSATTLLEKHPNLRLRDILDTLPRSVYEINPLKAWSRV  45


Spirulina   IINVVMVGLGWLGIAIAPWFLLPVVWVFTGTALTGFFVIGHDCGHRSFSR  98
Anabaena    LLSVVMVGLCYWSLAIAPWFLLLPAWFFTGTTLTGFFVIGHDCGHRSFSR  94
PCC 6803    LITLGAIAVGYLGIIYLPWYCLPITWIWTGTALTGAFVVGHDCGHRSFAK  99
PCC 6714    LITLGAIALGYLGIIYLPWYCLPFTWIWTGTALTGAFVVGHDCGHRSFAK  99
PCC 7002    LLSVAAVVGCYALLAIAPWYLLLPVWFLTGTTLTGFFVIGHDCGHRSFSR  95
                                                 *    *
                                                  *  *

Spirulina   NVWVNDWVGHILFLPIIYPFHSWRIGHNQHHKYTNRMELDNAWQPWRKE- 147
Anabaena    RNWVNNLVGHLFMMPLIYPFHSWRIKHNHHHKYTNNLDEDNAWHPIRPEV 144
PCC 6803    KRWVNDLVGHIAFAPLIYPFHSWRLLHDHHHLHTNKIEVDNAWDPWSVE- 148
PCC 6714    KRWVNDLVGHIAFAPLIYPFHSWRLLHDHHHLHTNKIEVDNAWDPWSVE- 148
PCC 7002    KNWVNNLVGHLAFLPLIYPFHSWRILHNHHHRYTNMNDEDNAWAPFTPEL 145
               *              *      **
                              *  **

Spirulina   EYQNAGKFMQVTYDLFRGRAWWIGSILHWASIHFDWTKFEGKQRQQVKFS 197
Anabaena    YASWGKTRQSAFKLFMRQRLWWVASVGHQAVVHFDWRKFKVKQQADVRFS 194
PCC 6803    AFQASPAIVRLFYRAIRGPFWWTGSIFHWSLMHFKLSNFAQRDRNKVKLS 198
PCC 6714    AFQASPAIVRLFYRAIRGPFWWTGSIFHWGLMHFKLSNFAERDRNKVKLS 198
PCC 7002    YDDSPAFIKAVYRA-IRGKLWWLASVIHQLKLHFMWFAFEGKQREQVRFS 194
                                  *   *

Spirulina   SLLVIGAAAIAFPTMILTIGVWGF-VKFWVIPWLVFHFWMSTFTLLHHTI 246
Anabaena    FSLVVIAGAVAFPTMFATLGIWGFFVKFWFVPWLGYHFWMSTFTLVHHTY 244
PCC 6803    IAVVFLFAAIAFPALIITTGVWGF-VKFWLMPWLVYHFWMSTFTIVHHTI 247
PCC 6714    IAVVFLFAAVAFPALIITTGVWGF-VKFWLMPWLVYHFWMSTFTIVHHTI 247
PCC 7002    ALFVIIAGAIAPPVMFYGLGVWG--VVKFWLMPWLGYHFWMSTFTLVHHTV 243
                                           *      **

Spirulina   ADIPFREPEQWHEAESQLSGTVHCNYSRWGEFLCHDINVHIPHHVTTAIP 296
Anabaena    PDVPFEAENKWHEAMAQLFGTIHCDYPKWVEVLCHDINVHVPHHLSTGIP 294
PCC 6803    PEIRFRPAADWSAAEAQLNGTVHCDYPRWVEVLCHDINVHIPHHLSVAIP 297
PCC 6714    PEIRFRPAEDWSAAEAQLNGTVHCDYPRWVEVLCHDINVHIPHHLSVAIP 297
PCC 7002    PEIPFSYRDKWNEAIAQLSGTVHCDYPKWVEVLCHDINVHVPHHLHTGIP 293
                                                *    **
                                                 *  **

Spirulina   WYNLRTPTPVYRKIGGEYLYPECDFSWGLMKQVVDHAICMMRITIIS-QS 345
Anabaena    SYNLRKAYSSIQQNWGDYL-HELRFSWSLM-K-LITDECQLYQTDVNYQP 341
PCC 6803    SYNLRLAHGSLKENWGPFLY-ERTFNWQLMQQISGQ--CHLYDPEHGYRT 344
PCC 6714    SYNLRLAHASLKQNWGPFLY-ERTFNWGLMQQISGQ--CHLYDPDNGYRT 344
PCC 7002    SYNLRKALASIKQNWGEYL-YETKFHWELM-K-AITEQCHLYVAEHNYIS 340


Spirulina   LTT-KRV           351
Anabaena    FKDYYAGR          349
PCC 6803    FGSLKKV           351
PCC 6714    FSSLK             349
PCC 7002    FAQ-HQKR          347
```

Fig. 3.2. Alignment of the amino acid sequence of the Δ12 desaturase of *Spirulina platensis* with those of Δ12 desaturases of *Anabaena variabilis*, *Synechocystis* sp. PCC 6803, *Synechocystis* sp. PCC 6714, and *Synechococcus* sp. PCC 7002 (22). Histidine residues conserved in the Δ12 desaturases are marked by asterisks. The histidine residues conserved in the Δ6, Δ9, Δ12, and Δ15 (ω-3) desaturases (19) are marked by double asterisks.

PCC 6714 and *Synechococcus* sp. PCC 7002 was calculated to be 56.5, 52.3, 52.3 and 57.2%, respectively. Seventeen histidine residues are conserved in the five Δ12 desaturases. Among them, eight histidine residues (Fig. 3.2) are conserved in the four desaturases that act at the Δ6, Δ9, Δ12, and ω-3 positions (19). As demonstrated in other enzymes with non-heme iron as the catalytic center, such as rubrerythrin (30), isopenicillin N synthase (31), stearoyl-acyl carrier protein desaturase (32), and lipoxygenase (33,34), it seems very likely that these histidine residues provide ligands to the iron that acts as the catalytic center.

The desD Gene for Δ6 Desaturase

The open reading frame (ORF) of the *desD* gene of *Synechosystis* sp. PCC 6803 was amplified by PCR with 5'-ATGCTAACAGCGGAAAGAAT-3' and 5'-GATGCTTTGCCCATGGCCTC-3' as the forward and reverse primers, respectively. The amplified product was subcloned into the TA cloning site of pCRII (Invitrogen, San Diego, CA). The genomic DNA library of *Spirulina platensis* that had been constructed in λDASHII was screened with a probe derived from the amplified DNA product, and the *desD* gene

```
Spirulina   MTSTTSKVTFGKSIGFRKELNRRVNAYLEAENISPRDNPPMYLKTAIILA   50
PCC 6803    MLTAERIKFTQKRGFRRVLNQRVDAYFAEHGLTQRDNPSMYLKTLIIVL   49


Spirulina   WVVSAWTFVVFGPDVLWMKLLGCIVLGFGVSAVGFNISHDGNHGGYSKYQ  100
PCC 6803    WLFSAWAFVLFAPVIFPVRLLGCMVLAIALAAFSFNVGHDANHNAYSSNP   99
                                                 *      *
                                                   *   *
Spirulina   WVNYLSGLTHDAIGVSSYLWKFRHNVLHHTYTNILGHDVEIHGDELVRMS  150
PCC 6803    HINRVLGMTYDFVGLSSFLWRYRHNYLHHTYTNILGHDVEIHGDGAVRMS  149
                            *    **        *     *
                                 **

Spirulina   PSMEYRWYHRYQHWFIWFVYPFIPYYWSIADVQTMLFKRQYHDHEIPSPT  200
PCC 6803    PEQEHVGIYRFQQFYIWGLYLFIPFYWFLYDVYLVLNKGKYHDHKIPPFQ  199
                                                        * *

Spirulina   WVDIATLLAFKAFGVAVFLIIPIAVGYSPLEAVIGASIVYMTHGLVACVV  250
PCC 6803    PLELASLLGIKLLWLGYVFGLPLALGFSIPEVLIGASVTYMTYGIVVCTI  249


Spirulina   FMLAHVIEPAEFLDPD-NL-HIDDEWAIAQVKTTVDFAPNNPIINWYVGG  298
PCC 6803    FMLAHVLESTEFLTPDGESGAIDDEWAICQIRTTANFATNNPFWNWFCGG  299
                *

Spirulina   LNYQTVHHLFPHICHIHYPKIAPILAEVCEEFGVNYAVHQTFFGALAANY  348
PCC 6803    LNHQVTHHLFPNICHIHYPQLENIIKDVCQEFGVEYKVYPTFKAAIASNY  349
               **           *  *
               **

Spirulina   SWLKKMSINPETKAIEQLTV                                368
PCC 6803    RWLEAMG-----KAS                                     359
```

Fig. 3.3. Alignment of the amino acid sequence of the Δ6 desaturase of *Spirulina platensis* with that of *Synechocystis* sp. PCC 6803 (29). Conserved histidine residues are marked by asterisks. The histidine residues conserved in the Δ6, Δ9, Δ12, and Δ15 (ω-3) desaturases (19) are marked by double asterisks.

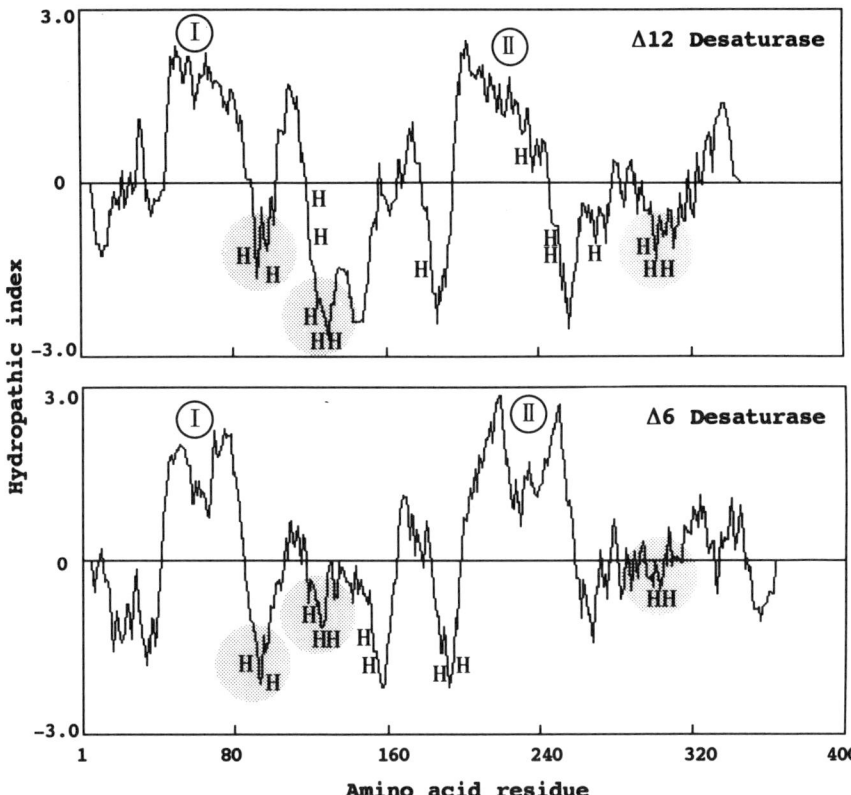

Fig. 3.4. Hydropathy plots and sites of histidine clusters in the Δ12 desaturase and Δ6 desaturase of *Spirulina platensis*. The three histidine (H) clusters conserved in the Δ6, Δ9, Δ12, and Δ15 (ω-3) desaturases (19) are shaded.

of *S. platensis* was cloned (its sequence has been deposited in the EMBL Data Library with the accession number X87094). Figure 3.3 shows the alignment of the deduced amino acid sequence of the Δ6 desaturase of *S. platensis* with that of *Synechocystis* sp. PCC 6803. The homology of the amino acid level between the two Δ6 desaturases is 52%, and 14 histidine residues are conserved in the two Δ6 desaturases. Seven of these histidine residues are conserved in all of the four desaturases that act at the Δ6, Δ9, Δ12, and ω-3 positions.

Figure 3.4 shows the predicted hydropathy profiles of the Δ12 and Δ6 desaturases of *S. platensis*. There are two hydrophobic domains, I and II, in both desaturases. It has been suggested that each domain spans the membrane twice, thus, each individual desaturase spans the membrane four times (19). Histidine residues are distributed throughout the sequences. However, the three histidine clusters conserved in all desaturases (19) are located at similar positions in both desaturases of *S. platensis*, and it seems likely that they are located on the cytoplasmic side of the membrane.

General Characteristics of *Spirulina platensis*

Spirulina platensis is a filamentous cyanobacterium, and its cells can be easily collected on nylon mesh. *S. platensis* grows under alkaline conditions with maximal growth at pH 10–11. These characteristics allow us to cultivate *S. platensis* in an open system and to collect the filamentous cells with a net, thereby freeing them of contaminating bacteria and fungi.

The history of *S. platensis* as a staple food for humans is of great interest (35). The cells contain a high proportion of protein (70% dry weight), several vitamins, and essential n-6 fatty acids. The strain that we used contains γ-linolenic acid, 18:3(6,9,12), as a major fatty acid. This compound has many pharmaceutical properties. It can relieve premenstrual syndrome (36) and is used as a treatment for a topic eczema. It also affects hyperlipidemia, which is frequently related to the development of arteriosclerosis and coronary heart disease, by lowering plasma levels of cholesterol and triglycerides.

Acknowledgments

The work summarized here was supported, in part, by Grants-in-Aid for Scientific Research on Priority Area (nos. 04273102 and 04273103) from the Ministry of Education, Science and Culture, Japan, to N.M.

References

1. Stanier, R.Y., and Cohen-Bazire, G. Phototrophic Prokaryotes: The Cyanobacteria (1977) *Annu. Rev. Microbiol. 31,* 225–274.
2. Omata, T., and Murata, N. Isolation and Characterization of the Cytoplasmic Membranes from the Blue-Green Alga (Cyanobacterium) *Anacystis nidulans* (1983) *Plant Cell Physiol. 24,* 1101–1112.
3. Block, M.A., Dorne, A.J., Joyard, J., and Douce, R. Preparation and Characterization of Membrane Fractions Enriched in Outer and Inner Envelope Membranes from Spinach Chloroplasts (1983) *J. Biol. Chem. 258,* 13281–13286.
4. Joyard, J., Block, M.A., and Douce, R. Molecular Aspects of Plastid Envelope Biochemistry (1991) *Eur. J. Biochem. 199,* 489–509.
5. Murata, N., Wada, H., and Gombos, Z. Modes of Fatty-Acid Desaturation in Cyanobacteria (1992) *Plant Cell Physiol. 33,* 933–941.
6. Murata, N., and Nishida, I. (1987) in *The Biochemistry of Plants,* Stumpf, P.K., Academic Press, Orlando, FL, vol. 9, pp. 315–347.
7. Sato, N., Murata, N., Miura, Y., and Ueta, N. Effect of Growth Temperature on Lipid and Fatty Acid Compositions in the Blue-Green Algae, *Anabaena variabilis* and *Anacystis nidulans* (1979) *Biochim. Biophys. Acta 572,* 19–28.
8. Sato, N., and Murata, N. Lipid Biosynthesis in the Blue-Green Alga, *Anabaena variabilis* II. Fatty Acids and Lipid Molecular Species (1982) *Biochim. Biophys. Acta 710,* 279–289.
9. Wada, H., and Murata, N. *Synechocystis* PCC 6803 Mutants Defective in Desaturation of Fatty Acids (1989) *Plant Cell Physiol. 30,* 971–978.

10. Holloway, P.W. (1983) in *The Enzymes*, Boyer, P. D., Academic Press, Orlando FL, vol. XVI, pp. 63–83.
11. McKeon, T.A., and Stumpf, P.K. Purification and Characterization of the Stearoyl-Acyl Carrier Protein Desaturase and the Acyl-Acyl Carrier Protein Thioesterase from Maturing Seeds of Safflower (1982) *J. Biol. Chem. 257*, 12141–12147.
12. Jaworski, J.G. (1987) in *The Biochemistry of Plants*, Stumpf, P.K., Academic Press, Orlando FL, vol. 9, pp. 159–174.
13. Wada, H., Schmidt, H., Heinz, E., and Murata, N. *In vitro* Ferredoxin-Dependent Desaturation of Fatty Acids in Cyanobacterial Thylakoid Membranes (1993) *J. Bacteriol. 175*, 544–547.
14. Sato, N., Seyama, Y., and Murata, N. Lipid-Linked Desaturation of Palmitic Acid in Monogalactosyl Diacylglycerol in the Blue-Green Alga (Cyanobacterium) *Anabaena variabilis* Studied *in vivo* (1986) *Plant Cell Physiol 27*, 819–835.
15. Kearns, E.V., Hugly, S., and Somerville, C.R. The Role of Cytochrome b_5 in $\Delta 12$ Desaturation of Oleic Acid by Microsomes of Safflower (*Carthamus tinctorius* L.) (1991) *Arch. Biochem. Biophys. 284*, 431–436.
16. Smith, M.A., Cross, A.R., Jones, O.T.G., Griffiths, W.T., Stymne, S., and Stobart, K. Electron-Transport Components of the 1-Acyl-2-Oleoyl-*sn*-Glycero-3-Phosphocholine Δ^{12}-Desaturase (Δ^{12}-Desaturase) in Microsomal Preparations from Developing Safflower (*Carthamus tinctorius* L.) Cotyledons (1990) *Biochem. J. 272*, 23–29.
17. Schmidt, H., and Heinz, E. Involvement of Ferredoxin in Desaturation of Lipid-Bound Oleate in Chloroplasts (1990) *Plant Physiol. 94*, 214–220.
18. Schmidt, H., and Heinz, E. Desaturation of Oleoyl Groups in Envelope Membranes from Spinach Chloroplasts (1990) *Proc. Natl. Acad. Sci. U.S.A. 87*, 9477–9480.
19. Murata, N., and Wada, H. Acyl-Lipid Desaturases and Their Importance in the Tolerance and Acclimation to Cold of Cyanobacteria (1995) *Biochem. J. 308*, 1–8.
20. Wada, H., Gombos, Z., Sakamoto, T. and Murata, N. Genetic Manipulation of Fatty Acids in Membrane Lipids in the Cyanobacterium *Synechocystis* PCC6803 (1992) *Plant Cell Physiol. 33*, 535–540.
21. Wada, H., Gombos, Z., and Murata, N. Enhancement of Chilling Tolerance of a Cyanobacterium by Genetic Manipulation of Fatty Acid Desaturation (1990) *Nature 347*, 200–203.
22. Sakamoto, T., Wada, H., Nishida, I., Ohmori, M., and Murata, N. Identification of Conserved Domains in the $\Delta 12$ Desaturases of Cyanobacteria (1994) *Plant Mol. Biol. 24*, 643–650.
23. Sakamoto, T., Wada, H., Nishida, I., Ohmori, M., and Murata, N. $\Delta 9$ Acyl-Lipid Desaturases of Cyanobacteria (1994) *J. Biol. Chem. 269*, 25576–25580.
24. Thiede, M.A., Ozols, J., and Strittmatter, P. Construction and Sequence of cDNA for Rat Liver Stearyl Coenzyme A Desaturase (1986) *J. Biol. Chem. 261*, 13230–13235.
25. Kaestner, K., Ntambi, J.M., Kelly, T.J., Jr., and Lane, M.D. Differentiation-Induced Gene Expression in 3T3-L1 Preadipocytes (1989) *J. Biol. Chem. 264*, 14755–14761.
26. Ntambi, J.M., Buhrow, S.A., Kaestner, K.H., Christy, R.J., Sibley, E., Kelly, T.J., Jr., and Lane, M.D. Differentiation-Induced Gene Expression in 3T3-L1 Preadipocytes (1988) *J. Biol. Chem. 263*, 17291–17300.
27. Stukey, J.E., McDonough, V.M., and Martin, C.E. The *OLE1* Gene of *Saccharomyces cerevisiae* Encodes the $\Delta 9$ Fatty Acid Desaturase and Can Be Functionally Replaced by the Rat Stearoyl-CoA Desaturase Gene (1990) *J. Biol. Chem. 265*, 20144–20149.
28. Sakamoto, T., Los, D.A., Higashi, S., Wada, H., Nishida, I., Ohmori, M., and Murata, N. Cloning of ω3 Desaturase from Cyanobacteria and Its Use in Altering the Degree of Membrane-Lipid Unsaturation (1994) *Plant Mol. Biol. 26*, 249–263.

29. Reddy, A.S., Nuccio, M.L., Gross, L.M., and Thomas, T.L. Isolation of a Δ^6-Desaturase Gene from the Cyanobacterium *Synechocystis* sp. Strain PCC6803 by Gain-of-Function Expression in *Anabaena* sp. Strain PCC7120 (1993) *Plant Mol. Biol. 27,* 283–300.
30. Donald, M.K., Jr., and Benet, C.P. Intrapeptide Sequence Homology in Rubrerythrin from *Desulfovibrio vulgaris*: Identification of Potential Ligands to the Diiron Site *Biochem. Biophys. Res. Commum. 181,* 337–341.
31. Li-June, M., and Lawrence, Q., Jr., NMR Studies of the Active Site of Isopenicillin N Synthase, A Non-Heme Iron (II) Enzyme (1991) *Biochemistry 30,* 11653–11659.
32. Brian, G.F., Shanklin, J., Somerville, C., and Münck, E. Stearoyl-Acyl Carrier Protein $\Delta 9$ Desaturase from *Ricinus communis* Is a Diiron-Oxo Protein (1993) *Proc. Natl. Acad. Sci. U.S.A. 90,* 2486–2490.
33. Chen, X.S., and Funk, C.D. Structure-Function Properties of Human Platelet 12-Lipoxygenase: Chimeric Enzyme and *in vitro* Mutagenesis Studies (1993) *FASEB J. 7,* 694–701.
34. Suzuki, H., Kishimoto, K., Yoshimoto, T., Yamamoto, S., Kanai, F., Ebina, Y., Miyatake, A., and Tanabe, T. Site-Directed Mutagenesis Studies on the Iron-Binding Domain and the Determinant for the Substrate Oxygenation Site of Porcine Leukocyte Arachidonate 12-Lipoxygenase (1994) *Biochem. Biophys. Acta 1210,* 308–316.
35. Richmond, A. (1986) *CRC Handbook of Microalgal Mass Culture,* CRC Press Inc., Boca Raton, FL, pp. 212–230.
36. Horrobin, D.F. The Role of Essential Fatty Acids and Prostaglandins in the Premenstrual Syndrome (1993) *J. Reprod. Med. 28,* 465–468.

Chapter 4

Enzymatic Enrichment of γ-Linolenic Acid from Black Currant Seed Oil

H.-J. Wille and J. Wang

Nestlé Research Center,
Lausanne, Switzerland

Introduction

The biological importance of γ-linolenic acid (GLA, 6,9,12-octadecatrienoic acid) of the n-6 series is well known (1,2). GLA is a precursor in the synthesis of series 1 prostaglandins and is created in vivo by enzymatic desaturation of linoleic acid (9,12-octadecadienoic acid). Certain factors such as stress, poor nutrition and aging impair the effectiveness of the 6-desaturase enzyme responsible for this conversion. Dietary supplementation with GLA is able to by-pass this impediment in the metabolic process.

Natural sources of GLA contain variable amounts of this acid (Table 4.1) but this rarely exceeds 25% and is even lower for oils other than borage oil. Thus there has always been an interest in producing higher concentrates of GLA. Different fractionation techniques have been developed to enrich GLA from natural sources. These include urea fractionation of fatty acids (3–7), separation on Y-zeolite and lipase-catalyzed reactions, such as selective hydrolysis of GLA-containing triacylglycerols (8), and selective esterification of GLA-containing fatty acid mixtures (9) derived from borage or evening primrose oil.

This paper reports an investigation concerning the ability of enzymes which catalyze the esterification of fatty acids to discriminate between α- and γ-linolenic acid. Another

TABLE 4.1 Average Fatty Acid Composition (%) of Several Main GLA-Containing Seed Oils

Fatty Acid	Borage	Blackcurrant	Evening Primrose
C16:0	9–11	6– 8	5– 7
C18:0	2– 4	1– 2	1– 2
C18:1, Δ9	14–18	9–13	5–10
C18:2, Δ9	35–40	44–51	73–78
C18:3, Δ6 (γ)	21–25	15–20	7–10
C18:3, Δ9 (α)	—	12–14	—
C18:4, Δ6	—	2– 4	—

goal of this study was to develop a complete process, moving from the hydrolysis of black currant seed oil (BCO) to the isolation of a GLA concentrate under mild conditions.

Experimental Procedures

Materials

Blackcurrant seed oil (BCO) of food quality was obtained from Food Ingredients Specialities Ltd. (Châtel St. Denis, Switzerland). Soya lecithin (Asol 100) was provided by Lucas Meyer (Hamburg, Germany). Phosphate buffer (pH 6.88, 0.025 M) and all other reagents were from E. Merck (Darmstadt, Germany). Lipase preparations used for hydrolysis were the lipase of *Candida cylindracea* from different suppliers. These were Type B (85 U/mg; Biocatalysts, Pontypridd, Wales), Type VII (12 U/mg; Sigma, St. Louis, MO), Type OF (360 U/mg; Meito Sangyo Co. Ltd.), Type MY (300 U/mg; Meito Sangyo Co. Ltd., Tokyo), Type F5 (Enzymatix, Cambridge, England) and Lot 189 (620 U/mg; Biogenzia Ltd., Lausanne, Switzerland). For selective esterification, lipases such as Lipozyme TM20 (Novo Nordisk A/S, Bagsvaerd, Danemark), Type PS (*Pseudomonas* sp., Amano), Type AP6 (*Aspergillus niger*, Amano), Type F-AP15 (*Rhizopus javanicus*, Amano, Japan), Type OF (Meito Sangyo Co. Ltd., Tokyo) and *Penicillium cyclopium*, *Penicillium roqueforti*, *Geotrichum cadidum*, *Rhizopus javanicus*, and Lipomod from Biocatalysts were evaluated.

Preparation of Fatty Acids

The hydrolysis reactions of BCO were carried out in an oil-in-water (o/w) emulsion for various time periods with magnetic stirring. The emulsion was prepared by mixing 20% by weight BCO, 1.2% lecithin and 78.8% aqueous phosphate buffer (0.025 M, pH 6.88) with a microfluidizer (Model 110T, Microfluidics). The lipase was first dissolved in the aqueous phosphate buffer and the insoluble residues were removed by centrifugation. Different lipases were evaluated following the same procedure. The hydrolysis reaction was started by adding the buffer solution containing the desired lipase (corresponding to 0.2 g of the lipase) to 10 mL of the emulsion (corresponding to 2 g of BCO) in a 25 mL Erlenmeyer flask immersed in a heated water bath. To stop the reaction, the mixture was centrifuged to break down the emulsion and the lipid phase was then extracted with diethyl ether. The diethyl ether solution of fatty acids was dried with anhydrous sodium sulfate and the solvent was evaporated. The fatty acid mixture obtained was kept in the freezer ($-25°C$) under nitrogen.

Lipase-Catalyzed Esterification of Fatty Acids with Methanol

Esterification reactions were carried out at 25°C in a flask with magnetic stirring. The reaction mixture was composed of 900 mg of the fatty acids, 11 mL of hexane, 1 mL of methanol, and 1200 mg of immobilized lipase or 300 mg lipase in powder form. At the end of the reaction, the immobilized lipase was separated from the reaction products by filtration. In the case of lipase powder, the lipase preparation was separated from the products by centrifugation.

Separation of the Unesterified Fatty Acids from the Methyl Esters

For the separation of the unesterified fatty acids from the methyl esters, an aqueous solution containing 1.1 g of sodium carbonate was added to 20 g of a hexane solution of the reaction products at 40°C. The resulting mixture was heated to 75°C with stirring. When the desired temperature was reached, heating was stopped and 20 g of an aqueous solution of sodium chloride was added to the mixture. The mixture was then centrifuged (3000 rpm, 10 min). The aqueous phase containing soaps was acidified with HCl and extracted with hexane. The hexane extract was evaporated to yield 1.5 g of the fatty acid fraction.

Analytical Procedures

The products resulting from the lipase-catalyzed esterification were separated by thin-layer chromatography (TLC) on silica gel G60 F254 with hexane:diethyl ether:acetic acid (80:20:2, v/v/v) as the developing solvent. The fractions corresponding to unesterified fatty acids were scraped off from the adsorbent layer. The fatty acids on the adsorbent were directly converted to methyl esters by treatment with acetyl chloride and methanol. Subsequently, each of the methyl ester fractions was analyzed by gas chromatography (GC) as previously described (3).

Results and Discussion

Preparation of Fatty Acids by Lipase-Catalyzed Hydrolysis of BCO in an Emulsion System

Fatty acids are conventionally obtained by saponification of an oil with a strong base in a hot aqueous-alcoholic medium or by hydrolysis at elevated temperature and pressure. Because polyunsaturated fatty acids are very sensitive to oxidation, enzymatic hydrolysis under mild conditions may be preferable. Lipase-catalyzed hydrolysis of oil can be performed at a low temperature, around 30°C. This enzymatic process does not cause undesired reactions of fatty acids and also improves the yield. In view of these advantages, a process for enzymatic hydrolysis of BCO in an emulsion system has been developed.

Lipase-catalyzed hydrolysis takes place at the interface between the organic phase (oil) and the aqueous phase (water + enzyme). The rate of hydrolysis depends, therefore, on mixing efficiency. A high rate of hydrolysis requires efficient mixing but this is difficult in practice. An emulsion medium would be preferable to create a large interface and improve the rate and degree of hydrolysis. Daeseok and Joon Shick used reversed micelles for solubilizing lipase in an organic solvent (10), while Lieberman and Follis employed gum arabic or polyvinyl alcohol to form normal

TABLE 4.2 Influence of the Reaction Medium on the Degree of Hydrolysis of BCO (20 h)

Lipase	Degree of hydrolisis in two-phase medium (%)	Degree of hydrolysis in the emulsion (%)
Type B	79.0	99.5
Type OF	81.1	99.2

micelles (11), but these were stable for only a few hours. On the other hand, it is difficult to separate the products after the reaction in such a micellar system.

In the present work, an o/w emulsion, stabilized by soya lecithin, has been used for the lipase-catalyzed hydrolysis of BCO. The emulsion is prepared by simply dispersing the oil (BCO) into an aqueous phosphate buffer in the presence of the lecithin. The resulting emulsion can be sterilized and is stable for many months. The hydrolysis reaction is initiated by adding an aqueous phosphate buffer containing the lipase (*Candida cylindracea*). After the reaction, the products can be separated by centrifugation. As shown in Table 4.2, lipase-catalyzed hydrolysis in an emulsion gives a yield of more than 95%.

The optimum composition of the emulsion is 20% BCO, 78.8% aqueous phosphate buffer, and 1.2% lecithin. The degree of hydrolysis decreases with the increase of the proportion of BCO in the emulsion (Table 4.3). A decrease in the proportion of lecithin lowers the stability of the emulsion and also leads to a lower degree of hydrolysis (Table 4.3).

Candida cylindracea lipases from different suppliers were tested for this reaction. As shown in Table 4.4, the lipases Type B from Biocatalysts and Type OF from Meito Sangyo gave the best results. With lipase Type B, the maximum degree of hydrolysis was obtained after 4 h reaction, whereas with Type OF this was achieved after 20 h.

Effect of Temperature and pH on Hydrolysis

Temperature and pH are parameters which influence lipase activity. The optimal temperature and pH for *Candida cylindracea* lipase-catalyzed oil hydrolysis were reported to be 26–45°C and 4.8–7.2 (12,13), respectively. In the present system, maximum degree of hydrolysis is obtained at a temperature of 37°C with lipases Type B, Lot 189, Type MY and Type F5 and at 20°C with lipases Type VII and Type OF. In fact, there was only a small variation in degree of hydrolysis (2–5%) within the temperature

TABLE 4.3 Influence of Composition of the Emulsion on the Degree of Hydrolysis (lipase: Type B from Biocatalysts; reaction time: 20 h)

Composition of the emulsion			Degree of hydrolysis (%)
Oil (%)	Phosphate buffer (%)	Lecithin (%)	
20	78.8	1.2	99.5
30	68.8	1.2	78
20	79	1.0	89

TABLE 4.4 Optimized Hydrolysis with Different Lipases

Lipase	Maximum degree of hydrolysis (%)
Type B (Biocatalysts)	99.5
Type VII (Sigma)	91.6
Lot 189 (Biogenzia Lemania)	96.0
Type OF (Meito Sangyo)	99.2
Type MY (Meito Sangyo)	91.1
Type F5 (Enzymatix)	97.6

range of 20–40°C. All lipases used here exhibit activity over a wide pH range. There was no influence on the conversion within the range of pH 6–8. Therefore, an aqueous phosphate buffer (pH 6.88) was used for all of the experiments.

Lipase Quantity

Generally an increase in lipase quantity markedly increases the degree of hydrolysis. As shown in Table 4.5, however, when more than 100 mg/g oil was used, the degree of hydrolysis remained unchanged. One possible explanation for this is that, because the enzymatic reaction takes place at the interface of water and oil, at high enzyme concentrations the rate is no longer influenced by the concentration of the enzyme, but is limited by the availability of the interface.

Quality of the Fatty Acids

The fatty acids obtained by lipase-catalyzed hydrolysis of BCO were compared with those obtained by chemical hydrolysis as previously described (3). Light absorption analysis has shown that the fatty acids from lipase-catalyzed hydrolysis are less colored than those from chemical hydrolysis. Determination of the peroxide value also indicated that the fatty acids obtained using enzymatic hydrolysis were of better quality than those obtained by chemical hydrolysis (1.5 vs. 8.0 mEq O_2/kg, respectively) (Fig. 4.1).

Enrichment of GLA by Lipase-Catalyzed Selective Esterification

The ability of some lipases to selectively esterify fatty acids has been used for the enrichment of GLA from the fatty acids of borage and evening primrose oils (10),

TABLE 4.5 Effect of Lipase Quantity on the Hydrolysis of BCO

Concentration of lipase (mg/g BCO)	Degree of hydrolysis (%)		
	Type VII	Type OF	Type MY
20	82.5	88.6	77.4
50	88.2	92.7	87.0
100	91.6	99.0	91.0

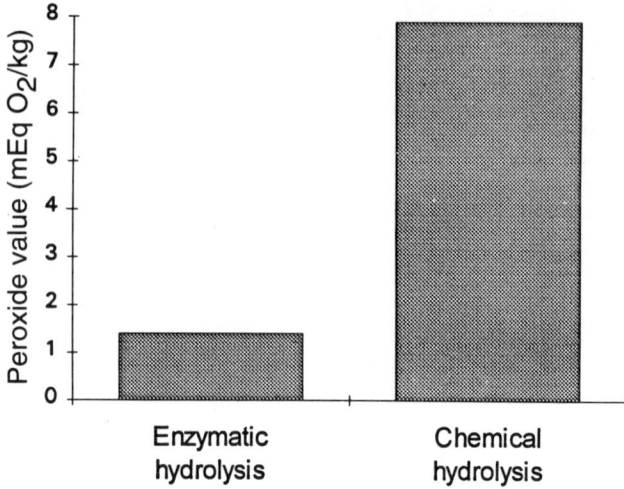

Fig. 4.1. Comparison of the quality of fatty acids obtained by enzymatic hydrolysis and chemical hydrolysis.

based on different esterification rates as a function of the degree of unsaturation. Unlike borage and evening primrose oil, BCO contains both α-linolenic acid (ALA) and GLA in similar quantities, as well as stearidonic acid, another biologically interesting fatty acid. The present study has shown that the lipase-catalyzed selective esterification can also separate GLA from α-linolenic acid. These two fatty acids have the same degree of unsaturation but different double bond positions. In addition, stearidonic acid can also be enriched in the fatty acid fraction.

The results given in Table 4.6 show that the reaction of BCO fatty acids with methanol, catalyzed by Lipozyme TM in the presence of hexane as solvent at ambient temperature for a period of 28 h, led to intensive esterification of all of the fatty acids except GLA and stearidonic acid. These two acids are enriched in the unesterified fatty acid fraction up to 81.2 and 13.8%, respectively, with 18% yield of the fatty acid fraction.

TABLE 4.6 Composition of Fatty Acids Before and After Esterification Catalyzed by Lipozyme TM

Fatty acids of BCO	Fatty acid composition (%) before fractionation	Fatty acid composition (%) after fractionation
C16:0	6.7	0.5
C18:0	1.4	0.1
C18:1	13.6	0.9
C18:2 (n-6)	45.7	2.0
C18:3γ (n-6)	15.2	81.2
C18:3α (n-3)	13.2	0.7
C18:4 (n-3)	3.0	13.8
Others	1.2	0.8

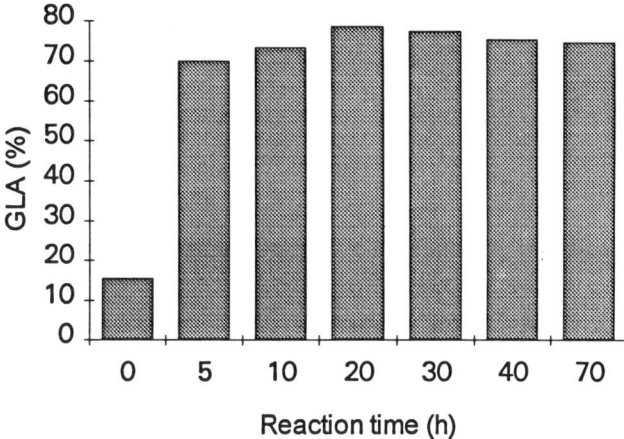

Fig. 4.2. Effect of the reaction time on the GLA enrichment by Lipozyme-catalyzed esterification with hexane as solvent at 25°C.

Because the selectivity of the esterification is due to the kinetic features of the lipase, the enrichment of GLA also depends on the reaction time. As shown in Fig. 4.2, the optimum enrichment is obtained within 20 h. A further increase in the reaction time may lead to a decrease in enrichment.

In addition, other lipases, as listed in the section on experimental procedures, were also evaluated for selective esterification. Except for the lipase from *Pseudomonas* sp., lipases such as *Rhizopus javanicus*, *Penicillium cyclopium*, *Penicillium roqueforti*, *Aspergillus niger*, Lipomod, and Type OF show selectivities similar to that of Lipozyme TM.

Separation of the Unesterified Fatty Acids from the Methyl Esters

The separation of the unesterified fatty acids from their esters is usually done by chromatographic procedures. Trials to carry out the separation by distillation or by liquid-liquid extraction failed. During oil refining, free fatty acids are separated from the triacylglycerols by neutralization with NaOH. In this case, the strongly alkaline conditions may cause hydrolysis of the methyl esters. In addition, to obtain the fatty acid fraction, a large amount of HCl solution is required to acidify the alkaline aqueous phase. To avoid these disadvantages, an alternative method has been developed in the present study. The hexane solution containing the unesterified fatty acids and the methyl esters was stirred with an aqueous solution of Na_2CO_3 to transform the free fatty acids into soaps, which remain in the aqueous phase. After the addition of an aqueous solution of NaCl, the two phases were separated by centrifugation. The aqueous phase containing the soaps was acidified with HCl to yield the fatty acid fraction enriched in GLA and stearidonic acid.

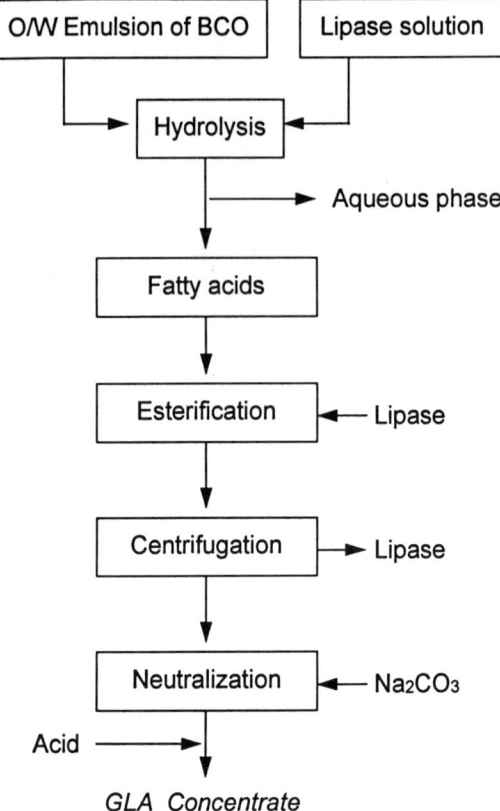

Fig. 4.3. Simplified flow-sheet of the process for enzymatic enrichment of GLA.

Conclusions

A complete process, as summarized in Fig 4.3, has been developed for the enrichment of GLA from BCO under mild conditions. Lipase-catalyzed hydrolysis of BCO was carried out in a special o/w emulsion system, and the resulting fatty acids showed an improved quality in comparison with that produced by alkaline hydrolysis. It was demonstrated that some lipases discriminate ALA from GLA. Consequently, this technique allows us to enrich GLA from BCO fatty acids. The separation of unesterified fatty acids from their methyl esters was achieved by transforming the fatty acids into soaps with salts such as sodium carbonate.

Acknowledgments
The authors thank L. Sandoz and Ch. Capponi for their contribution to this work.

References

1. Horrobin, D.F. Nutrition and Medical Importance of Gamma Linolenic Acid (1992) *Prog. Lipid Res. 31,* 163–194.
2. Gunstone, F.D. Gamma Linolenic Acid—Occurrence and Physical and Chemical Properties (1992) *Prog. Lipid Res. 31,* 145–161.
3. Traitler, H., Wille, H.-J., and Studer, A. Fractionation of Blackcurrant Seed Oil (1988) *J. Am. Oil Chem. Soc. 65,* 755–760.
4. Traitler, H., and Studer, A., U.S. Patent 4,776,984 (1988).
5. Wille, H.-J., Traitler, H., and Lagarde, M. Preparation of Stearidonic Acid Concentrates (1991) *Fat Sci. Technol. 93,* 362–368.
6. Traitler, H., and Wille, H.-J. Isolation of Pure Fatty Acids from Fats and Oils (1992) *Fat Sci. Technol. 94,* 506–511.
7. Traitler, H., Wille, H.-J., and Studer, A. Fractionierung mehrfach ungesättigter Fettsäuren aus verschiedenen natürlichen Rohstoffen (1986) *Fette Seifen Anstrichmittel 88,* 378–382.
8. Syed Rahmatullah, M.S.K., Shukla, V.K.S., and Mukherjee, K.D. Enrichment of γ-Linolenic Acid from Evening Primrose Oil and Borage Oil *via* Lipase-Catalyzed Hydrolysis (1994) *J. Am. Oil Chem. Soc. 71,* 569–573.
9. Syed Rahmatullah, M.S.K., Shukla, V.K.S., and Mukherjee, K.D. γ-Linolenic Acid Concentrates from Borage and Evening Primrose Oil *via* Lipase-Catalyzed Esterification (1994) *J. Am. Oil Chem. Soc. 71,* 563–577.
10. Daesok, H., and Joon Shick, H. Characteristics of Lipase-Catalyzed Hydrolysis of Olive Oil in AOT-Isooctane Reversed Micelles (1986) *Biotechnol. Bioeng. 28,* 1250–1255.
11. Lieberman, R.B., and Ollis, D.F. Hydrolysis of Particulate Tributyrin in a Fluidized Lipase Reactor (1975) *Biotechnol. Bioeng. 17,* 1401–1419.
12. Khor, H.T., Tan, N.H., and Chua, C.L. Lipase-Catalyzed Hydrolysis of Palm Oil (1986) *J. Am. Oil Chem. Soc. 63,* 538–540.
13. Macrae, A.R. (1983) in *Microbial Enzyme and Biotechnology,* Fogarty, W.M., Elsevier Applied Science, London, pp. 225–250.

Chapter 5

Transport of Long-Chain Polyunsaturated Fatty Acids Across the Human Placenta: Role of Fatty Acid-Binding Proteins

Asim K. Dutta-Roy*, Fiona M. Campbell, Samson Taffesse, and Margaret J. Gordon

Receptor Research Laboratory,
Rowett Research Institute,
Aberdeen, Scotland, U.K.

Introduction

Linoleic acid, (LA, 18:2n-6) and α-linolenic acid (ALA, 18:3n-3) are the two main dietary essential fatty acids (EFA) (1). LA and ALA are not interconvertible, but they can be further elongated and desaturated by the same enzyme systems to n-6 and n-3 long-chain polyunsaturated fatty acids (LCPUFA) in the body (2). LA and ALA are primarily present in the diet in vegetable oils, whereas preformed LCPUFA may also be consumed in foods of animal origin. The importance of LCPUFA has been related to their structural action, their specific interaction with membrane proteins or their ability to serve as precursors of second messenger systems (3–5). Therefore, both LA and ALA must be converted to their further metabolites to exert the full range of biological actions. Among LCPUFA, arachidonic acid (AA, 20:4n-6) and docosahexaenoic acid (DHA, 22:6n-3) are found in high concentrations in the structural lipids of central nervous system as well as other mammalian tissues (6,7). The first and rate-determining step in LCPUFA synthesis is Δ6-desaturation. The Δ6-desaturation step is therefore critical for full utilization of dietary LA and ALA in the body. The formation of γ-linolenic acid (GLA), the immediate Δ6-desaturated metabolite of LA, is reported to be reduced in a number of diseases (6–8), indicating an abnormality in EFA metabolism in the body. In such conditions, dietary supplementation of GLA could be useful as a means of by-passing the rate-limiting Δ6-desaturation step to maintain optimum LCPUFA levels in the body.

The developing fetus and the placenta require EFA/LCPUFA for the formation of structural components of cell membranes, for participation in intracellular signaling, and in the provision of triacylglycerol stores necessary for postnatal life (4,9–13). Because of the fundamental role of EFA and their LCPUFA as structural elements and functional modulators, it has been hypothesized that maternal/fetal EFA/LCPUFA status is an important determinant of health and disease in infancy and later life (9,10). As in the adult, the human fetus is unable to synthesize the EFA which must be supplied by the mother through the placenta (9,14). Placental transport of LCPUFA is crucial for fetal growth and development because fetal synthesis is also very low (11,15–19). Because human placental tissue lacks both the Δ6 and Δ5-desaturase activities (19–22), any LCPUFAs in the fetal circulation are the desaturated metabolites produced in the mother. The deposition of LCPUFA in the fetus is rapid during growth, and it is believed that a failure to accomplish a specific component of brain growth due to inadequacy of critical membrane lipids may result in irrevocable damage (9,14). In humans, the vulnerable period of brain development and maximal rate of LCPUFA deposition occur in the third trimester and the first 6–9 months postnatally (9). During this period, DHA and AA are deposited in large amounts in the fetal brain and retina (9,10,14). Accretion of large amounts of LCPUFA in the growing fetus (9,10) and the presence of DHA, AA, and GLA in human milk (23,24) suggest the importance of these LCPUFA for human growth and development. Evidence from various studies suggests that retinal function and learning ability may be permanently impaired if there is a reduction in the accumulation of sufficient DHA during development (9,10,14). The rate of deposition of LCPUFA in the developing fetus depends on the fatty acid uptake by the placenta from maternal circulation. LCPUFA are provided by the maternal plasma because the activity of metabolic enzymes required for their synthesis is almost nonexistent in the fetuses of mammals (15–19). Recent studies in humans and other animals suggest that a mild deficiency in EFA intake could limit fetal growth processes, while maternal dietary supplementation of EFA could prevent intrauterine growth retardation (IUGR) (25,26). Therefore, EFA supplementation during pregnancy could affect pregnancy outcomes.

The placenta is the organ responsible for the transfer of practically all nutrients and waste products between mother and fetus (27). The continuous layer of the syncytiotrophoblast cells constitutes the main barrier to maternal-fetal transport for many nutrients, including complex lipids (28,29). However, a large supply of the hydrolyzed fatty acids as well as unesterified fatty acids (FFA) from the maternal circulation rapidly appears in the uterine vein and provides an important component of the total supply of fatty acids to the placenta (9,14,17). The delivery of fatty acids from the maternal circulation to the developing fetus has been studied using whole perfused placenta (9,17,19), but many of the details of the transport mechanism have yet to be elucidated. Many studies have described the fact that levels of LCPUFA (major fatty acids, DHA, AA, and minor fatty acids, GLA, DGLA) are higher in the fetal than in the maternal plasma (9,17), but the biochemical mechanism responsible remains obscure. The critical importance of placental transfer of LCPUFA rather than fetal and/or placental synthesis by desaturation and elongation of transferred dietary LA and ALA to the accumulation of LCPUFA in the developing tissue is now well recognized, because the feto-placental synthesis of LCPUFA is either very low or nonexistent (9,11,15–22). Therefore, it is pertinent to investigate whether the human placenta is capable of preferentially transporting EFA/LCPUFA from the maternal circulation, and if so, what are the biochemical processes involved in the specific fatty acid transfer between mother and fetus. To date, several reviews have been published that comprehensively cover the earlier work on placental fatty acid transport and metabolism (9–11,16,17). The aim of this article is to bring together recent developments on placental EFA/LCPUFA uptake and metabolism and the evolving concepts concerning the roles of fatty acid-binding proteins in these processes.

Placental Fatty Acid Transport and Metabolism

Unesterified free fatty acids (FFA) in the maternal circulation are the major source of fatty acids for transport across the placenta (11,19,21) because triglycerides are not transported intact (30,31). LDL receptors on the maternal microvillous membrane of the syncytiotrophoblast could also account for EFA/LCPUFA present in the LDL and cholesteryl ester fractions, but the metabolic fate of these fatty acids within the placenta is uncertain. FFAs are generated either by intravascular lipolysis of lipoproteins or by the hydrolysis of triglycerides in the adipose tissue. Maternal placental lipoprotein lipase (LPL) must be active to facilitate placental uptake of FFA from circulating triglycerides (11,19). The LPL activity is present only in the microvillous membrane of the placental trophoblast (32). In the guinea pig, LPL activity increases approximately 11-fold during the last stages of gestation and seems to be implicated in fatty acid transfer between mother and fetus (32). The placental LPL, however, hydrolyzes triglycerides from maternal VLDL (32,33) but not the triglycerides present in chylomicrons (9,34,35). The preferential hydrolysis of posthepatic triglycerides (VLDL) in the maternal circulation by the placental LPL may thus result in an increased availability of LCPUFA for placental uptake and serve as both a protection of the fetus from the immediate impact of an unusual fatty acid composition in a meal and as a facilitator of LCPUFA availability to the fetus. Therefore, the enrichment of LCPUFA in the FFA pool for placental uptake may be important for feto-placental growth and development.

Once hydrolyzed, the FFA bind to albumin in the maternal circulation and represent an important, readily available FFA source to the fetus through the placenta (19,36–37). Yet despite its overall significance in the transfer of fatty acids across the maternal-fetal axis, the mechanism by which FFA cross the human placental membrane is poorly understood. FFA uptake has been studied extensively in several tissues, and a variety of mechanisms of FFA uptake have been proposed, including passive diffusion, and by specific binding to plasma membrane fatty acid-binding protein ($FABP_{pm}$) (38). There are now several reports providing evidence of the involvement of $FABP_{pm}$ in the uptake of FFA into a variety of mammalian tissues: hepatocytes, adipocytes, cardiomyocytes and jejunal mucosal cells (39–42). Experimental evidence has also recently been provided on the $FABP_{pm}$-mediated FFA uptake by the heart (43). $FABP_{pm}$ expression and the kinetics of FFA uptake are now known to be affected by the physiological status of the cells (44), suggesting the importance of this protein in cellular growth and differentiation. Placental $FABP_{pm}$ may therefore play an important role in extracting fatty acids from the maternal circulation to provide an adequate supply of LCPUFA during fetal growth and development. Recently, we have reported the presence of a $FABP_{pm}$ in both sheep and human placental membranes (45,46). Antibodies to $FABP_{pm}$ inhibited the binding of LCPUFA to the placental membranes, suggesting the involvement of the protein in fatty acid uptake in the placenta. Placental

$FABP_{pm}$ appeared to be different in amino acid composition and pI value from the hepatic or gut $FABP_{pm}$ (46). However, further studies are required to define the precise role of the protein in the LCPUFA sequestration process.

Once they are taken up in the cell, the intracellular transport of long-chain fatty acids is mediated by fatty acid-binding proteins ($FABP_c$) within the cytosol. A human placenta contains two types of cytoplasmic $FABP_c$ (~15 kDa): liver type (L-$FABP_c$) and heart type (H-$FABP_c$) (47). Regulation of the expression of these two proteins in the placenta is thought to be related to fetal development (47). Fatty acid uptake and internalization by living cells may involve a sequence of steps: dissociation from albumin, transport across the plasma membranes (via $FABP_{pm}$) and transport within the cytoplasm (via $FABP_c$), and its metabolism (48–50). Although cytoplasmic $FABP_c$ have been extensively characterized, their exact function is not well understood. Based upon their tissue expression, binding affinities, regulation, in vitro effects on fatty acid transfer and the enzymes involved in fatty acid and carbohydrate metabolisms, it has been postulated that these proteins play an important controlling role in the cytoplasmic transport and metabolism of long-chain fatty acids (48–50). In addition, these proteins are thought to have more diverse functions, including, for example, a role in the modulation of cell growth (48–52).

The presence of two types of cytoplasmic FABP in the kidney at two different locations has also been reported (48,49). However, no such information is available regarding placental $FABP_c$ (47). The different types of placental $FABP_c$ may be involved in the channeling of specific fatty acids to β-oxidation, in the synthesis of structural and storage lipid in the placenta, in the transfer to fetal circulation or in placental growth and regulation. L-$FABP_c$ has also been implicated in cell growth and regulation by virtue of its binding to various growth stimulatory and inhibitory eicosanoids as well as to selenium (51,52). However, further work is required on the location, function and binding specificity of these two placental FABPs before definitive conclusions can be made. Figure 5.1 summarizes the putative roles of the fatty acid-binding proteins in placental fatty acid uptake and metabolism. The increasing knowledge of the factors which modulate the expression of these proteins would give us a better understanding of their role in feto-placental growth and development.

Fatty Acid Binding Activity of Human Placental Membranes

The fatty acid-binding characteristics of human placental membranes have been investigated in our laboratory to examine the existence of any preferential binding of EFA/LCPUFA to placental membranes. Binding of [^{14}C]oleic acid, [^{14}C]linoleic acid, [^{14}C]α-linolenic acid, and [^{14}C]arachidonic acid to human placental membranes was determined as described elsewhere (45). The binding characteristics of these fatty acids suggest that the process of FFA transport across the plasma membrane is carrier mediated with the characteristics of facilitated diffusion. The binding of [^{14}C] fatty acid to the membranes is time and temperature-dependent, and the

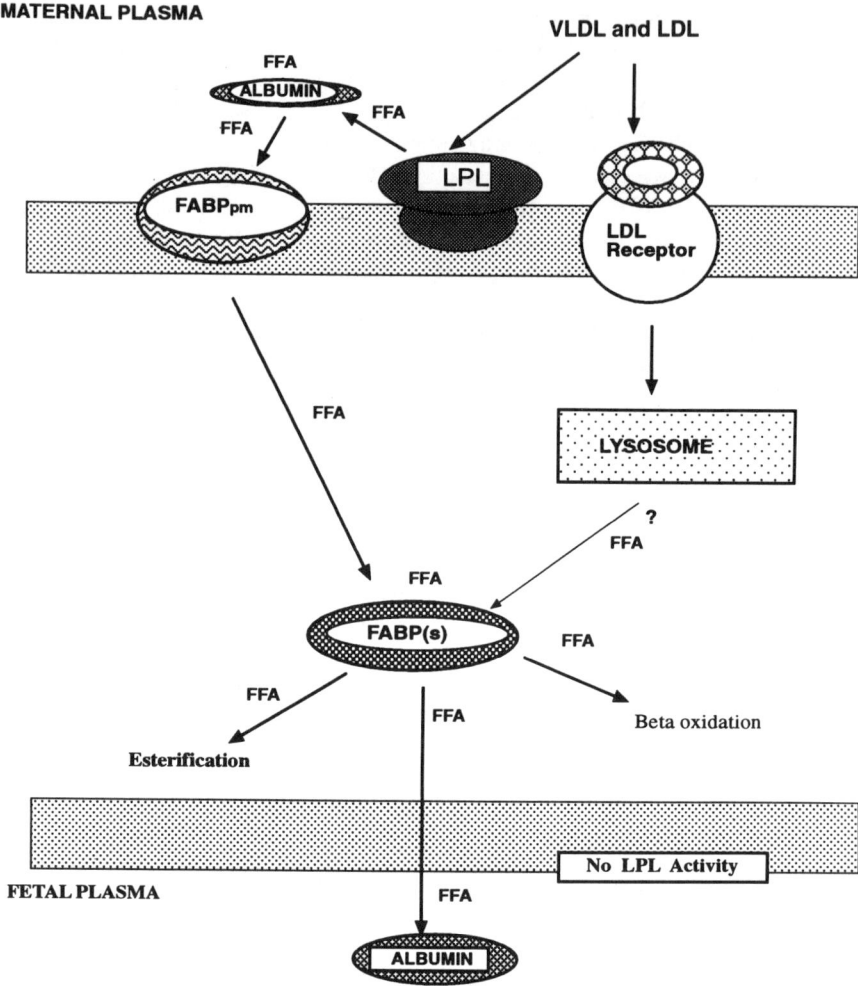

Fig. 5.1. Schematic presentations of the putative roles of the plasmalemmal and cytoplasmic fatty acid-binding proteins (FABP$_{pm}$ and FABP$_c$) in fatty acid uptake and metabolism in the placenta. FABP$_{pm}$ may sequestrate EFA/LCPUFA and their plasmalemmal translocation, and cytoplasmic FABPs may be responsible for transcytoplasmic movement of poorly soluble fatty acids to their sites of esterification, β-oxidation or to the fetal circulation via basal membranes. Abbreviations: VLDL, very low density proteins; LDL, low-density lipoproteins; LPL, lipoprotein lipase.

shape of the binding curves for the fatty acids indicates that the binding of fatty acid is not a linear function of the unbound fatty acid concentrations present in the incubation mixture, suggesting a saturability of binding. In these studies, radiolabeled fatty acid was presented to the placental membranes in the form of complexes with albumin in various molar ratios to determine the fatty acid binding at different unbound fatty acid concentrations. Saturation of binding of all four fatty acids was achieved at a molar ratio of fatty acid to albumin of 1:1. Similar saturation binding of FFA has been observed in other tissues (38–42). The maximum binding for oleate, linoleate, α-linolenate and arachidonate were 5.1 ± 0.1, 2.8 ± 0.2, 0.5 ± 0.1, and 2.06 ± 0.4 nmol/mg protein, respectively, at 1:1 molar ratio of FA:BSA, at 37°C. Addition of a 20-fold excess of unlabeled fatty acid to the incubation mixture at the beginning of the incubation reduced the binding of the corresponding fatty acid, indicating the competitive nature of the binding of the radiolabeled fatty acid. For oleate binding, the displacement was the smallest (37%) compared with that of linoleate and α-linolenate (62 and 69%, respectively). The maximum specific binding of [^{14}C]oleate, [^{14}C]linoleate, [^{14}C]α-linolenate and [^{14}C]arachidonate to the membranes attained at 20 min of incubation at 37°C was 1.88 ± 0.1, 1.74 ± 0.1, 0.35 ± 0.01 and 1.77 ± 0.2 nmol/mg protein, respectively. When the specific binding is expressed as a ratio of the total [^{14}C]fatty acid binding, linoleate, α-linolenate and arachidonate exhibit a significantly higher ratio of specific binding (0.63 ± 0.11, 0.78 ± 0.01, and 0.86 ± 0.02 respectively) compared with oleate, 0.37 ± 0.03, ($P < 0.01$), at equilibrium and also at 20 min of incubation at 37°C. This is probably due to the relatively higher nonspecific binding of oleate compared with the nonspecific binding of linoleate, α-linolenate and arachidonate to placental membranes. The binding of EFA/LCPUFA to human placental membranes is highly reversible compared with that of oleate, but the physiological significance of this observation is not yet clear. However, one may speculate that the placenta has a great requirement for EFA/LCPUFA in the growth and development of the feto-placental axis and that this could be met by the preferential uptake of EFA/LCPUFA via the $FABP_{pm}$. Similarly, it has recently been reported that the uptake of linoleate by keratinocytes is higher than that of oleate, and these cells also require greater amounts of EFA for the synthesis of stratum corneum membrane lipids (53).

The binding specificity of each radiolabeled fatty acid to placental membranes was also examined by conducting incubations in the presence of a 20-fold excess of unlabeled ligands such as oleic acid, linoleic acid, α-linolenic, γ-linolenic, arachidonic, elaidic, linoelaidic acid, α-tocopherol and sulphobromo-phenophthalein (BSP). When unlabeled AA or GLA was used at similar concentrations the maximum degree of inhibition of binding of [^{14}C]LA and ALA was around 90–95%. Competition studies therefore suggest that the fatty acid binding sites have a stronger preference for LCPUFA than the parent EFA (LA and ALA). The order of preference was GLA = AA > ALA > LA >>>>> OA.

The presence of elaidic acid (*trans* 9-18:1) in the incubation medium reduced 68–70% of binding of radiolabeled fatty acids, whereas the inhibition of binding of linoleate and α-linolenate by oleate was only around 45%. This indicates a weaker competition between LA and OA. Linoelaidic acid (*trans,trans*-9,12-18:2) strongly inhibited the binding of [^{14}C] linoleate and [^{14}C] α-linolenate by 82 and 69%, respectively, but inhibited oleate binding to a lesser extent (46%). *Trans* fatty acids are not synthesized *in situ*, but they do occur in both fetal and placental tissues, suggesting that they are transported through the placenta from the maternal circulation (54). Our data suggest that the *trans* fatty acids may compete with the essential fatty acids for fatty acid-binding sites in human placental membranes, thereby inhibiting the transport of LCPUFA to the placenta. *Trans* fatty acids are also thought to competitively inhibit the synthesis of LCPUFA, e.g., at the desaturation and chain-elongation steps. They may therefore cause an abnormal eicosanoid metabolism as well as a perturbance of membrane structure and function (54).

The competition experiments described here have also shown that the binding sites have heterogeneous binding affinities for different fatty acids. The lack of strong inhibition of the binding of EFA to placental membranes by oleate may be due to the existence of either single binding sites with preferential affinities for EFA/LCPUFA (n-3 and n-6 fatty acids) compared with oleate or the presence of two different binding sites, one with high affinity for linoleate and α-linolenate, and the other for oleate but with a low affinity.

To examine the specificity of fatty acid binding, BSP and α-tocopherol were used. BSP and α-tocopherol did not inhibit the binding of any of the radiolabeled fatty acids, suggesting that the binding sites are highly specific for fatty acids. BSP, a non-bile acid cholephil (like bilirubin), is efficiently extracted from the blood by the liver through a specific liver plasma membrane protein (55), whereas the mechanism of α-tocopherol uptake by tissues is quite different from that of fatty acid (56).

The interpretation of these competition studies may be limited because both the binding and competition assays represent an equilibrium between albumin and the protein and lipids of the placental membranes. Therefore, several complications could arise due to the differences in binding of the fatty acids and competitors to albumin, or to the differences in the partitioning of fatty acids in the lipid bilayer and in the binding of fatty acids to protein. However, some of these concerns are not sustainable because the association constants of these fatty acids with bovine serum albumin are in a similar range (57). Thus a redistribution of these fatty acids among binding sites on albumin when the fatty acids are mixed is unlikely to account for these differences in competition for the binding sites in the placental membranes. This is further supported by Schurer et al. (53) who demonstrated the differences in fatty acid uptake by different cell lines using similar fatty acids and albumin mixture (53). Moreover, specific antisera raised against the $FABP_{pm}$ inhibited the binding of these fatty acids, again suggesting that specific binding was mediated through the protein.

Our finding on the preferential uptake of specific fatty acids mediated by placental $FABP_{pm}$ has recently been reinforced by Haggarty et al. (22) who also showed that the human placenta is able to selectively transfer the EFA to the fetal circulation in preference to the nonessential fatty acid using a physiological mixture of fatty acids and fatty acid-free albumin in the perfused placenta. Furthermore, treating the membranes with trypsin reduced the specific binding of oleate, linoleate and α-linolenate by 65 ± 4.1, 60 ± 5.6, and 75 ± 7.8% ($P < 0.05$, $n = 3$), respectively. Heat-treatment of membranes at 50°C for 6 h also abolished specific binding of [^{14}C] fatty acid completely. The trypsin-treated membranes were prepared by incubating membranes (100 µg) with 316 BAEE units of trypsin for 2 h at 37°C, as described (44). Heat denaturation of membranes was accomplished by incubating membranes at 50°C for 6 h. These studies suggest that the specific binding of all of the radiolabeled fatty acids to the membranes was due to a membrane protein, because trypsin and heat treatment decreased specific [^{14}C]fatty acid binding.

Recently, we have purified and characterized a FABP$_{pm}$ (~40 kDa) from human placental membranes (46). Antisera raised against the FABP$_{pm}$ were used in the studies to determine the involvement of this protein in the binding of EFA/LCPUFA to human placental membranes and BeWo cells (human trophoblast cell line). Preincubation of the membranes or the BeWo cells with polyclonal antiserum inhibited the binding of these fatty acids by more than 50% compared with that of membranes/cells pretreated with preimmune serum. These data suggest that FABP$_{pm}$ may be involved in the placental EFA/LCPUFA uptake.

Conclusions

The biomagnification of LCPUFA from the maternal to fetal tissues is generally thought to be the result of the combined effects of placental fatty acid uptake, selective fatty acid oxidation, and lipid synthesis in the placenta, as well as fetal liver LCPUFA synthesis. However, more evidence is now emerging concerning the critical importance of maternal LCPUFA metabolism and the subsequent preferential transfer of these fatty acids by the placenta to the fetus (9,22,45,46,58). The biochemical mechanism(s) underlying the placental uptake of EFA/LCPUFA and their subsequent transport to the fetus is not yet known. EFA/LCPUFA bound to albumin are preferentially transported by human placental membranes. Binding characteristics show that the fatty acid-binding sites in the human placenta behave like other physiological receptors. Competition studies suggest the existence of heterogeneous affinities and binding capacities for the fatty acids. Binding sites seem to have a strong preference for LCPUFA; for the binding of [^{14}C] fatty acids [OA, LA, ALA, and AA], the order of competition was GLA = AA >>> LA > ALA >>>> OA, whereas BSP and α-tocopherol did not show any competition with any of the [^{14}C] fatty acids. Elaidic acid also competed very strongly for the [^{14}C] fatty acid binding. This study suggests the preferential binding of LCPUFA (GLA, and AA) to the human placental membranes over their parent molecule, and this could be impaired by *trans* fatty acids.

The data presented here demonstrate that placental FABP$_{pm}$ may be involved in the sequestration of EFA/LCPUFA by the placenta. Studies are now required to understand the role of FABP$_{pm}$ in the transport and metabolism of LCPUFA in human placenta. These studies should include the factors responsible for regulating the expression of FABP$_{pm}$ and cytoplasmic FABP and their relationship with the kinetics of placental fatty acid transport and metabolism.

Acknowledgment

This work was supported by the Scottish Office Agriculture and Fisheries Department.

References

1. Tinoco, J. Dietary Requirements and Functions of Alpha Linolenic Acid in Animals (1983) *Prog. Lipid Res. 21,* 1–45.
2. Sprecher, H. Biochemistry of Essential Fatty Acids (1981) *Prog. Lipid Res. 20,* 13–22.
3. Sinclair, A.J., and Crawford, M.A. The Accumulation of Arachidonic Acid and Docosahexaenoic Acid in the Developing Rat Brain (1972) *J. Neurochem. 19,* 1753–1758.
4. Dutta-Roy, A.K. Insulin Mediated Processes in Platelets, Monocytes / Macrophages and Erythrocytes: Effects of Essential Fatty Acid Metabolism (1994) *Prostaglandins Leukotrienes Essen. Fatty Acids 51,* 385–399.
5. Huang, Y.-S., and Nassar, B.A. (1990) in *Omega 6 Essential Fatty Acids: Pathophysiology and Roles in Clinical Medicine,* Horrobin, D.F., Liss, A.R., New York, pp. 127–144.
6. Hrboticky, N., Mackinnon, M.J., Puterman, M.L., and Innis, S.M. Effect of Linoleic Acid-Rich Infant Formula Feeding on Brain Synaptosomal Lipid Accretion and Enzyme Thermotropic Behaviour in the Piglet (1989) *J. Lipid Res. 30,* 1303–1311.
7. Spector, A.A., and Yorek, M. A. Membrane Lipid Composition and Cellular Functions (1985) *J. Lipid Res. 26,* 1015–1035.
8. Holman, R., and Johnson, S. Changes in Essential Fatty Acid Profile of Serum Phospholipids in Human Diseases (1981) *Prog. Lipid Res. 20,* 67–73.
9. Innis, S.M. Essential Fatty Acids in Growth and Development (1986) *Prog. Lipid Res. 30,* 39–103.
10. Uauy, R., Treen, M., and Hoffman, D. Essential Fatty Acid Metabolism and Requirements During Development (1989) *Semin. Perinatol. 13,* 118–130.
11. Crawford, M.A., Hassam, A.G., and Stevens, P.A. Essential Fatty Acid Requirements in Pregnancy and Lactation with Special Reference to Brain Development (1981) *Prog. Lipid Res. 20,* 30–40.
12. Dutta-Roy, A.K., Kahn, N.N., and Sinha, A.K. Interaction of Receptors for Prostaglandin E_1/Prostacyclin and Insulin in Human Erythrocytes and Platelets (1990) *Life Sci. 49,* 1129–1139.
13. Dutta-Roy, A.K. Prostaglandin E_2 Receptors of Monocytes/Macrophages: Regulation by Insulin and Interleukin-1a (1993) *Immunol. Methods 2,* 203–210.
14. Yavin, E.,and Green, P. (1994) in *Fatty Acids and Lipids: Biological Aspects,* World Rev. Nutr. Diet., Galli, C., Simopoulos, A. P., and Tremoli, E., Basel, Krager, pp. 134–138.
15. Scott, B.L., and Bazan, N.G. Membrane Docosahexaenoic Acid Is Supplied to the Developing Brain and Retina by the Liver (1989) *Proc. Natl. Acad. Sci. U.S.A. 86,* 2903–2907.
16. Nouvelot, A., Delbart, C., and Bourre, J.M. Hepatic Metabolism of Dietary Alpha Linolenic in Suckling Rats, and Its Possible Importance in Polyunsaturated Fatty Acid Uptake by the Brain (1986) *Nutr. and Metab. 30,* 316–323.
17. Coleman, R.A. The Role of the Placenta in Lipid Metabolism and Transport (1989) *Semin. Perinatol. 13,* 180–191.
18. Bourre, J.M., Pascal, G., Durand, G., Masson, M., Dumont, O., and Piciotti, M. Alterations in the Fatty Acid Composition of Rat Brain Cells (Neurons, Astrocytes, and Oligodendrocytes) and of Subcellular Fractions (Myelin and Synaptosomes) Induced by a Diet Devoid of n-3 Fatty Acids (1984) *J. Neurochem. 43,* 342–348.
19. Kuhn, H., and Crawford, M. Placental Essential Fatty Acid Transport and Prostaglandin Synthesis (1986) *Prog. Lipid Res. 25,* 345–353.

20. Chambaz, J., Ravel, D., Manier, M.C., Pepin, D., Mulliez, N., and Bereziat, G. Essential Fatty Acids Interconversion in the Human Fetal Liver (1985) *Biol. Neonate 47*, 136–140.
21. Bereziat, G., Thomas, G., Cardot, P., and Chambaz, J. (1992) in *Essential Fatty Acids and Infant Nutrition,* Ghisolfi, J., and Putet, G., John Libbey, Paris, pp. 45–55.
22. Haggarty, P., Page, K., Abramovich, D., and Ashton, J. Placental Transfer of Fatty Acids from the Maternal to Fetal Circulation Studied in the Perfused Human Placenta (1995) *Proc. Nutr. Soc.* (in press).
23. Crawford, M.A., Costello, K., Doyle, W., Leighfield, M.J., Lennon, E.A., and Meadows, N. Potential Diagnostic Value of the Umbilical Artery As a Definition of Neural Fatty Acids Status of the Fetus during Its Growth: The Umbilical Artery As a Diagnostic Tool (1990) *Biochem. Soc. Trans. 18*, 761–766.
24. Clandinin, M. T., Chappell, J. E., and van Aerde, E. E. Requirements of Newborn Infants for Long Chain Polyunsaturated Fatty Acids (1989) *Acta Paediatr. Scand. 351S*, 63–71.
25. Menon, K., and Dhopeshwarkar, G.A. Essential Fatty Acid Deficiency and Brain Development (1982) *Prog. Lipid Res. 21*, 309–326.
26. Robillard, P.Y., and Christon, R. Lipid Intake during Pregnancy in Developing Countries. Possible Effects of Essential Fatty Acid Deficiency on Fetal Growth (1993) Prostaglandins, Leukotrienes *Essen. Fatty Acids 48*, 139–142.
27. Page, K. (1993) in *The Physiology of the Human Placenta,* UCL Press, London.
28. Brunette, M.G., Auger, D., and Lafond, J. Effect of Parathyroid Hormone on PO_4 Transport through the Human Placenta Microvilli (1989) *Pediatr. Res. 25*, 15–18.
29. Stephenson, T.J., Stammers, J.P., and Hull, D. Effects of Altering Umbilical Flow and Umbilical Free Fatty Acid Concentration on Transfer of Free Fatty Acids across the Rabbit Placenta (1991) *J. Dev. Physiol. 15*, 221–227.
30. Elphick, M.C., Edson, H.C., Lawler, J., and Hull, D. Source of Fetal-Stored Lipids During Maternal Starvation in Rabbits (1978) *Biol. Neonate 34*, 146–149.
31. Shand, J. H., and Noble, R. C. The Role of Maternal Triglycerides in the Supply of Lipids to the Ovine Fetus (1979) *Res. Vet. Sci. 26*, 117–123.
32. Thomas, C. R., and Lowy, C. The Interrelationships between Circulating Maternal Esterified and Non-Esterified Fatty Acids in Pregnant Guinea Pigs and Their Relative Contributions to the Fetal Circulation (1987) *J. Dev. Physiol. 9*, 203–214.
33. Thomas, C.R., Lowy, C., St. Hilliaire, R.J., and Brunzell, J. D. (1984) in *Fetal Nutrition, Metabolism and Immunology. The Role of the Placenta,* Miller, R.K., and Thiede, H. A., Plenum Press, New York, pp. 135–146.
34. Rothwell, J.E., and Elphic, M. C. Lipoproten Lipase Activity in Human and Guinea Pig Placenta (1982) *J. Dev. Physiol. 4*, 153–159.
35. McBride, O.W., and Burton, G.J. Uptake of Free Fatty Acids and Chylomicrons Glycerides by Guinea Pig Mammary Gland in Pregnancy and Lactation (1964) *J. Lipid Res. 5*, 453–458.
36. Hummel, L., Schwartze, A., Schirmeister, W., and Wagner, H. Maternal Plasma Triglycerides As a Source of Fetal Fatty Acids (1976) *Acta Biol. Med. Germ. 35*, 1635–1641.
37. Ramsay, T. G., Karousis, J., White, M. E., and Wolverton, C. K. Fatty Acid Metabolism by the Porcine Placenta (1991) *J. Anim. Sci. 69*, 3645–3654.
38. Sorrentino, D., and Berk, P. D. (1993) in *Hepatic Transport and Bile Secretion: Physiology and Pathophysiology,* Tavaloni, N., and Berk, P.D., Raven Press, New York, pp. 197–210.
39. Stremmel, W., Kleinert, H., Fitscher, B.A., Gunwan, J., Klaassen-Schluter, C., Moller, K., and Wegener, M. Mechanism of Cellular Fatty Acid Uptake (1992) *Biochem. Soc. Trans. 20*, 814–817.

40. Stremmel, W., Strohmeyer, G., Borchard F., Kochwa S., and Berk, P.D. Isolation and Partial Characterization of a Fatty Acid Binding Protein in Rat Liver Plasma Membranes (1985) *Proc. Natl. Acad. Sci. U.S.A. 82*, 4–8.
41. Abumrad, N.A., Park, J.H., and Park, C.R. Permeation of Long-Chain Fatty Acids into Adipocytes (1984) *J. Biol. Chem. 259*, 8945–8953.
42. Stremmel, W., Lotz, G., Strohmeyer, G., and Berk, P.D. Identification, Isolation, and Partial Characterization of a Fatty Acid Binding Protein from Rat Jejunal Microvillous Membranes (1985) *J. Clin. Invest. 75*, 1068–1076.
43. Goresky, C.A., Stremmel, W., Rose, C.P., Guiguis, S., Schwab, A.J., Diede, H. E., and Ibrahim, E. The Capillary Transport System for Free Fatty Acids in the Heart (1994) *Circ. Res. 74*, 1015–1026.
44. Zhou, S.L., Stump, D., Sorrentino, D., Potter, B.J. , and Berk, P. Adipocyte Differentiation of 3T3-L1 Cells Involves Augmented Expression of a 43-kDa Plasma Membrane Fatty Acid-Binding Protein (1992) *J. Biol. Chem. 267*, 14456–14461.
45. Campbell, F. M., Gordon, M.J., and Dutta-Roy, A. K. Plasma Membrane Fatty Acid Binding Protein ($FABP_{pm}$) from the Sheep Placenta (1994) *Biochim. Biophys. Acta 1214*, 187–192.
46. Campbell, F. M., Gordon, M. J., and Dutta-Roy, A. K. Plasma Membrane Fatty Acid-Binding Protein from Human Placenta: Identification and Characterization. (1995) *Biochem. Biophys. Res. Commun. 209*, 1011–1017.
47. Das, T., Gaurishankar, S. A., and Mukerjea, M. Characterization of Cardiac Fatty Acid-Binding Protein from Human Placenta (1993) *Eur. J. Biochem. 211*, 725–730.
48. Veerkamp, J. H., Peeters, R.A., and Maatman, R.G.H.J. Structural and Functional Differences of Cytoplasmic Fatty Acid-Binding Proteins (1991) *Biochim. Biophys. Acta 1081*, 1–24.
49. Glatz, J.F.C., Vork, M.M., Cistola, D.P., van der Vusse, G.J. Cytoplasmic Fatty Acid-Binding Protein: Significance for Intracellular Transport of Fatty Acids and Putative Role on Signal Transduction Pathways (1993) *Prostaglandins, Leukotrienes Essen. Fatty Acids 48*, 33–41.
50. Dutta-Roy, A.K., Huang, Y., Dunbar, B., and Trayhurn, P. Purification and Characterization of Fatty Acid-Binding Proteins from Brown Adipose Tissue of the Rat (1993) *Biochim. Biophys. Acta 1169*, 73–79.
51. Dutta-Roy, A.K., Gopalswamy, N., and Trulzsch, D.V. Prostaglandin E_1 Binds to Z Protein of Rat Liver. (1987) *Eur. J. Biochem. 162*, 615–619.
52. Raza, H., Pogubala, J.R., and Sorof, S. Specific High Affinity Binding of Lipooxygenase Metabolites of Arachdionic Acid by Liver Fatty Acid Binding Protein. (1989) *Biochem. Biophys. Res. Commun. 161*, 448–455.
53. Schurer, N.Y., Stremmel, W., Grundmann, J.-U., Schliep, V., Kleinert, H., Bass, N.M., and Williams, M.L. Evidence for a Novel Keratinocyte Fatty Acid Uptake Mechanism with Preference for Linoleic Acid: Comparison of Oleic Acid Uptake by Cultured Human Keratinocytes, Fibroblasts and a Human Hepatoma Cell Line (1994) *Biochim. Biophys. Acta 1211*, 51–60.
54. Koletzko, B., and Muller, J. Cis- and trans -Isomeric Fatty Acids in Plasma Lipids of Newborn Infants and Their Mothers (1990) *Biol. Neonate 57*, 172–178.
55. Sorrentino, S., Potter, B.J., and Berk, P.D. (1990) in *Progress in Liver Disease*, Popper, H., and Schaffner, F., Saunders, Philadelphia, pp. 203–224.
56. Dutta-Roy, A.K., Gordon, M.J., Campbell, F.M., Duthie, G.G., and James, W.P.T. Vitamin E Requirements, Transport and Metabolism: Role of α-Tocopherol-Binding Proteins (1994) *J. Nutr. Biochem. 5*, 562–570.

57. Spector, A.A., Ashbrook, J.K., and Fletcher, J.A. Binding of Long Chain Fatty Acids to Bovine Serum Albumin (1969) *J. Lipid Res. 10,* 56–67.
58. Lafond, J., Simneau, L., Savard, R., and Gagnon, M.-C. Linoleic Acid Transport by Human Placental Synctiotrophoblast Membranes (1994) *Eur. J. Biochem. 226,* 707–713.

Chapter 6

Absorption of γ-Linolenic Acid from Borage, Evening Primrose, and Black Currant Seed Oils: Fatty Acid Profiles, Triacylglycerol Structures, and Clearance Rates of Chylomicrons in the Rat

Carl-Erik Høy and Michael Søberg Christensen

Department of Biochemistry and Nutrition,
Technical University of Denmark,
DK-2800 Lyngby, Denmark

Introduction

In the formation of long-chain polyunsaturated fatty acids of the n-6 series, the rate-limiting step is the Δ6-desaturation of 18:2n-6 into 18:3n-6 (1). Numerous biological effects of 18:3n-6 mediated by prostanoids or by the influence of the fatty acid *per se* on membrane structure have been demonstrated, e.g., effects on inflammation, premenstrual syndrome, hypertension and cholesterol metabolism. This has recently been reviewed extensively by Horrobin (2).

Due to the effects of 18:3n-6 there is a considerable interest in natural sources of this fatty acid. The predominant natural sources are plant oils such as borage oil, evening primrose oil, and black currant seed oil.

In the digestion and absorption of an oil, the intestinal degradation is influenced by the fatty acid profile, the triacylglycerol (TAG) structure, and the species composition. The lipases involved in the degradation of triglycerides are regiospecific, and their action results in the formation of *sn*-1/2-DG and *sn*-2/3-DG, and finally *sn*-2-MG. The most important lipase participating in degradation and absorption of triglycerides is pancreatic lipase, which degrades the TAG into *sn*-2-MG and free fatty acids (3). Other lipases may contribute to varying extents to the degradation of TAG. In the stomach, the lingual lipase (4) and gastric lipase (5) are active. These lipases in particular hydrolyze short- and medium-chain fatty acids from the *sn*-3-position and thus are important during digestion and absorption of butterfat, cocoa butter and human milk. Once formed, the MG and the free fatty acids are absorbed by the enterocytes. In the enterocytes, a reacylation by the 2-MG pathway takes place, leading to the formation of TAG, which is then assembled with phospholipids, cholesterol and apoproteins into chylomicrons (CM). The CM are released into the lymphatic duct and further into the circulation, where they are degraded by lipoprotein lipase (6). The fatty acids are taken up in part by the endothelial tissues to be used for oxidation or for synthesis of phospholipids which are components of biological membranes. Following degradation of approximately 70% of the TAG in the CM, remnant particles are formed which are cleared by the liver.

All processes involved in the intestinal degradation of TAG and reacylation as well as in the systemic clearance of TAG are regiospecific. The triglyceride structure of the dietary fat may therefore influence the metabolism of fatty acids both in the intestine and in the circulation. Such effects have previously been described by Kritchevsky et al. (7) who demonstrated that the atherogenic potential of peanut oil was related to its TAG-structure rather than to the fatty acid profile, with C20 and C22 fatty acids being located in the *sn*-3-position. Filer et al. (8) demonstrated that the growth support of maternal milk was related to its particular TAG-structure with 16:0 almost exclusively located in the *sn*-2-position. We have recently demonstrated that the TAG-structure affects the lymphatic absorption of medium-chain fatty acids (9,10), the initial rate of absorption of marine oils (11), the clearance of CM as well as the ratio of distribution of cholesterol between the hepatic and the extrahepatic tissue (12). The total digestibility of fish oil and peanut oil, as determined by fecal fat contents, however, has been found by others not to be influenced by the TAG-structure (13,14).

In this paper we report the regiospecific TAG-structures of borage oil, evening primrose oil and black currant seed oil, the absorption profiles of major fatty acids from these oils as determined by collection of the mesenteric lymph, the TAG structure of the CM formed during absorption, and finally the clearance of the CM from the circulation.

Methods

Oils

Borage oil, evening primrose oil and black currant seed oil were analyzed as follows: The oils were methylated (15) and the fatty acid profile was determined by gas-liquid chromatography (GLC) using a HP5880 (Hewlett-Packard Instruments) with FID and a 0.32 mm i.d. × 25 m fused silica column, SP2380 (Supelco Inc.). Split-injection was applied. Temperature programming was as follows: Initial temperature 120°C followed by programming at 4°C increase/min to 160°C, constant temperature for 2 min, programming at 8°C increase/min to 200°C, constant temperature for 10 min, followed by programming at 30°C increase/min to 225°C. The triacylglycerol structure of the oil was determined by Grignard degradation with allylmagnesium bromide (16) followed by isolation of the *sn*-2-MG by thin-layer chromatography, methylation and GLC. This method determines the fatty acid profiles of the *sn*-2-MG and the *sn*-1/3- positions. However, the method establishes neither the distribution between the *sn*-1- and the *sn*-2-positions nor the composition of the TAG-species. Nevertheless, the method is more convenient and reliable than degradation with pancreatic lipase, which may discriminate polyunsaturated fatty acids in the *sn*-1/3- positions; in these highly unsaturated oils, this could lead to erroneous results. Acylmigration as controlled by degradation of 1,3-dipalmitoyl, 2-oleyl-glycerol was less than 2%.

Absorption of Oils

Male albino Wistar rats were anesthetized with pentobarbital and subjected to cannulation of the main mesenteric lymph duct (11). A feeding tube was inserted into the stomach. The rats were placed in restraining cages with free access to tap water and a continous infusion of saline (0.15 M) at 2 mL/h. The day following the surgery, the absorption study was initiated by collection of lymph for 1 h. A bolus of oil (0.5 mL) was then injected into the stomach followed by 0.5 mL saline (0.15 M). Lymph fractions were collected in 1 h fractions for the first 8 h followed by one fraction from 8 to 24 h after administration. The total lipid from each lymph fraction was extracted with chloroform:methanol (2:1, v/v) following addition of internal standards (C13:0 and C17:0 methyl esters). The total fatty acid profile was determined by GLC. Regiospecific analysis of the TAG-structure was performed as described above.

Labeling of Chylomicrons

Donor rats were cannulated as described above. Following recovery, an emulsion made of 0.3 mL oil, 20 µCi [^{14}C]-oleic acid, 40 µCi [^{3}H]-cholesterol, and 10 ng di-pentadecanoyl-phosphatydylcholine was administered through the feeding tube followed by saline. After 30 min, the lymph was collected for 8 h into tubes containing EDTA-Na$_2$, gentamycin and glutathione. The lymph from two rats was pooled. Cells were removed by low speed centrifugation. The chylomicrons were isolated by ultracentrifuge flotation (12).

Clearance Studies

Rats were subjected to cannulation of the jugular vein and carotid artery. The labeled chylomicrons were introduced intravenously into the jugular vein at time 0. At 3, 5, 8, 12, 20, 25, and 30 min, blood samples of 0.4 mL were drawn from the carotid artery and compensated by saline injection (0.15 M). Plasma was prepared and the labels were counted by liquid scintillation. Following this, the rats were killed and the liver, heart, kidney, spleen, and brain were excised and rinsed for blood. The lipids were extracted and the organ uptake of radioactivity counted by liquid scintillation (data not shown).

Results and Discussion

Oils

Borage oil had the highest content of 18:3n-6 and the lowest of 18:2n-6. Evening primrose oil was rich in 18:2n-6, but was lowest in 18:3n-6. Only black currant seed oil was intermediate with respect to 18:2n-6 and 18:3n-6. Black currant oil contained considerable levels of 18:3n-3 as well as 18:4n-3 (Fig. 6.1).

From the regiospecific analyses of the three oils and the fatty acid profiles of the TAG, the ratio of major fatty acids located in the *sn*-2-position relative to the total contents was calculated (Fig. 6.2). A content above 33% in the *sn*-2-position indicates that the oil examined was structured with respect to the fatty acid considered. This demonstrated that most unsaturated fatty acids were evenly esterified among the three positions of the TAG, probably due to the high contents of unsaturated fatty acids in the oils examined. Borage oil, however, was specifically structured with

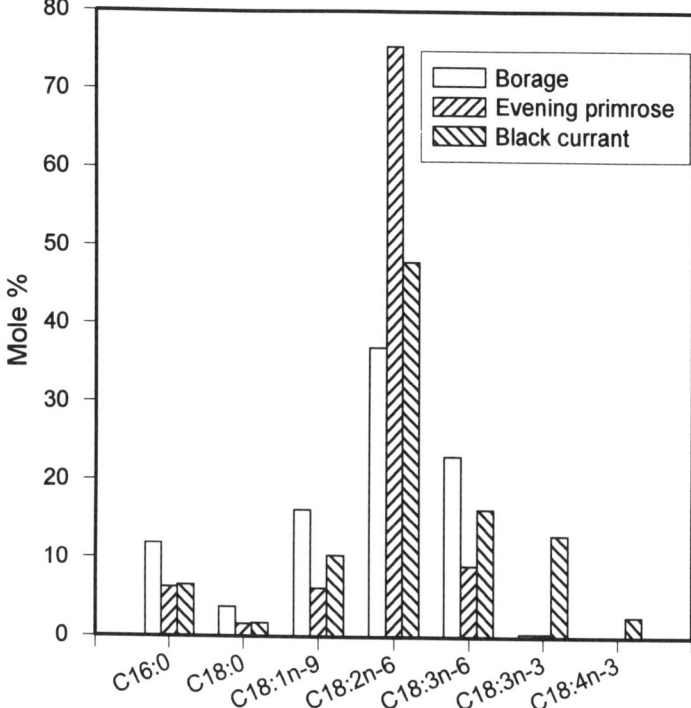

Fig. 6.1. Major fatty acids in borage oil, evening primrose oil, and black currant seed oil. Mole % determined by GLC.

regard to 18:3n-6, because approximately 60% of the 18:3n-6 was esterified in the *sn*-2-position. In black currant seed oil, a slight accumulation (47%) of 18:1n-9 in the *sn*-2-position was also observed. It has previously been established that evening primrose oil consists of relatively few TAG-species compared with borage oil (17). Our methodology does not allow a separation into species, but reflects the total distribution of fatty acids in all species.

Absorption

During the first 3–4 h after administration of the oils, the mole % of 18:3n-6 and of 18:2n-6 in the lymph lipids rose to maximum levels, reflecting the levels in the oils administered (Figs. 6.3A and 6.3B). The amount of 18:3n-6 in the lymph declined after 7 h. The total amounts of all fatty acids (mg/h) transported through the lymphatics were similar for the three diets (Fig. 6.4), indicating that the oils were equally well absorbed and reflecting that all three oils contained mainly C16 and C18 fatty acids, which in general are well absorbed. The small amounts of C20 and C22 fatty acids present in the borage oil neither affect the total absorption nor introduce a time lag in the absorption profile.

From the individual fractions collected, the accumulated transport was calculated for each fatty acid. This included exogenous as well as endogenous contributions.

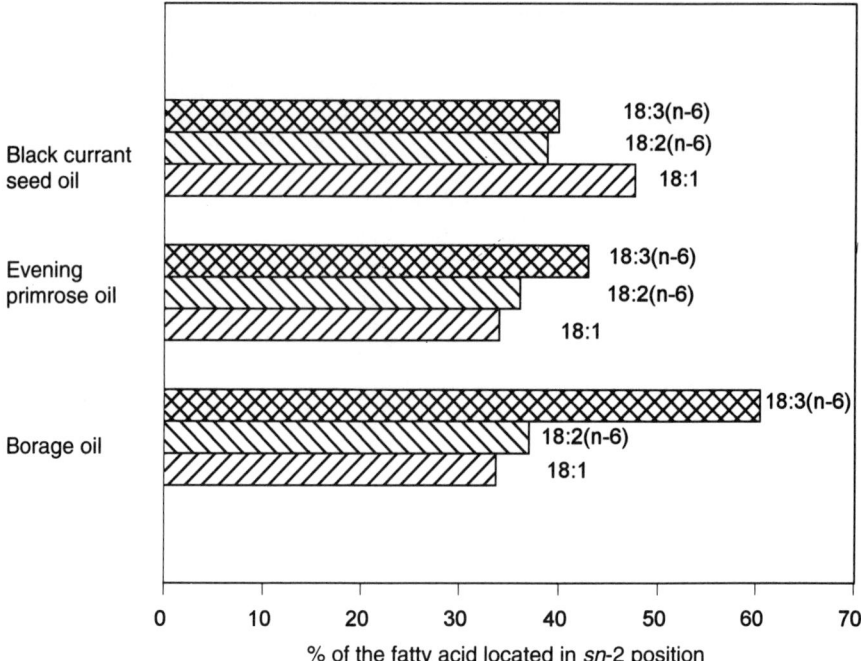

Fig. 6.2. Regiospecific distribution of major unsaturated fatty acids in borage oil, evening primrose oil, and black currant seed oil. A content above 33% indicates that the fatty acid is accumulated in the *sn*-2-position.

By estimating the absorption of fat from the composition of the lymph, the transfer of fatty acids to the portal blood during absorption is neglected. The magnitude of this transfer depends on the chain length of the fatty acid and whether esterified or free fatty acids are considered. Bernard and Carlier (18) found that approximately 10% of the oleic and linoleic acid absorbed was transported through the portal blood. For the oils considered in this experiment, similar transfers to the portal blood may be expected. The accumulated transports of all fatty acids (Fig. 6.5) were similar for all three oils for the first 8 h, indicating that they were digested at equal rates. Only negligible amounts of endogenous 18:3n-6 appeared in the lymph before administration of the oils. The absorption curves (Figure 6.6A) reflected the relative occurrence in the oils, with borage oil resulting in the largest and evening primrose oil in the smallest amount of fatty acid transported. Previous investigations (19) have established that the depositions of 18:3n-6 and the formation of 20:3n-6 simply reflect the dietary levels in agreement with our observation on the absorptions.

For 18:2n-6, the accumulated transport (Fig. 6.6B) included an endogenous contribution, which cannot be determined by the methods applied in this experiment. In the rats given evening primrose oil, by far the largest transport of 18:2n-6 was found, which also reflected the very high dietary level. For the borage oil and the black currant seed oil groups, lower and similar transports were observed. The accumulated transport of 20:4n-6 (Fig. 6.6C) was the same for all three oils although

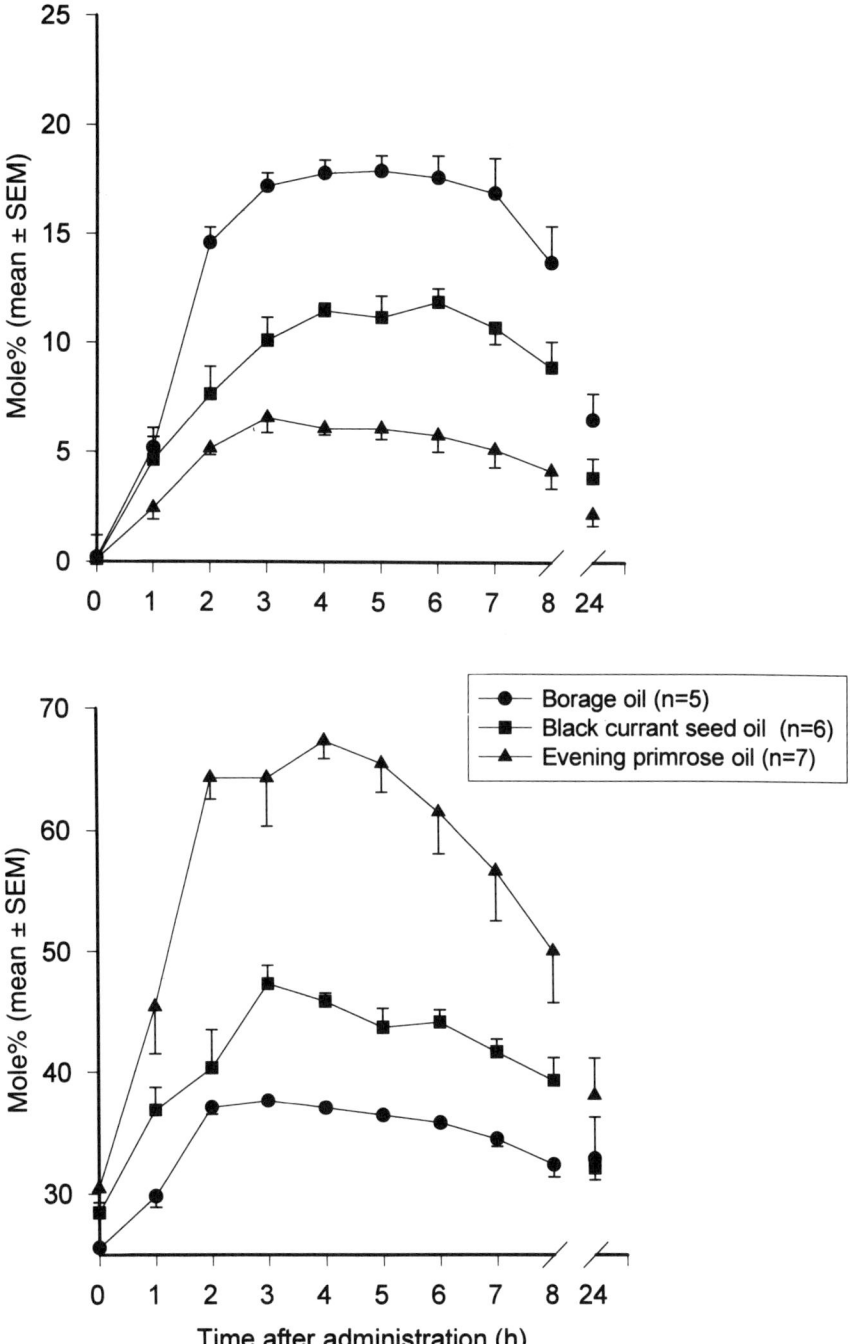

Fig. 6.3. Lymphatic contents (mole % of total fatty acids in the lymph) of 18:3n-6 (A) and 18:2n-6 (B) vs. time following administration of borage oil, evening primrose oil, and black currant seed oil.

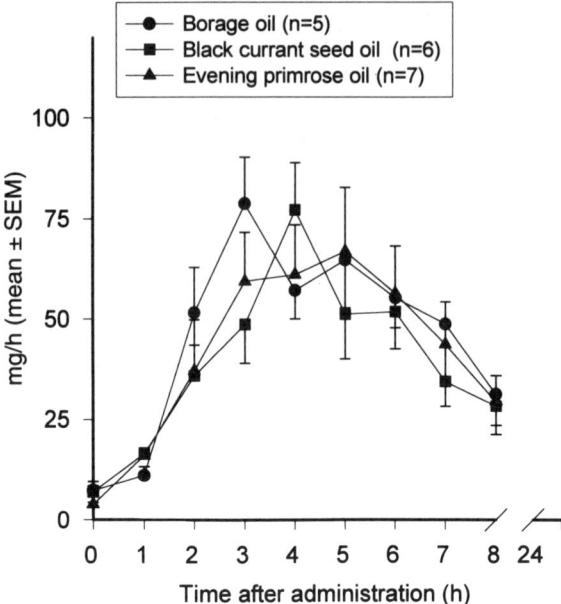

Fig. 6.4. Total lymphatic contents of fatty acids during absorption of fat following gastric administration of borage oil, evening primrose oil, and black currant seed oil.

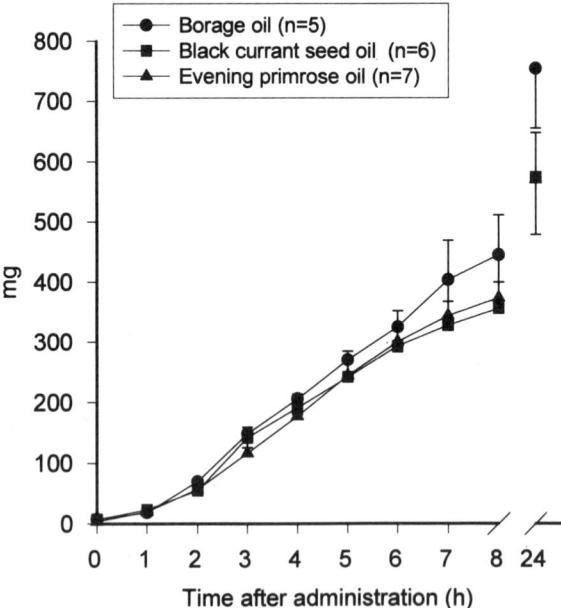

Fig. 6.5. Accumulated lymphatic transport of fatty acids following gastric administration of borage oil, evening primrose oil, and black currant seed oil.

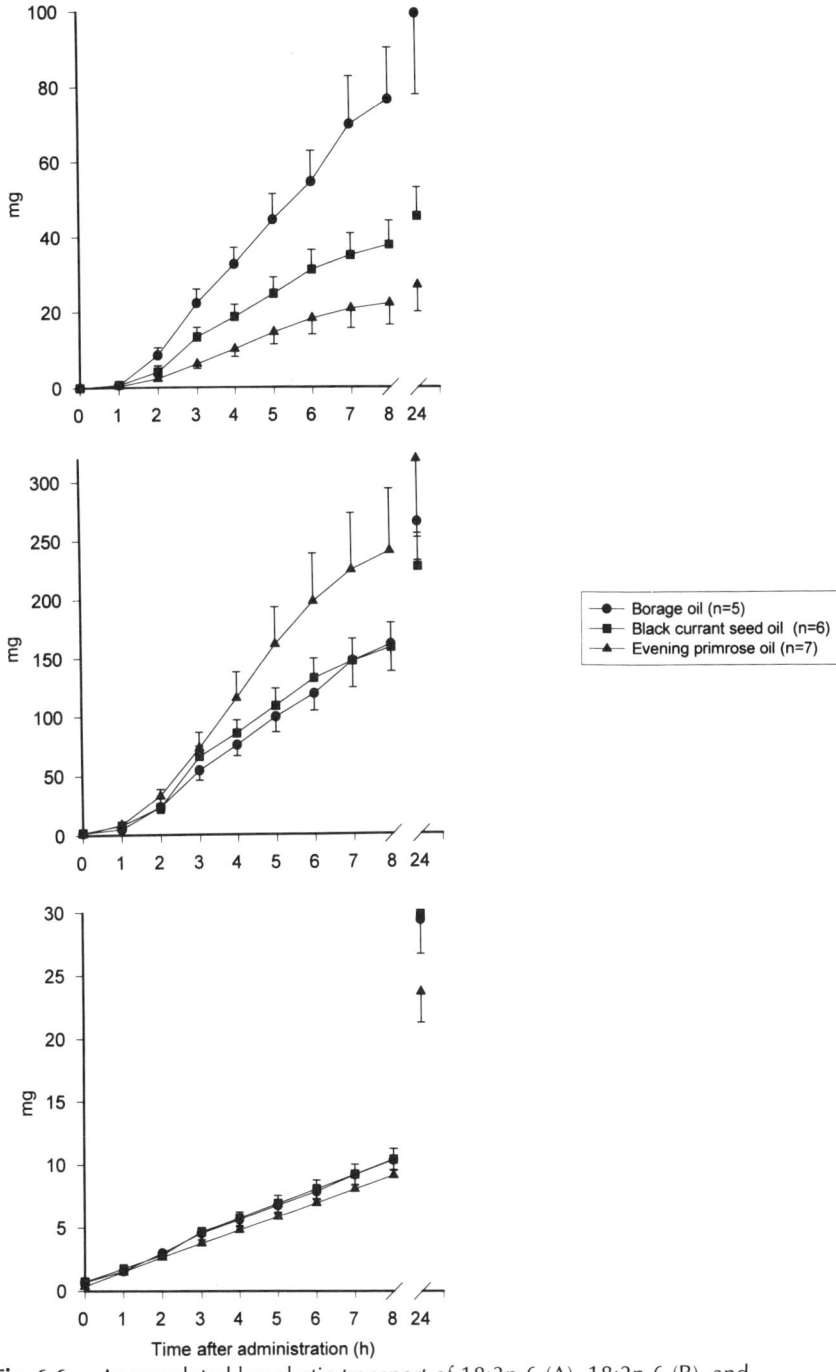

Fig. 6.6. Accumulated lymphatic transport of 18:3n-6 (A), 18:2n-6 (B), and 20:4n-6 (C) following gastric administration of borage oil, evening primrose oil, and black currant seed oil.

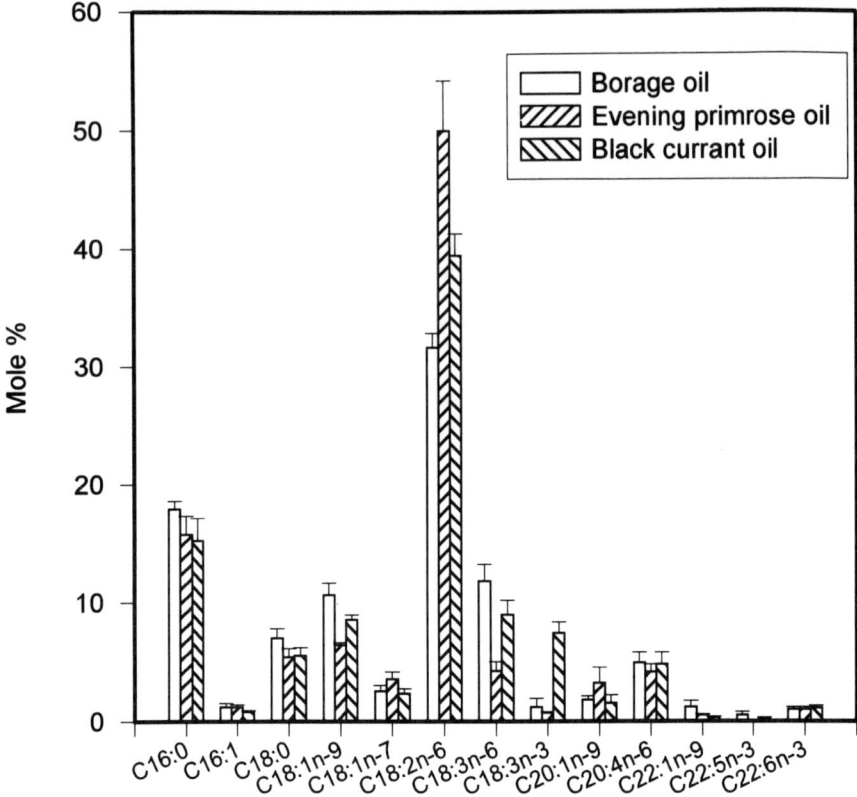

Fig. 6.7. Fatty acid profile (mole %, $n = 2$) of chylomicrons at 8 h following administration of borage oil, evening primrose oil, and black currant seed oil.

there was a tendency for the oils with the highest contents of 18:3n-6 to transport slightly more 20:4n-6, possibly reflecting formation of 20:4n-6. The major part of the 20:4n-6, however, probably originated from the bile or the plasma.

Chylomicrons

The fatty acid profile of chylomicrons varied with time, reflecting the absorption of fat and the release of triglycerides into the lymph. At 8 h (Fig. 6.7), the fatty acids reflected the oils given, but significant endogenous contributions of 20:4n-6 and 22:6n-3 were observed. The ratios between the contents of 18:3n-6 were similar to those of the dietary contents. The contents of 16:0 and 18:0 were considerably higher than for the dietary oils, presumably also reflecting endogenous recirculation of bile phospholipids or uptake and release of fatty acids from the circulation.

In the chylomicrons, a positional redistribution of fatty acids in the TAGs compared with the dietary oils was evident (Fig. 6.8 vs. Fig. 6.2), making the TAGs very random. Only in the chylomicrons from the borage oil group was a specific TAG

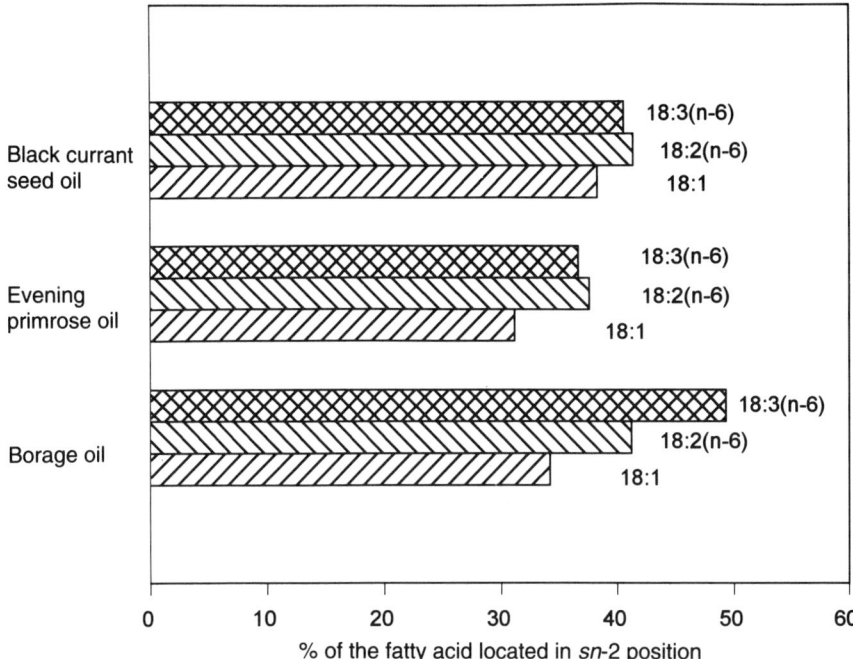

Fig. 6.8. Regiospecific distribution of major unsaturated fatty acids in chylomicrons following administration of borage oil, evening primrose oil, and black currant seed oil. A content above 33% indicates that the fatty acid is accumulated in the *sn*-2-position.

structure observed, with 18:3n-6 being located mainly in the *sn*-2-position. Compared with borage oil, in which 60% of the 18:3n-6 was located in the *sn*-2-position, there was a decrease to 50% in chylomicrons. This agrees with the previous observation for model substrates that 75% of the fatty acids in the *sn*-2-position is maintained during absorption (20), indicating that a rearrangement during absorption may be expected although the major pathway is by the 2-MG reacylation. The preferential incorporation of endogenous fatty acids into the *sn*-2- and *sn*-3-positions (21) may contribute to this effect. In all three groups, the 18:2n-6 was nearly evenly distributed among the three positions of the TAG from the chylomicrons.

Clearance of Chylomicrons

The chylomicrons (Figs. 6.9A and 6.9B) were rapidly removed from the circulation as indicated by the disappearance of labeled oleic acid and cholesterol. The removal rates observed were in accordance with the results of Chen et al. (22). However, oleic acid was removed at a faster rate than cholesterol in agreement with the formation of remnant particles. No differences in the metabolism of the chylomicrons from the three groups were observed, indicating that they were degraded and removed at similar rates; this is in agreement with the observation by Raedersdorff

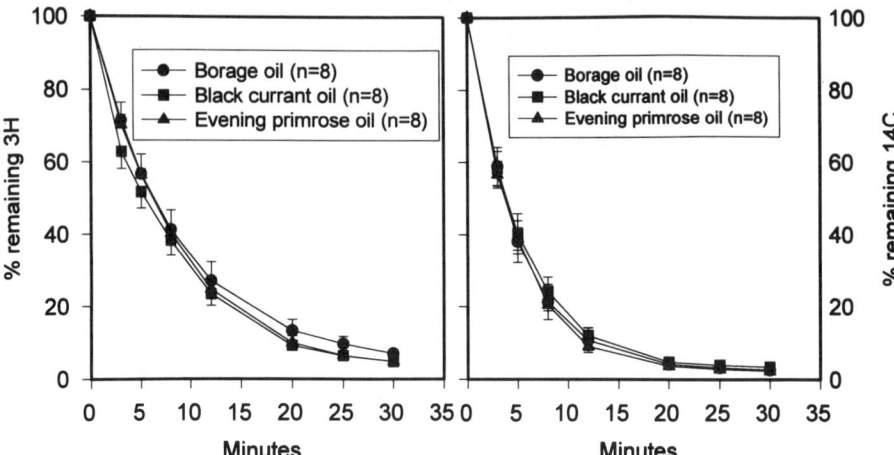

Fig. 9. Clearance of chylomicrons, [^{3}H]-cholesterol (A) and [^{14}C]oleic acid (B). Percentage of remaining label vs. time following following systemic injection of labeled chylomicrons.

and Moser (19) that the deposition of 18:3n-6 reflects the dietary intake. Our experiments thus indicate that the chylomicrons formed during intake of the three oils have similar substrate properties towards lipoprotein lipase.

Summary

We examined borage oil, black currant seed oil, and evening primrose oil with respect to fatty acid profile and fatty acid composition. We found that only borage oil was specifically structured with respect to 18:3n-6, this fatty acid being preferentially esterified in the *sn*-2-position. During absorption, the composition of the lymph largely reflected the fatty acid profiles of the oils administered. The total absorptions as indicated by the transport of fatty acids in the lymph were similar for the three oils and indicated that all three oils were well absorbed. In the chylomicrons, a redistribution of 18:3n-6 from the *sn*-2-position to the *sn*-1/3-positions in the borage oil-fed rats was found. The chylomicrons from the three groups were cleared at similar rates.

References

1. Marcel, Y.L., Christiansen, K., and Holman, R.T. The Preferred Metabolic Pathway from Linoleic Acid to Arachidonic Acid *in vitro* (1968) *Biochim. Biophys. Acta 164,* 25–34.
2. Horrobin, D.F. Nutritional and Medical Importance of Gamma-Linolenic Acid (1992) *Prog. Lipid Res. 31,* 163–194.

3. Mattson, F.H., and Beck, L.W. The Specificity of Pancreatic Lipase for the Primary Hydroxyl Groups of Glycerides (1956) *J. Biol. Chem. 219,* 735–740.
4. Bläckberg, L., Hernell, O., Fredrikzon, B., and Akerblom, H.K. On the Source of Lipase Activity in Gastric Contents (1977) *Acta Pædiatr. Scand. 66,* 473–477.
5. Levy, E., Goldstein, R., Freier, S., and Shafrir, E. Characterization of Gastric Lipolytic Activity (1981) *Biochim. Biophys. Acta 664,* 316–326
6. Nilsson-Ehle, P., Garfinkel, A.S., and Schotz, M.C. Lipolytic Enzymes and Plasma Lipoprotein Metabolism (1980) *Annu. Rev. Biochem. 49,* 667–693.
7. Kritchevsky, D., Davidson, L.M., Weight, M., Kriek, N.P.J., and du Plessis, J.P. Influence of Native and Randomized Peanut Oil on Lipid Metabolism and Aortic Sudanophilia in the Vervet Monkey (1982) *Atherosclerosis 42,* 53–58.
8. Filer, L.J., Mattson, F.H., and Fomon, S.J. Triglyceride Configuration and Fat Absorption by the Human Infant (1969) *J. Nutr. 99,* 293–298.
9. Jensen, M.M., Christensen, M.S., and Høy, C.-E. Intestinal Absorption of Octanoic, Decanoic and Linoleic Acids. Effect of Triglyceride Structure (1994) *Ann. Nutr. Metab. 38,* 104–116.
10. Christensen, M.S., Müllertz, M. and Høy, C.-E. Absorption of Triglycerides with Defined or Random Structure by Rats with Biliary and Pancreatic Diversion (1995) *Lipids 30,* 521–526.
11. Christensen, M.S., Høy, C.-E., and Redgrave, T.G. Lymphatic Absorption of n-3 Polyunsaturated Fatty Acids from Marine Oils with Different Intramolecular Fatty Acid Distributions (1994) *Biochim. Biophys. Acta 1215,* 198–204.
12. Christensen, M.S., Mortimer, B.-C., Høy, C.-E., and Redgrave, T.G. Clearance of Chylomicrons Following Fish Oil or Seal Oil Feeding (1995) *Nutr. Res. 15,* 359–368.
13. de Schrijver, R., Vermeulen, D., and Backx, S. Digestion and Absorption of Free and Esterified Fish Oil Fatty Acids in Rats (1991) *Lipids 26,* 400–404.
14. de Schrijver, R., Vermeulen, D., and Viane, E. Lipid Metabolism Responses in Rats Fed Beef Tallow, Native or Randomized Fish Oil and Native or Randomized Peanut Oil (1991) *J. Nutr. 121,* 948–955.
15. Christopherson, S.W., and Glass, R.L. Preparation of Milk Fat Methyl Esters by Alcoholysis in an Essentially Nonalcoholic Solution (1969) *J. Dairy Sci. 52,* 1289–1290.
16. Becker, C.C., Rosenquist, A., and Hølmer, G. Regiospecific Analysis of Triacylglycerols Using Allyl Magnesium Bromide (1993) *Lipids 28,* 147–149.
17. Redden, P.R., Huang, Y.-S., Lin, X., and Horrobin, D.F. Separation and Quantification of the Triacylglycerols in Evening Primrose and Borage Oils by Reversed-Phase High-Performance Liquid Chromatography (1995) *J. Chromatogr. A694,* 381–389.
18. Bernard, A., and Carlier, H. Absorption and Intestinal Catabolism of Fatty Acids in the Rat: Effect of Chain Length and Unsaturation (1991) *Exp. Physiol. 76,* 445–455.
19. Raedersdorff, D., and Moser, U. Borage or Evening Primrose Oil Added to Standardized Diets are Equivalent Sources for Gamma-Linolenic Acid in Rats (1992) *Lipids 27,* 1018–1023.
20. Åkesson, B., Gronowitz, S., Herlöff, B., and Ohlson, R. Absorption of Synthetic, Stereochemically Defined Acylglycerols in the Rat (1978) *Lipids 13,* 338–343.
21. Breckenbridge, W.C., Yeung, S.K.F., and Kuksis, A. Biosynthesis of Triacylglycerols by Rat Intestinal Mucosa in vivo (1976) *Can. J. Biochem. 54,* 145–152.
22. Chen, I.S., Le, T., Subramanian, S., Cassidy, M.M., Sheppard, A.J., and Vahouny, G.V. Comparison of the Clearance of Serum Chylomicron Triglycerides Enriched with Eicosapentaenoic Acid or Oleic Acid (1987) *Lipids 22,* 318–321.

Chapter 7

Metabolism of [3-^{13}C] γ-Linolenic Acid in the Suckling Piglet and Rat

S.C. Cunnane, J. Vogt, S.S. Likhodii, G. Moine,[a] R. Muggl,[a]
K.-H. Tovar,[b] G. Kohn,[b] and G. Sawatzki[b]

> Department of Nutritional Sciences, Faculty of Medicine, University of Toronto, Toronto, Canada M5S 1A8
> [a]Vitamins and Fine Chemicals Division, Roche, Basel, Switzerland, and
> [b]Research International Department, Milupa AG, Friedrichsdorf, Germany

Introduction

Analytical methods used to investigate the metabolism of γ-linolenic acid (18:3n-6, GLA) to n-6 long chain polyunsaturated fatty acids (LC-PUFAs) have thus far been limited primarily to measurement by gas chromatography (GC) of changes in fatty acid composition of tissues or blood, or to tracing of the metabolism of carbon-14 (^{14}C)-labeled GLA. The GC method has some applications in human studies, but they are largely restricted to analysis of blood samples that can be difficult to obtain in infants and are infrequently collected at multiple time points to determine peak changes in utilization. Radio tracer studies in humans are becoming ethically unacceptable, especially when stable isotope analogues are potentially available.

This chapter describes two recent studies attempting to develop new approaches to monitoring the metabolism of PUFAs by stable isotope methodology. The impetus for these studies arose because of the need for more detailed and accurate information concerning the metabolism of PUFAs in humans, especially infants. For instance, it is important to know whether LC-PUFAs beyond linoleic acid (18:2n-6) and α-linolenic acid (18:3n-3) should be present in breast-milk substitutes given to term and preterm infants. If it is advised that infant formulas contain LC-PUFAs, does GLA offer a significant advantage over linoleate or is a dietary source of arachidonate (20:4n-6, AA) advisable in the preweaning period? GC-based analyses, with their access limited to small blood samples from infants, are not ideal to address these questions, yet they are all that is currently available. A new method capable of providing noninvasive analyses of breath CO_2 excretion that permits noninvasive assessment of fatty acid levels and metabolism in different organs as well would have considerable application in this field.

We realized that ^{13}C tracer methods employing isotope ratio mass spectrometry (IRMS) or nuclear magnetic resonance (NMR) spectroscopy would both be applicable to such a goal. However, it was also apparent that few studies of the metabolism of ^{13}C-labeled PUFA have been conducted and, even in animal models, none had attempted to monitor the metabolism of ^{13}C-labeled fatty acids noninvasively. We started with two animal models, each with its own advantages and disadvantages—the suckling rat and piglet. Although the suckling rat pup is small and not necessarily comparable to the human infant, it requires much less of the tracer, thereby allowing acquisition of detailed time course data even though artificial feeding is difficult. In contrast, the piglet is larger and is widely considered a good model for early human development. It readily consumes formula diets differing in fatty acid composition, but it requires much more of the tracer, especially for NMR purposes.

For these studies, ^{13}C-enriched GLA was custom-synthesized at Hoffmann-La Roche (Basel, Switzerland) with the ^{13}C placed at C-3. This permitted detection by ^{13}C NMR of the conversion of GLA to n-6 LC-PUFAs, particularly AA. Ideally, this conversion would also be visible when measured by *in vivo* ^{13}C NMR.

γ-Linolenic Acid and Longer-Chain Polyunsaturated Fatty Acids in the Brain

GLA was chosen for this initial study because, in evaluating the synthesis of AA in neonates, it bypasses the rate-limiting Δ6 desaturase step between linoleate and AA. Hence, interference or delays in the metabolism of linoleate might be reduced. In the context of infant nutrition and development, the addition of GLA to human milk formulas might be a more efficient way to address the problem of achieving and maintaining appropriate tissue levels of AA in human infants consuming milk formulas compared with provision of linoleate without any n-6 LC-PUFAs.

GLA would also provide a probe for determining whether the majority of brain AA in infants originates *in situ* or from the milk, adipose tissue stores or synthesis in the liver. Brain levels of GLA are usually <0.2% of total fatty acids, but it is not known whether this is because of low uptake or rapid conversion to n-6 LC-PUFAs. Supplementation of the diet with GLA increases the level of AA in rat liver and other organs (1,2) but this does not seem to affect the amount of AA accumulating in the developing rat brain. [1-^{14}C] GLA is incorporated into ^{14}C-AA in brain and other organ lipids more easily than ^{14}C-linoleate in the suckling rat (3). In the case of the developing brain, however, the relative importance of the liver in this conversion has not been clearly established (4,5).

^{13}C Tracer Methods for Polyunsaturated Fatty Acid Metabolism

^{13}C Tracer methods have potentially wide application in studies of fatty acid metabolisms in humans. IRMS is well established as a precise and sensitive analytical tool for stable isotope studies. It is the only practical and established method for breath ^{13}CO$_2$ analysis. Analysis of ^{13}C excretion in breath after oral dosing of adult male volunteers with ^{13}C-linoleate, oleate (18:1n-9) or stearate (18:0) showed that complete β-oxidation of linoleate exceeded that of stearate (6). Little if any further use of this noninvasive methodology to address ^{13}C PUFA metabolism at different ages, in diseases or under different dietary fat intakes has been reported since this 10-year-old study.

Coupling a GC to a combustion interface prior to determining ^{13}C enrichments in an IRMS has recently become a valuable method for fatty acid tracer studies involving ^{13}C. Combustion interfaces between standard GC and IRMS instruments are now available commercially, and results on both analytical quality of the data that can be obtained (7,8) and the application of this method to ^{13}C studies in animal models have been reported (9). It is crucial to recognize that this method provides data only on ^{13}C *enrichment* of a single fatty acid. Without knowledge of the *mass* of that fatty acid in the lipid or tissue of interest, it is not possible to determine whether high ^{13}C *enrichment* equals high ^{13}C *mass*; very often the enrichment is high in a small pool but the total amount of ^{13}C in that small pool may be much less than in a larger pool of a related or product fatty acid. This method brings a valuable new dimension to fatty acid analysis but, as for fatty acid analysis by percentage composition, the results have to be interpreted carefully and are highly dependent on changes in pool size of the fatty acid(s) in question.

^{13}C NMR of crude lipid extracts of tissues or of purified lipids provides valuable and unique insight into the exact carbon-by-carbon location of a ^{13}C-enriched tracer carbon (10). If the ^{13}C-enriched site changes in structure during the metabolism, e.g., from an aliphatic (CH_2) to an olefinic carbon (C=C) or from a carbonyl (C=O) to an aliphatic carbon, this change is readily demonstrated using ^{13}C NMR. C-3 of GLA is an aliphatic carbon and resonates at about 24.7 ppm in lipid extracts. After chain-elongation and desaturation, the C-3 becomes an olefinic carbon (C-5) in AA which resonates at about 129 ppm. Therefore, locating the ^{13}C specifically at C-3 in GLA provided us with a simple and specific marker in NMR spectra of the relative rate of GLA accumulation *vs.* its conversion to AA or other metabolites.

We have previously applied this valuable feature of ^{13}C NMR to assess the metabolism of different ^{13}C-labeled fatty acid tracers on a carbon-by-carbon basis. With [2-^{13}C] acetate as a substrate for fatty acid synthesis, it is clear in ^{13}C NMR spectra of liver lipid extracts that the ^{13}C differentially enters different carbon sites; even-numbered carbons are more highly enriched and, as expected, carbons toward the CH_3 terminal of PUFA remain unenriched (10). We have also shown that a large proportion of the metabolism of uniformly (U) ^{13}C-labeled eicosapentaenoic acid (20:5n-3) involves loss of the first four carbons with apparent production of a 16-carbon fatty acid product (11).

One other useful outcome of the NMR-based analysis of tissue samples is that sample preparation is minimal, i.e., total lipid extracts provide good resolution of most carbons of fatty acids and cholesterol. Hence, ^{13}C enrichment can be monitored in a broad range of metabolites without purification of the lipid class in question. In some cases, the ^{13}C-enriched product may be one that is unidentified or may have been unexpected. For instance, in addition to the enrichment expected in brain AA and docosahexaenoic acid (22:6n-3), metabolism of [U-^{13}C] linoleate (18:2n-6) and α-linolenate (18:3n-3) by suckling rats also yields substantial ^{13}C enrichment in brain *cholesterol* (9). This occurs in a highly regular pattern of pairs of ^{13}C-enriched carbons reflecting initial ^{13}C enrichment in acetyl CoA (12). Although previous studies using radiolabeled PUFAs have demonstrated similar results, they have not shown where the radiolabel is located in the cholesterol. We were able to determine the exact cholesterol labeling pattern in brain total lipid extracts using one- and two-dimensional NMR techniques (12).

^{13}C NMR also has *in vivo* applications that provide the opportunity to monitor the presence and metabolism of a tracer noninvasively and, potentially, in humans. It has already been successfully developed as a noninvasive probe for glucose metabolism in humans (13). Differences in human subcutaneous adipose tissue composition have been demonstrated in vegetarians and in cystic fibrosis patients using *in vivo* ^{13}C NMR (14,15). We have shown that an oral dose of [U-^{13}C] linoleate and α-linolenate produces ^{13}C enrichment in suckling rat brain that is visible *in vivo* and lasts for at least 8 d (Fig. 7.1). Initially, the enrichment was mainly in the aliphatic carbons of brain lipids, reflecting rapid utilization for ketogenesis and subsequent brain lipid synthesis (16,17). However, later on, olefinic carbon enrichment that reflected the slower conversion of linoleate and α-linolenate to LC-PUFAs in the brain was also visible.

Hence, IRMS provides data on precise amounts of ^{13}C metabolized to particular products including CO_2, whereas NMR provides the specific location of the ^{13}C. NMR is probably the only practical way to trace fatty acid metabolism *in vivo* in real time. These two methods are therefore complementary and should be exploited to provide new insights into human fatty acid metabolism.

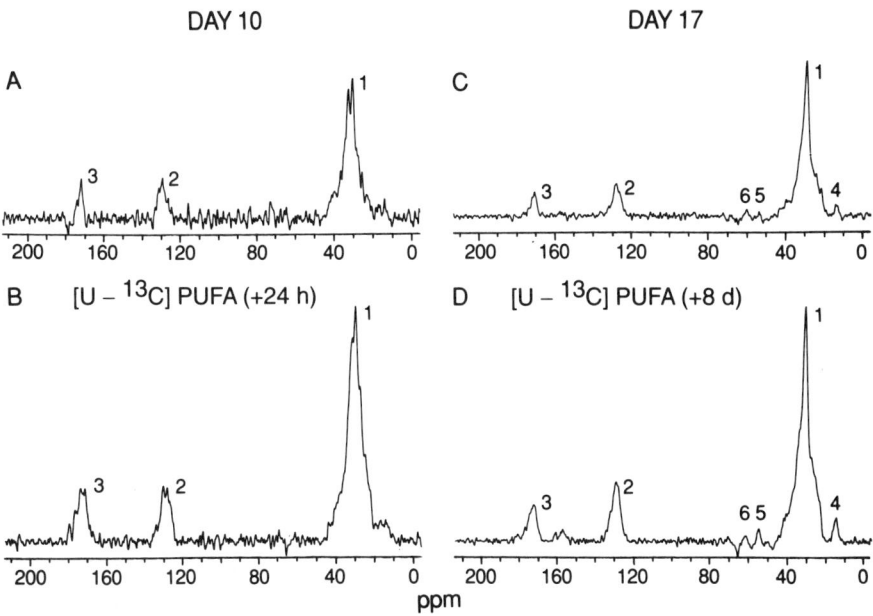

Fig. 7.1. *In vivo* ^{13}C NMR spectra of the head of live suckling rats before (A,C) and after (B,D) oral dosing with [U-^{13}C]-labeled PUFA. Peaks are identified as (1) methyl carbons, (2) olefinic carbons, (3) carboxyl carbons, (4) terminal methyl carbon, (5) phosphatidylcholine, and (6) glycerol carbons. Note the increased signal/noise ratio in the spectra from rats injected with the tracer; at 24 h postdosing (B); the main change was an increase in peak 1 relative to peaks 2 and 3, whereas 8 d later (D) both peaks 1 and 2 were increased relative to peak 3. *Source:* Cunnane et al. (9).

Breath ^{13}C Analysis

Analysis of the ^{13}C appearing in breath CO_2 after dosing with a ^{13}C-labeled fatty acid represents the carbon that is completely β-oxidized. Few studies have addressed the metabolism and β-oxidation of ^{13}C-labeled PUFAs in humans, and yet it is becoming increasingly clear that a full understanding of the metabolic importance of PUFAs awaits more complete knowledge of their β-oxidation, e.g., their role in energy metabolism (18,19). For instance, whole-body fatty acid balance studies in laboratory animals now clearly show that at the commonly accepted minimally adequate level for linoleate intake (2 energy %), complete oxidation accounts for about 75% of the whole-body utilization of dietary linoleate; only 6% is converted to n-6 LC-PUFAs while the rest is stored as linoleate itself, mostly in adipose tissue (20). If the majority of linoleate is β-oxidized, is part of the essentiality of linoleate in some way connected to its oxidation or is the current requirement for linoleate overestimated? If the latter is the case, one would expect oxidation to be lower at a lower linoleate intake. However, even at 0.3% of energy, at least 50% of dietary linoleate is still completely oxidized (21). With repeated cycles of 24-h fasting followed by 72-h refeeding, complete oxidation of linoleate exceeds 85% in male rats and can reach 100% in pregnancy (22,23). Hence, oxidation is quantitatively the most important route of linoleate metabolism in rats and is markedly dependent not only on linoleate intake but also on the physiological and nutritional status of the animal.

Comparable studies have not yet been done in humans, making it difficult to extrapolate, but attention has to be focused on oxidation of PUFAs in humans, especially in infants and individuals undergoing voluntary or medically supervised energy restriction. In addition to holding potentially important information about PUFA metabolism, breath CO_2 measurements are noninvasive and well accepted for human studies; hence, their merits and limitations for understanding PUFA metabolism in humans have to be fully explored and defined.

In Vivo ^{13}C NMR

In vivo ^{13}C NMR methods are now well established in several centers in North America and Europe for the purpose of monitoring metabolism in living human volunteers. At the moment, virtually all of this research addresses the metabolism of ^{13}C-labeled glucose. Despite the fact that fatty acids in adipose tissue are also readily observed by *in vivo* NMR (15,24–26), very little research on fatty acid metabolism has been conducted using ^{13}C NMR. One reason for this is that the lean tissues that are active in fatty acid metabolism, e.g., heart, liver and brain, have very poor natural abundance of ^{13}C fatty acid signals because they contain relatively low amounts of "mobile" fatty acids, e.g., those in the free form or in triglycerides. Another reason is that adipose tissue masks the signal from these lean tissues, making it difficult to observe ^{13}C signals emitting from only the underlying lean tissues. A third reason is that fatty acids labeled with ^{13}C at a specific carbon other than the carboxyl carbon (C-1) have not become available until recently and are very expensive given the degree of dilution in an adult human.

Our first *in vivo* investigation of metabolism of ^{13}C-labeled PUFA was in suckling rats so as to obtain the highest possible body concentration but at a minimal level of adipose tissue masking of lean tissue signals (9). We used [U-^{13}C]-labeled linoleate and α-linolenate and, despite the ^{13}C-^{13}C coupling that occurs when adjacent carbons have high levels of ^{13}C enrichment, we were able to observe significant increases in ^{13}C NMR signals in lipids of the brain in living rat pups. Many technical and methodological issues still have to be resolved before *in vivo* ^{13}C NMR is used to monitor fatty acid metabolism in humans, but it is feasible in small animals, which should give us the incentive to refine the methods and eventually pursue human studies.

The Piglet Model

The piglet is well established as a model for studying the nutritional biochemistry of the human infant (27–30). Innis et al. (31,32) have modeled fatty acid metabolism in human infants on the hand-reared suckling piglet and have determined the influence of changes in dietary fatty acid intake on brain fatty acid composition. Their studies have shown that a high ratio of linoleate to α-linolenate in the piglet formula milk compromises brain accumulation of docosahexaenoate (31). Raised intake of docosahexaenoate also compromises accumulation of n-6 LC-PUFAs (32). The authors suggest that accumulation of LC-PUFAs in the piglet brain may depend more on the linoleate/α-linolenate ratio in the milk formulas than on the presence of LC-PUFAs in the formula. The importance of these contributions is undermined by the absence of tracer studies to monitor the source and rates of brain uptake of LC-PUFAs.

Among models for human infant brain development, the piglet brain is close in size to that of the newborn term infant and thus can also be used as a good physical model for potential *in vivo* NMR studies in human infants. The relatively large size of the piglet brain also provides a reasonable signal/noise ratio which is a crucial limitation for *in vivo* NMR studies. Thus, we used this model to address whether uptake of [3-^{13}C]-GLA by the piglet brain could be detected noninvasively using *in vivo* ^{13}C NMR.

In our study, the piglets were early weaned at 3 d of age and transferred to a pen where they consumed a commercial sow's milk formula from a liquid formula feeder designed for preweanling piglets (Shur-Gain, St. Mary's, ON). This type of feeder has a trough into which the milk is pumped from an insulated reservoir at intervals and for a duration set by the operator. With initial hand feeding and a little prompting, the piglets learn to use this feeder within 6–12 h. The piglets were group fed at the same time from a single trough. The milk reservoir was insulated to keep the milk cooler and restrict bacterial growth. The entire feeder system was cleaned and disinfected once every 24 h. Only on rare occasions was there any diarrhea and usually for <12 h. The commercial milk formula contained 24% protein and 28% fat blended from coconut and soybean oils, and it was virtually devoid of LC-PUFAs. Using a timer, the milk formula was automatically dispensed into the trough once hourly, 24 h/d at a rate of 20–40 mL/h/piglet depending on age. A separate water bowl was also available at all times.

All piglets were studied at 11–12 d of age. Thus, those consuming the formula milk had been adapted to it for 8–9 d and were compared with sow-reared piglets of the same age. A comparison of the fatty acid composition of total lipids of the liver from the sow-reared and formula-fed piglets reflected the differences in milk fatty acids, with the sow-reared piglets having a lower proportion of oleate but a higher proportion of most PUFAs compared with piglets consuming the milk formula. Sow-reared piglets had significantly higher LC-PUFAs in the liver and more palmitate (16:0) and linoleate in brain total lipids (Table 7.1).

In vivo ^{13}C NMR

In vivo ^{13}C NMR was performed on several control piglets and one formula-fed piglet given an oral dose of 500 mg [3-^{13}C] GLA 24 h earlier. A horizontal 2.1-T magnet with an internal bore diameter of 17 cm was used for this study. The piglets were anesthetized for the duration of each *in vivo* NMR experiment with halothane (4% priming dose; 1% for maintaining anesthesia) and lay in the prone position in a Plexiglas support fitted to the cylindrical bore of the magnet. Warm air was piped into the bore of the magnet to keep the temperature at about 28°C. A two-turn, home-built surface coil tuned for ^{13}C and a concentric figure-eight coil tuned for ^1H decoupling were fitted onto the piglet's head to acquire the ^{13}C NMR signals noninvasively. After tuning and optimizing the homogeneity of the magnetic field around the area of interest (shimming), the signal acquisition phase of each *in vivo* NMR experiment lasted 1–2 h. The spectra obtained were for the head only and were acquired directly over the cerebral cortex. They were not localized specifically on the brain due to the loss of signal/noise ratio during this process.

TABLE 7.1 Fatty Acid Composition (%) of Total Lipids of the Brain and Liver in 11- to 12-d-old Piglets That Were Sow-Reared (Sow) or Consumed a Commercial Sow's Milk Formula Devoid of LC-PUFA (Formula)

	Liver		Brain	
	Sow	Formula	Sow	Formula
16:0	16.0 ± 0.6[1]	15.1 ± 0.7	19.5 ± 0.4	18.8 ± 0.4[a]
18:0	23.4 ± 0.6	23.4 ± 1.0	20.6 ± 0.3	21.1 ± 0.3
18:1n-9	9.2 ± 0.5	16.2 ± 1.3[a]	17.4 ± 1.1	18.4 ± 1.3
18:2n-6	14.8 ± 0.3	12.2 ± 0.8[a]	1.6 ± 0.1	1.2 ± 0.1[a]
20:3n-6	0.7 ± 0.1	0.9 ± 0.1	0.7 ± 0.04	0.6 ± 0.02
20:4n-6	19.6 ± 0.8	16.6 ± 0.6[a]	11.8 ± 0.3	11.4 ± 0.4
22:4n-6	1.3 ± 0.1	1.0 ± 0.04[a]	5.0 ± 0.2	4.9 ± 0.1
22:5n-6	1.4 ± 0.1	1.8 ± 0.06[a]	3.4 ± 0.2	4.0 ± 0.2
18:3n-3	0.4 ± 0.1	—	—	—
20:5n-3	—	0.2 ± 0.03	—	—
22:5n-3	1.9 ± 0.2	1.1 ± 0.1[a]	0.4 ± 0.04	0.3 ± 0.0
22:6n-3	4.7 ± 0.3	3.5 ± 0.3[a]	8.9 ± 0.3	8.6 ± 0.4

[1]Mean ± SD (*n* = 5/group).
[a]*P* < 0.01 *vs.* SOW group (Student's *t*-test).

The narrow line widths and broad bases of the main peaks in the ^{13}C NMR spectra obtained from control piglets (not ^{13}C-dosed) indicated that they contained signals arising from both the brain and from triglycerides in the surrounding tissues (Fig. 7.2). Although localization would have increased the relative amount of the signal detected from the brain, the signal/noise ratio would have been lower because brain tissue is much lower in mobile lipid molecules, e.g., free fatty acids and triglycerides, than the surrounding adipose tissue. Furthermore, the ^{13}C enrichment reported previously for a similar study of rat brain using unlocalized ^{13}C NMR (9) was quantitatively almost all in the brain compared with surrounding tissues. Hence, localization on the brain seemed unnecessary at this time.

The spectrum from the piglet dosed 24 h previously with 500 mg [3-^{13}C] GLA showed no detectable difference with several control spectra (Fig. 7.2). ^{13}C NMR of the extracted brain lipids from this piglet showed no detectable change in the C-3 resonance of GLA (data not shown) or the C-5 resonance of AA (Fig. 7.3). This explains the lack of detectable change in these signals in the spectra obtained *in vivo*.

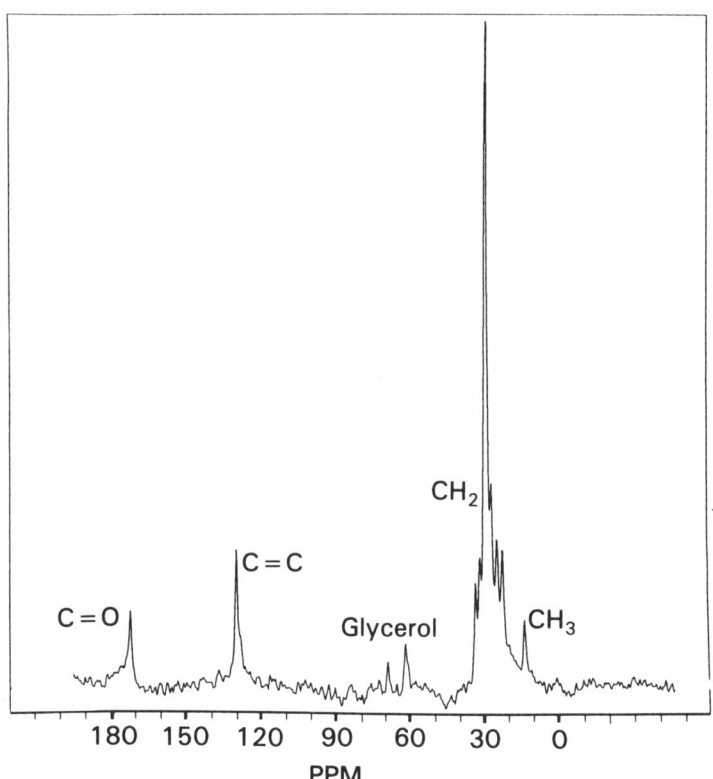

Fig. 7.2. An *in vivo* ^{13}C NMR spectrum of the brain and surrounding tissues of a live piglet under halothane anesthesia. The broad base on each of the major peaks (C=O, carboxyl; C=C, olefinic; CH$_2$ and CH$_3$, methyl carbons) arises from lipids in the brain, but the main signal is derived from fatty acids outside the brain, primarily in the scalp.

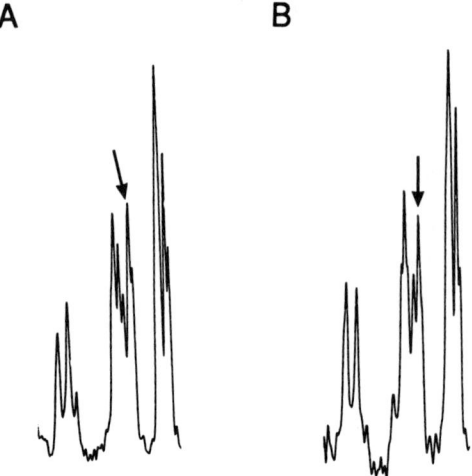

Fig. 7.3. Expansion of a ^{13}C NMR spectrum of piglet brain total lipids in chloroform solution showing the olefinic region. The arrow indicates the location of the C-5 resonance of arachidonate at 128.7 ppm. Twenty-four hours after an oral dose of 500 mg of [3-^{13}C] GLA given to sow-fed piglets (B), this resonance was not significantly different than in control piglets (A).

However, ^{13}C NMR spectra of the liver lipids clearly showed the expected increase in these resonances along with the presence of numerous other small resonances in the aliphatic (CH_2), olefinic (C=C), and carbonyl (C=O) regions of the lipid spectrum (see ^{13}C NMR of Brain and Liver Lipid Extracts), thus clearly demonstrating that [3-^{13}C]-GLA had been metabolized to AA. However, neither were detectable in the brain within 24 h of dosing.

Breath ^{13}C

Breath $^{13}CO_2$ measurements were made on our piglets after dosing with [3-^{13}C]-GLA. The breath samples were collected hourly for 8 h and then at 24 and 48 h after dosing. The breath collection chamber was connected to a metabolic cart from which air was drawn at about 12 L/min. Air was sampled into a 50 mL syringe and transferred to an evacuated tube for ^{13}C analysis by IRMS. Excretion of $^{13}CO_2$ over a 48 h period after receiving the 200-mg dose of [3-^{13}C] GLA was 22.6% of the dose given in the sow-reared piglets and 8.0% of the dose in the piglets consuming the formula (Fig. 7.4). In the sow-reared piglets, a plateau in ^{13}C excretion in the breath was not reached within 48 h of dosing, but in the formula-fed piglets, it was reached within 24 h of dosing.

^{13}C NMR of Brain and Liver Lipid Extracts

^{13}C NMR spectra of liver total lipid extracts had two particular regions of interest, the resonance for C-3 of GLA (24.7 ppm), and the resonance for C-5 of AA (128.9 ppm). Control spectra of liver total lipids had no detectable signal at C-3 of GLA. Piglets receiving the [3-^{13}C]-GLA had clear evidence in NMR spectra of liver total lipid extracts of ^{13}C labeling at C-3 of GLA (24.7 ppm) and a big increase at the resonance

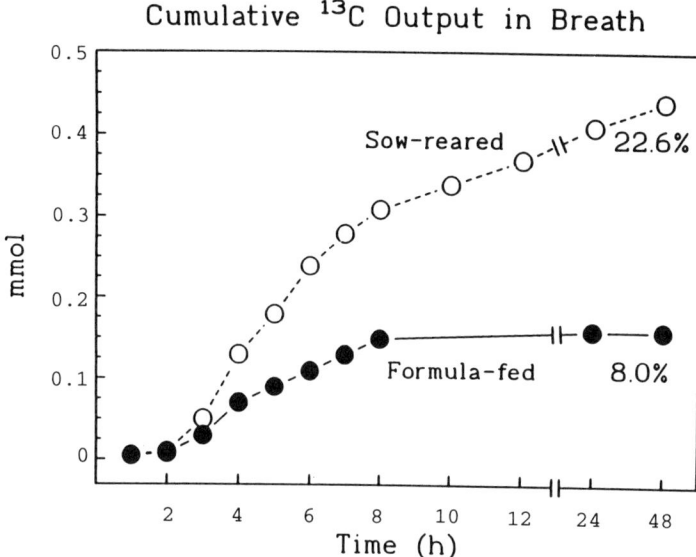

Fig. 7.4. ^{13}C excretion in breath CO_2 over a 48-h period after oral dosing with 200 mg of [3-^{13}C]-GLA in sow-reared piglets (○) or piglets consuming a commercial sow's milk formula (●). Each point is the mean of duplicate measurements on two piglets.

for C-5 of AA (about 129 ppm) (Fig. 7.5). In the vicinity of the main GLA peak, there were other smaller peaks suggestive of GLA in different lipid classes that would have slightly shifted the C-3 signal. There was also ^{13}C enrichment at several resonances around 29 ppm where C-5 of dihomo-γ-linolenate (20:3n-6) would be expected to resonate (Fig. 7.5). The identity of the peak for C-5 of dihomo-γ-linolenate remains uncertain because this peak has not been previously assigned. Unexpectedly, peaks in the carbonyl region of the liver lipids also had several sites of ^{13}C enrichment, indicating that some C-3 from GLA was recycled into fatty acid synthesis *de novo* and hence appeared at C-1 of some new fatty acids.

Despite the clear evidence for extensive metabolism of ^{13}C-GLA by the liver, spectra of piglet brain lipids after dosing with 500 mg [3-^{13}C]-GLA remained devoid of ^{13}C enrichment either at 24.7 ppm (C-3 of GLA) or at 129 ppm (C-5 of AA) (Figs. 7.3 and 7.6). In view of the high cost of this tracer and the lack for evidence that even large amounts of GLA lead to ^{13}C enrichment in n-6 LC-PUFA in the brain, the comparison between formula-fed and sow-reared piglets was done using an oral dose of 200 mg [3-^{13}C]-GLA.

Formula Milk Compared with Sow Rearing

One of our aims was to assess whether a sow's milk replacer formula containing virtually no LC-PUFA would affect metabolism of GLA compared with sow rearing. In

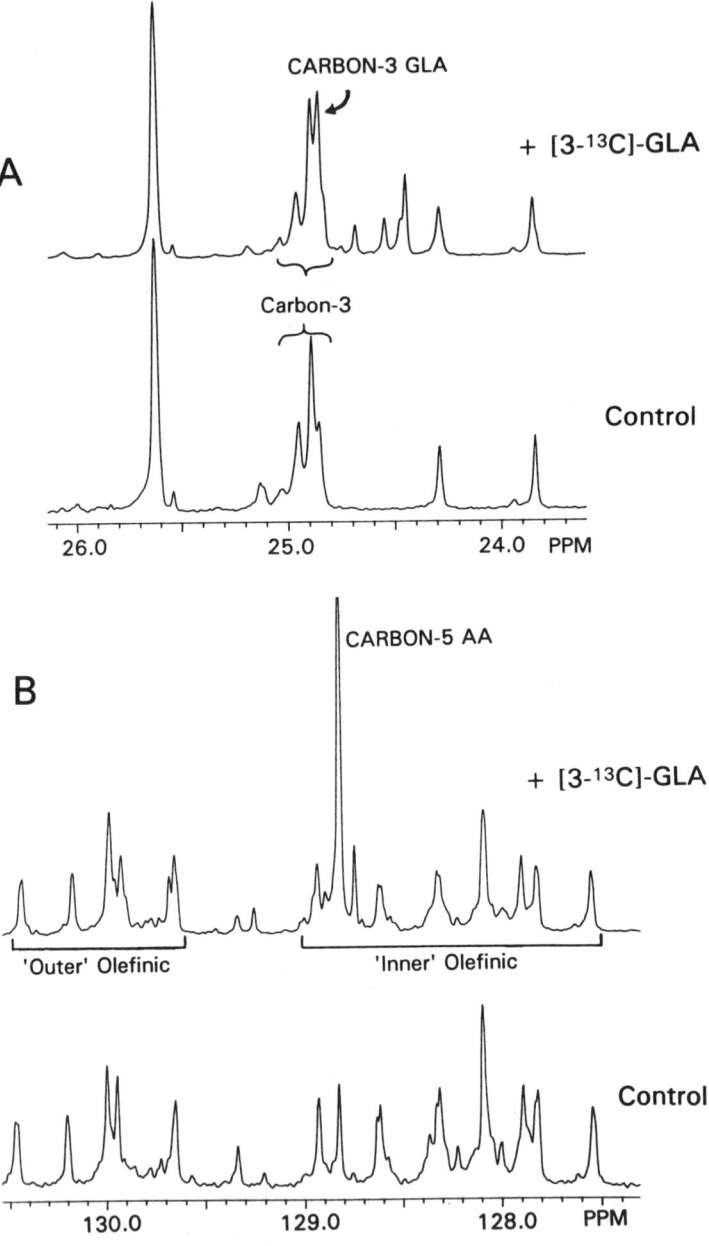

Fig. 7.5. Expansion of a ^{13}C NMR spectrum of piglet total liver lipids in chloroform solution showing the carbon-3 (A) and olefinic region (B) before and 24 h after an oral dose of 500 mg [3-^{13}C]-GLA. The liver lipids were from a 12-d-old piglet which had been consuming a commercial sow's milk formula devoid of LC-PUFA for 8 d.

liver lipids of formula-fed piglets, ^{13}C enrichment 48 h after oral dosing with 200 mg of [3-^{13}C]-GLA was greater than in the sow-reared piglets. In brain total lipids, ^{13}C enrichment did not differ significantly between the two groups and did not change significantly from control (natural abundance) values (Table 7.2). In both brain and liver lipids, ^{13}C enrichment from ^{13}C-GLA was mainly in phospholipids (as expected) but detectable labeling of brain cholesterol (sow-reared only) and liver cholesterol (both groups) did occur (Table 7.3).

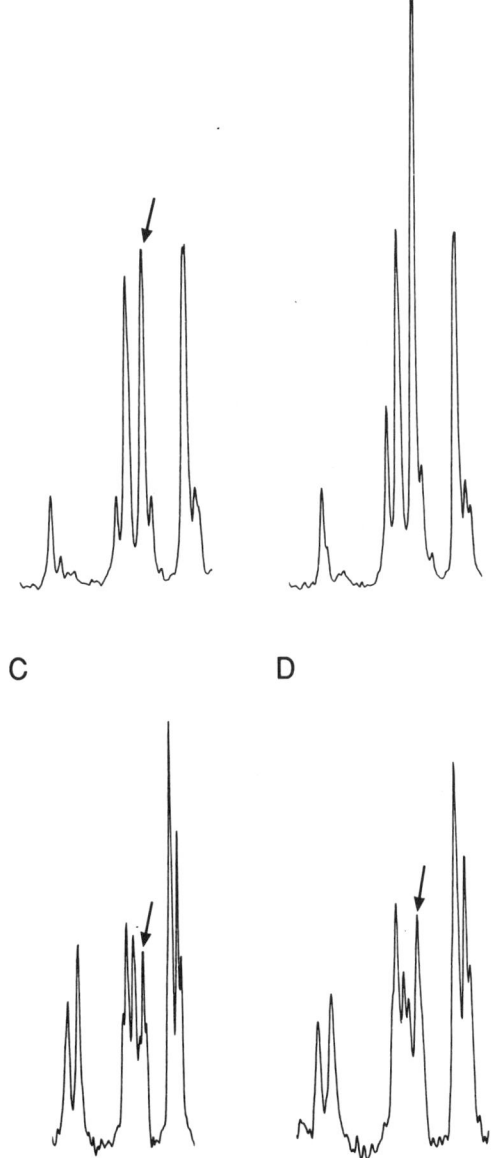

Fig. 7.6. Expansions of ^{13}C NMR spectra of piglet total brain and liver lipids in chloroform solution showing the olefinic region. The arrow indicates the location of the resonance of C-5 of arachidonate at 128.7 ppm. Forty-eight hours after an oral dose of 200 mg of [3-^{13}C] GLA, this resonance was significantly higher in the liver (B vs. A) but not in the brain (D vs. C).

TABLE 7.2 ^{13}C Levels (atom % ^{13}C and atom % excess [APE]) in Total Lipids of the Brain and Liver of 11 to 12-d-old Piglets That Were Sow-Reared (Sow) or That Consumed a Commercial Sow's Milk Formula (Formula) and Were Not Gavaged (Control) or Were Gavaged with 200 mg of [3-^{13}C] GLA 48 h Earlier (^{13}C-GLA)

		Sow[1]	Formula[2]
Brain	Control	1.10217 ± 0.00082[3]	1.10191 ± 0.00109
	^{13}C-GLA	1.10208 ± 0.00105	1.10338 ± 0.00167
	APE X 10^{-3}	–0.09 ± 0.2	1.5 ± 1.3
Liver	Control	1.09848 ± 0.00183	1.09724 ± 0.00117
	^{13}C-GLA	1.10283 ± 0.00287	1.11461 ± 0.00017
	APE X 10^{-3}	4.4 ± 2.9	17.4 ± 0.2[a]

[1]Controls ($n = 7$); ^{13}C-GLA ($n = 4$).
[2]Controls ($n = 10$); ^{13}C GLA ($n = 3$).
[3]Mean ± SD.
[a]$P < 0.01$ vs. respective Sow liver and Formula brain (Student's t-test).

The Suckling Rat Model

Lipid metabolism has been extensively studied in the suckling rat (16,17). The suckling rat brain contains the desaturases required for synthesis of LC-PUFA (33) and also actively utilizes keto acids from the circulation to synthesize cholesterol and fatty acids. Suckling rats can be fed artificially (34,35), and changes in the fat blend used in the milk formula do affect liver and brain fatty acid composition (16,35). We have shown that the brain of suckling rats contains ^{13}C-labeled LC-PUFA after an oral dose of [U-^{13}C] linoleate and α-linolenate (9). Hence, this is a well-established model in which to study the synthesis of n-6 LC-PUFA from ^{13}C-GLA. In view of the lack of appearance of ^{13}C-labeled AA in the piglet brain 48 h after large oral doses of ^{13}C-GLA, we decided to do a detailed time-course experiment of [3-^{13}C]-GLA metabolism in the suckling rat to determine whether the optimum time point for tissue analysis in the piglet might have been later than 48 h postdosing.

TABLE 7.3 Atom % Excess (APE X 10^{-3}) ^{13}C in Total Phospholipids (PL) and Cholesterol (CH) of the Brain and Liver of 11 to 12-d-old Piglets That Were Sow-Reared (Sow) or That Consumed a Commercial Sow's Milk Formula (Formula) and Were Gavaged with 200 mg of [3-^{13}C]-GLA 48 h Earlier

	Sow[1]	Formula[2]
Brain PL	1.4 ± 1.9[3]	2.0 ± 0.8
Liver PL	6.6 ± 3.0	22.6 ± 9.5[a]
Brain CH	0.0 ± 0.6	0.2 ± 0.1
Liver CH	0.2 ± 0.9	4.4 ± 3.3

[1]($n = 5$–8).
[2]($n = 3$–4).
[3]Mean ± SD.
[a]$P < 0.01$ vs. Sow liver.

Six-day-old suckling rats were dosed directly into the stomach with 20 mg of [3-^{13}C] GLA and killed at 11 time points over 8 d. Total lipid extracts were recovered by standard procedures (9). The C-3 signal for GLA was easily seen in spectra of liver lipids 12–24 h after dosing with [3-^{13}C] GLA (Fig. 7.7). The NMR signal for C-5 of liver AA at 128.9 ppm was highest 48 h after dosing. No ^{13}C enrichment was detected at any time point at the C-3 resonance of GLA in spectra of brain total lipids. However, in NMR spectra of brain lipid extracts, C-5 of AA was maximally enriched at 48 h postdosing (Fig. 7.7).

Peak ^{13}C enrichment in liver phospholipids occurred 24–48 h postdosing and was 2–3 times higher than natural abundance levels in GLA, but increased only by 9% for ^{13}C-AA. Taking liver total fatty acid pool size into consideration, the *mass* of ^{13}C in AA was seven times higher than in GLA at 24 h and 16 times higher at 48 h postdosing (Fig. 7.8). In brain phospholipids, ^{13}C enrichment was maximal 48–96 h postdosing and ^{13}C *mass* enrichment in AA was 43–130 times higher at these time points (Fig. 7.8). However, ^{13}C-GLA was also present in free fatty acids of the brain but we were unable to quantitate the exact amount.

Thus, most of the ^{13}C-AA accumulating in the suckling rat brain appears to have been derived from ^{13}C-AA synthesized in the liver; both the C NMR (Fig. 7.7) and

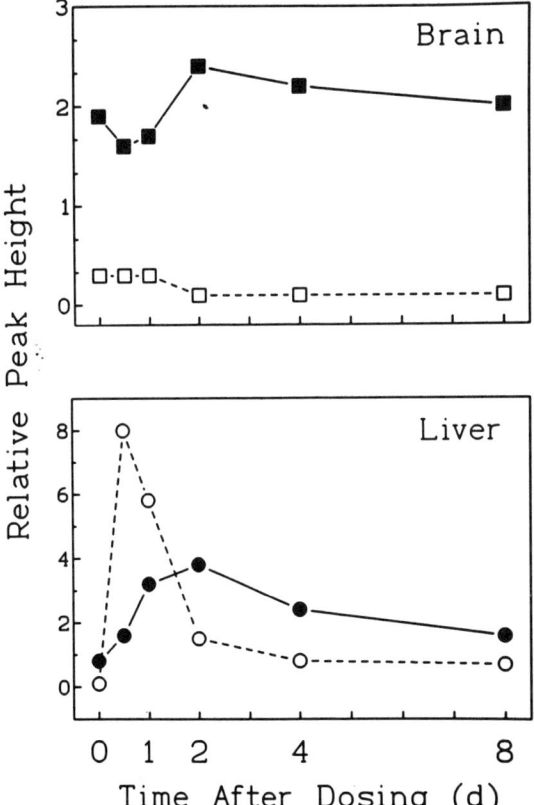

Fig. 7.7. The time course of ^{13}C enrichment in ^{13}C NMR spectra at carbon-3 of γ-linolenate (□) and C-5 of arachidonate (■) in brain lipid extracts and at carbon-3 of γ-linolenate (○) and C-5 of arachidonate (●) in liver lipid extracts. Suckling rats were dosed with [3-^{13}C]-γ-linolenate on d 6, and the time course lasted to d 14. Peak heights were compared relative to the peak for n-3 carbons of n-3 polyunsaturates that cannot be enriched by carbon recycling from the tracer.

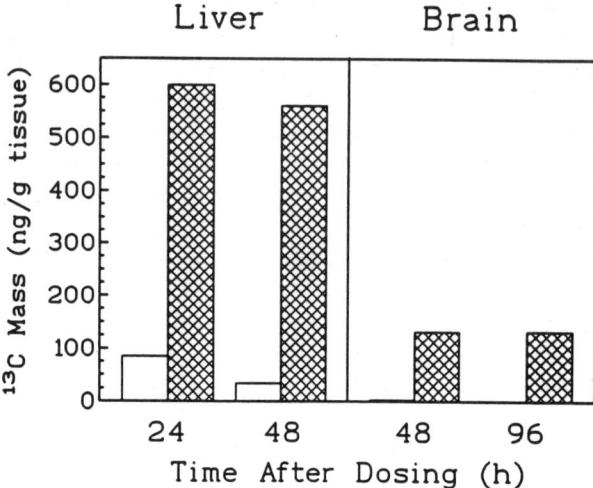

Fig. 7.8. ^{13}C mass enrichment in GLA (unshaded) and AA (shaded) of liver and brain lipids of the suckling rat after oral dosing with [1-^{13}C]-GLA.

the GC-combustion IRMS (Fig. 7.8) are in agreement on this point. Data acquired by GC-combustion IRMS clearly showed that a trace of [3-^{13}C]-GLA did access brain phospholipids but, in view of the small pool of GLA in total brain lipids, the mass of [3-^{13}C]-GLA entering the brain in this period was very low and only 1–2% of the mass of ^{13}C-labeled AA in the brain.

Conclusion

Only low amounts of intact GLA (if any) appear to reach the suckling rat or piglet brain. On the assumption that linoleate would have no greater access to the brain than GLA, our results suggest that the developing rat brain derives most of its AA either directly from the diet (maternal milk at the age studied here), from adipose tissue stores or from its synthesis in the liver. Alternatively, some brain AA could be synthesized *in situ* if dihomo-γ-linolenate penetrates the brain. Therefore, the liver would still seem to be an obligatory site from which the brain derives at least some of its n-6 LC-PUFA. The present results suggest that the low levels of GLA in the mammalian brain appear to be due to relatively low access of GLA to the brain and are less likely to be due to rapid conversion of dietary GLA to AA. In piglets, sowrearing seems to make an oral dose of GLA more dispensable (less incorporation into tissue lipids and greater complete β-oxidation), possibly because of the presence of n-6 LC-PUFA in sow milk.

There were also clear species differences in the utilization of ^{13}C-GLA for synthesis of brain AA in the suckling rat compared with the sow-reared or formula-fed piglet; GLA appears to penetrate brain lipids of 10-d-old suckling rats in low amounts, but we obtained no evidence that it accessed the brain of the 11- to 12-d-old suckling pig within 48 h of dosing. AA synthesized from dietary GLA does access the developing rat brain but did not accumulate in the piglet brain in NMR-detectable quantities. One possibility is that neurological development in these two species may have reached different stages at the same postnatal age, and hence their utilization of GLA would differ.

The stable isotope methodology used here provides preliminary evidence for the usefulness of NMR and continuous flow IRMS in monitoring metabolism of ^{13}C-labeled PUFA. The capability to directly analyze breath samples and to provide a high degree of precision and sensitivity are the two main advantages of IRMS for these studies. Access to information on ^{13}C labeling on a carbon-by-carbon basis was clearly demonstrated for NMR of tissue lipid extracts. The *in vivo* NMR methodology still suffers from a lack of sensitivity and a strong masking effect from subcutaneous adipose tissue. The fact that very little ^{13}C-labeled PUFA accessed the piglet brain under the conditions of our study may limit the application of this noninvasive method in piglets, but we are optimistic that it will prove useful in species such as the rat pup which can be studied at higher magnetic field strength.

Acknowledgments

Milupa AG (Freidrichsdorf, Germany), Van den Bergh Foods (Baltimore, MD) and the National Institutes of Health (grant no. GM49209) provided financial support for this research. Chemists led by Dr. G. Moine in the Division of Vitamins and Fine Chemicals, Roche, Basel, Switzerland synthesized the [3-^{13}C]-GLA. Dr. Claude Lemaire (MRI Laboratory, Toronto Western Hospital) is thanked for collaborating over the *in vivo* ^{13}C NMR study in piglets. The laboratory of Dr. Sheila Cohen (Merck, Nutley, NJ) is thanked for providing a detailed PCA extraction protocol. Mary-Ann Ryan provided excellent technical assistance. Collaborators including Dr. David Kyle (Martek Biosciences), Drs. Steven Brookes and Kerr Craig (Europa Scientific) and Dr. Tom Brenna and Tom Corso (Cornell University) are thanked for their extensive help in these and related studies.

References

1. Garcia, P.T., and Holman, R.T. Competitive Inhibitions in the Metabolism of Polyunsaturated Fatty Acids Studied via the Composition of the Phospholipids, Triglycerides and Cholesterol Esters of Rat Tissues (1965) *J. Am. Oil Chem. Soc. 42*, 1137–1141.
2. Horrobin, D.F. Gamma-Linolenic Acid: An Intermediate in Essential Fatty Acid Metabolism with Potential as an Ethical Pharmaceutical and as a Food (1990) *Rev. Contemp. Pharmacother. 1*, 1–45.
3. Hassam, A.G., Sinclair, A.J., and Crawford, M.A. The Incorporation of Orally-Fed Radioactive Gamma-Linolenic Acid and Linoleic Acid into the Liver and Brain Lipids of Suckling Rats (1975) *Lipids 10*, 417–420.
4. Hassam, A.G., Rivers, J.P.W., and Crawford, M.A. Metabolism of Gamma-Linolenic Acid in Essential Fatty Acid Deficient Rats (1977) *J. Nutr. 107*, 519–524.
5. Crawford, M.A. The Role of Essential Fatty Acids in Neural Development: Implications for Perinatal Nutrition (1993) *Am. J. Clin. Nutr. 57 (Suppl.)*, 703S–710S.

6. Jones, P.J.H., Pencharz, P.B., and Clandinin, M.T. Whole Body Oxidation of Dietary Fatty Acids: Implications for Energy Utilization (1985) *Am. J. Clin. Nutr. 42*, 769–777.
7. Sheaff, R.C., Si, H.-M., Keswick, L.A., and Brenna, J.T. Conversion of α-Linolenate to Docosahexaenoate Is Not Depressed by High Dietary Levels of Linoleate in Young Rats: Tracer Evidence Using High Precision Mass Spectrometry (1995) *J. Lipid Res. 36*, 998–1008.
8. Goodman, K.J., and Brenna, J.T. High Sensitivity Tracer Detection Using High-Precision Gas Chromatography-Combustion-Isotope Ratio Mass Spectrometry and Highly Enriched [U-^{13}C]-Labelled Precursors (1992) *Anal. Chem. 64*, 1088–1095.
9. Cunnane, S.C., Williams, S.C.R., Bell, J.D., Craig, K., Brookes, S., Iles, R.A. and Crawford, M.A. Utilization of [U-^{13}C] Polyunsaturates in the Synthesis of Cholesterol and Long Chain Fatty Acids in the Developing Rat Brain (1994) *J. Neurochem. 62*, 2429–2436.
10. Cunnane, S.C. Carbon-by-Carbon Discrimination of ^{13}C Enrichment in Liver Fatty Acids (1992) *FEBS Lett. 306*, 273–275.
11. Cunnane, S.C., McDonagh, R.J., Narayan, S., and Kyle, D.J. Metabolism of [U-^{13}C] Eicosapentaenoic Acid in the Rat (1993) *Lipids 28*, 273–277.
12. Likhodii, S.S., and Cunnane, S.C. Utilization of [U-^{13}C]-Labelled Polyunsaturates for Brain Cholesterol Synthesis in the Developing Rat: A ^{13}C NMR Study (1995) *Mag. Res. Med. 34*, 803–813.
13. Beckmann, N. (1995) in *^{13}C NMR Spectroscopy of Biological Systems*, Academic Press, New York, pp. 7–64.
14. Moonen, C.T.W., Dimand, R.J., and Cox, K.L. The Noninvasive Determination of Linoleic Acid Content of Human Adipose Tissue by Natural Abundance ^{13}C NMR (1988) *Mg. Reson. Med. 6*, 140–157.
15. Dimand, R.J., Moonen, C.T.W., Chu, S.C., Bradbury, E.M., Kurland, G., and Cox, K.L. The Noninvasive Determination of Linoleic Acid Content of Human Adipose Tissue by Natural Abundance ^{13}C NMR (1988) *Pediatr. Res. 24*, 243–250.
16. Yeh, Y.Y., Streuli, L., and Zee P. Ketones Serve as Important Precursors of Brain Lipids in the Developing Rat (1977) *Lipids 12*, 957–964.
17. Edmond, J., Auestad, N., Robbins, R.A., and Bergstrom, J.D. Ketone Body Metabolism in the Neonate: Development and the Effect of Diet (1985) *Fed. Proc. 44*, 2359–2364.
18. Su, W., and Jones, P.J.H. Dietary Fatty Acid Composition Influences Energy Accretion in Rats (1993) *J. Nutr. 123*, 2109–2114.
19. Jones, P.J.H., and Schoeller, D.A. Polyunsaturated:Saturated Ratio of Dietary Fat Influences Energy Substrate Utilization in the Human (1988) *Metabolism 37*, 145–151.
20. Anderson, M.J., and Cunnane, S.C. Whole Body Utilization and Organ Compartmentation of Linoleate in Rats Consuming a Low but Adequate Level of Dietary Linoleate, in *Proceedings of the Second ISSFAL Conference*, Washington, June, 1995.
21. Becker, W., and Bruce, A. Retention of Linoleic Acid in Carcass Lipids of Rats Fed Different Levels of Essential Fatty Acids (1986) *Lipids 21*, 121–126.
22. Chen, Z.-Y., and Cunnane, S.C. Refeeding After Fasting Markedly Increases Oxidation of n-6 and n-3 Fatty Acids (1993) *Metabolism 42*, 1205–1211.
23. Chen, Z.-Y., Menard, C.R., and Cunnane, S.C. Moderate, Selective Depletion of Linoleate and α-Linolenate in Weight-Cycled Rats (1995) *Am. J. Physiol. 268*, R498–R505.
24. Cerdan, S., and Seelig, J. NMR Studies of Metabolism (1990) *Ann. Rev. Biophys. Chem. 19*, 43–67.

25. Canioni, P., Alger, J.R., and Shulman, R.G. Natural Abundance ^{13}C NMR Spectroscopy of Liver and Adipose Tissue of the Living Rat (1983) *Biochemistry 22*, 4974–4980.
26. Fan, T.W.-M., Clifford, A.J., and Higashi, R.M. In vivo ^{13}C NMR Analysis of Acyl Chain Composition and Organisation of Perirenal Triacylglycerides in Rats Fed Vegetable and Fish Oils (1994) *J. Lipid Res. 35*, 678–689.
27. Book, S.A., and Bustad, L.K. The Fetal and Neonatal Pig in Biomedical Research (1974) *J. Anim. Sci. 38*, 997–1002.
28. Glauser, E.M. Advantages of Piglets as Experimental Animals in Pediatric Research (1966) *Exp. Med. Surg. 24*, 181–190.
29. Purvis, J.M., Clandinin, M.T., and Hacker, R.R. Fatty Acid Accretion During Perinatal Brain Growth in the Pig. A Model for Fatty Acid Accretion in the Human Brain (1982) *Comp. Biochem. Physiol. [B] 72*, 195–199.
30. Odle, J., Lin, W., Wieland, T.M., and van Kempen, T.A.T.G. Emulsification and Fatty Acid Chain Length Affect the Kinetics of [^{14}C]-Medium Chain Triacylglycerol Utilization by Neonatal Piglets (1994) *J. Nutr. 124*, 84–93.
31. Hrboticky, N., MacKinnon, M.J., and Innis, S.M. Effect of a Vegetable Oil Formula Rich in Linoleic Acid on Tissue Fatty Acid Accretion in the Brain, Liver, Plasma, and Erythrocytes of Infant Piglets (1990) *Am. J. Clin. Nutr. 51*, 173–182.
32. Arbuckle, L.D., and Innis, S.M. Docosahexaenoic Acid and Developing Brain and Retina of Piglets Fed High or Low α-Linolenate Formula with and without Fish Oil (1992) *Lipids 27*, 89–93.
33. Cook, H.W. In vitro Formation of Polyunsaturated Fatty Acids by Desaturation in Rat Brain: Some Properties of the Enzymes in Developing Brain and Comparisons with Liver (1978) *J. Neurochem. 30*, 1327–1334.
34. Auestad, N., Korsak, R.A., Bergstrom, J.D., and Edmond, J. Milk Substitutes Comparable to Rat's Milk: Their Preparation, Composition, and Impact on Development and Metabolism in the Artificially-Reared Rat (1989) *Br. J. Nutr. 61*, 495–518.
35. Winters, B.L., Yeh, S.-M., and Yeh, Y.-Y. Linolenic Acid Provides a Source of Docosahexaenoic Acid for Artificially Reared Rat Pups (1994) *J. Nutr. 124*, 1654–1659.

Chapter 8

In Vivo and *In Vitro* Metabolism of Linoleic and γ-Linolenic Acids

Yung-Sheng Huang,[a] David E. Mills,[b] Richard C. Cantrill,[c] and Jean-Pierre Poisson[d]

[a]Medical Nutritional Research and Development, Ross Products Division, Abbott Laboratories, Columbus, OH 43215
[b]Department of Health, Scienfitic Laboratory Division, Albuquerque, NM 87196
[c]Efamol Research Institute, Kentville, Nova Scotia, B4N 4H8, Canada
[d]University of Bourgogne, B.P. 138, 21004 Dijon, France

Introduction

In mammals, dietary linoleic acid (18:2n-6) is metabolized by Δ6-desaturase to form γ-linolenic acid (GLA, 18:3n-6), which is rapidly elongated to form dihomo-γ-linolenic acid (DGLA, 20:3n-6). DGLA is then desaturated by Δ5-desaturase to form arachidonic acid (AA, 20:4n-6). DGLA and AA are precursors of 1- and 2-series of prostaglandins (PGs) and thromboxanes (TXs), respectively, which regulate a wide range of physiological functions. In this pathway, the desaturation of LA to GLA is considered to be the rate-limiting step (1). Thus, the essentiality of LA depends on the ability of animals to convert this acid to other long-chain polyunsaturated fatty acids (PUFAs). In humans, the activity of Δ6-desaturase is lower than many other mammals (2). It has been shown that this enzyme is further reduced by other factors such as aging, poor health (e.g., diabetes, viral infection), lifestyle factors (e.g., alcohol, stress), and certain dietary elements (e.g., intake of high levels of cholesterol, saturated fats, and *trans* fatty acids) (3). Under these circumstances, the formation of long-chain PUFAs is reduced, and the nutritional value of dietary LA is significantly compromised. Clinical data have related the deficiency of PUFAs to the etiology of many degenerative chronic diseases (3). Indeed, direct consumption of GLA, bypassing the depressed Δ6-desaturase, has been shown to lower blood cholesterol, blood pressure and body fat. GLA also enhances the immune response, alleviates the neuropathic symptoms of diabetes and partially reverses the age-related abnormalities of tissue lipids (see review in reference 3).

Because LA and GLA represent the precursor and product of the Δ6-desaturase reaction, respectively, the tissue levels of PUFAs might be expected to reflect the type of fatty acid supplemented in the diet. This is not so. A moderate increase in LA intake has been shown to significantly raise the plasma level of AA, but had no significant effect on the levels of GLA and DGLA (4). Dietary supplementation of GLA, on the other hand, raised plasma levels of GLA and DGLA, but not AA (4). This finding is not limited to normal healthy subjects. Boberg et al. (5) reported that GLA consumption increased the levels of GLA and DGLA in serum cholesterol esters and triglycerides and in the levels of DGLA in platelet phospholipids without any variation in the level of AA in hypertriglyceridemic patients. Viikari and Lethonen (6) reported significant increases in the levels of GLA in plasma TG, cholesterol esters and PL and in the levels of DGLA in PL in hyperlipidemic subjects. Moreover, Bourguignon et al. (7) observed a significant increase in the levels of GLA in cholesterol esters and in the levels of DGLA in both cholesterol esters and phospholipids in schizophrenic patients with a daily intake of 200 mg of GLA for 3 mon. These findings clearly indicate that differences in LA and GLA metabolism are modulated not only by $\Delta 6$-desaturase activity but also by other factors. The purpose of this chapter is to review the published data from the *in vivo* and *in vitro* studies and examine the possible mechanism(s) which differentially modulate the metabolic fates of LA and GLA.

In Vitro Metabolism of Linoleic and γ-Linolenic Acids

The ability to desaturate ($\Delta 6$ and $\Delta 5$) and elongate fatty acids differs greatly among cultured cell lines. For example, a human monocyte-like cell line, U937 cells, is active in both $\Delta 6$- and $\Delta 5$-desaturation. When these cells are incubated with LA and GLA, the levels of DGLA and AA rise significantly (8) (Fig. 8.1). The fact that the levels of GLA are low in cells incubated with either LA or GLA suggests that GLA, whether converted from the LA or taken up directly from the medium, is rapidly elongated to form DGLA, and subsequently AA.

Cultured human intestinal cells (Caco-2) have low $\Delta 6$-desaturase activity, because incubation with LA does not lead to significant amounts of long-chain n-6 fatty acids (9). However, incubation with GLA significantly raises the proportions of DGLA and

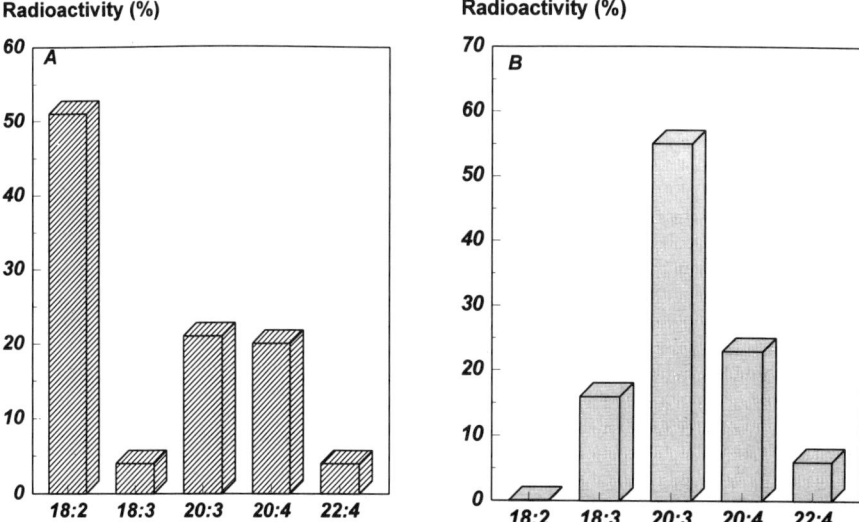

Fig. 8.1. Radioactivity distribution of n-6 fatty acids in U937 cells incubated with (A) [1-^{14}C]18:2n-6 and (B) [1-^{14}C]18:3n-6. *Source:* Howie et al. (8).

AA in the cells. These findings suggest that both elongation and Δ5-desaturation are active in Caco-2 cells. However, the level of AA and the ratio of AA/DGLA are significantly lower in the differentiated cells than in the undifferentiated cells, suggesting that the Δ5-desaturase activity is attenuated by this process (Fig. 8.2).

Cultured human fibroblasts (NIH-3T3) are active in Δ6-desaturation and elongation of fatty acids, but are not active in Δ5-desaturase activity. When these cells are incubated with α-linolenic acid (ALA, 18:3n-3) and its Δ6-desaturation product, stearidonic acid (SDA, 18:4n-3), analogs of LA and GLA, respectively, the levels of 20:4n-3 but not eicosapentaenoic acid (EPA, 20:5n-3) increase in cellular phospholipids (PL) (10).

Other cell lines may be deficient in either Δ6- or Δ5-desaturase activity. Bailey and colleagues (11,12) have shown that conversion of LA to GLA is either reduced or absent in a variety of cancer cell lines. Primary cultures of resident mouse peritoneal macrophages possess an extremely active enlongase but only modest Δ5-desaturase activity (13–15).

Factors Modulating the *In Vitro* Linoleic Acid and γ-Linolenic Acid Metabolism

In view of the above evidence, there are three major factors modulating the *in vitro* metabolism of LA and GLA: the presence of enzymes (Δ6-desaturase, elongase, and Δ5-desaturase), the enzyme activities as affected by the state of differentiation of cells, and the availability of acceptor PL molecular species. These will be addressed in more detail later.

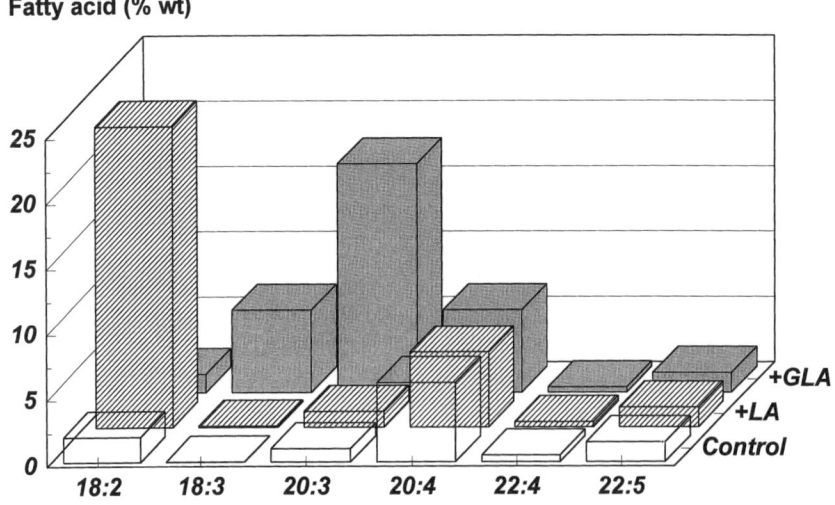

Fig. 8.2. Distribution of n-6 fatty acids in Caco-2 cells incubated with linoleic acid (LA) or γ-linolenic acid (GLA). *Source:* Huang et al. (9).

In Vivo Metabolism of Linoleic and γ-Linolenic Acids

Animal species vary in their dietary requirements for essential fatty acids (EFA) based on their ability to metabolize them (16,17) (Fig. 8.3). In the cat, the activity of Δ6-desaturase is virtually absent (18). When LA is supplemented, it cannot be effectively converted to AA. Because AA has an important role in reproduction (19), AA is a dietary essential for the cat. On the other hand, in many other animals species equipped with both Δ6-desaturase and Δ5-desaturase activities, LA can be metabolized to form long-chain PUFAs, and therefore LA is essential. In other words, depending on which animal species is studied, the metabolic fates of LA and GLA differ.

In an early study, we compared the *in vivo* metabolism of [1-^{14}C]18:2n-6 and [1-^{14}C]18:3n-6 following their adminstration by gavage to rats. After 24 h, most of the radioactivity was recovered in PL (mainly phosphatidylcholine, PC), and to a lesser extent, in triacylglycerol (TG) fractions. In rats administered [1-^{14}C]18:2n-6, most of the radioactivity remained as 18:2n-6, and only a small proportion was associated with its Δ6-desaturation product, GLA. In rats given [1-^{14}C]18:3n-6, on the other hand, a substantial proportion of the radiolabeled GLA was elongated to DGLA, and further metabolized to AA (Fig. 8.4). These results were consistent with the view that activity of Δ5-desaturase is the rate-limiting step in n-6 fatty acid metabolism (2).

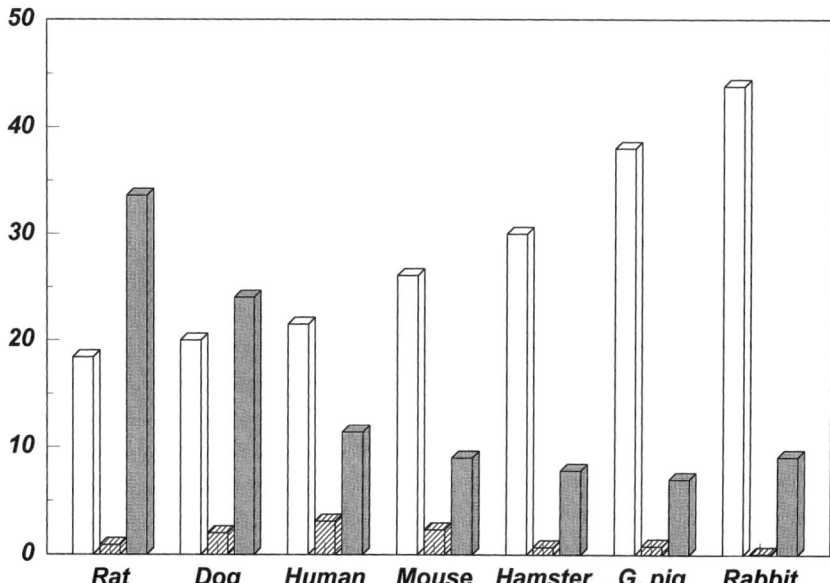

Fig. 8.3. Distribution of 18:2n-6 (□), 20:3n-6 (cross-hatched) and 20:4n-6 (shaded) of plasma phospholipids in different animal species. *Source:* Horrobin et al. (16).

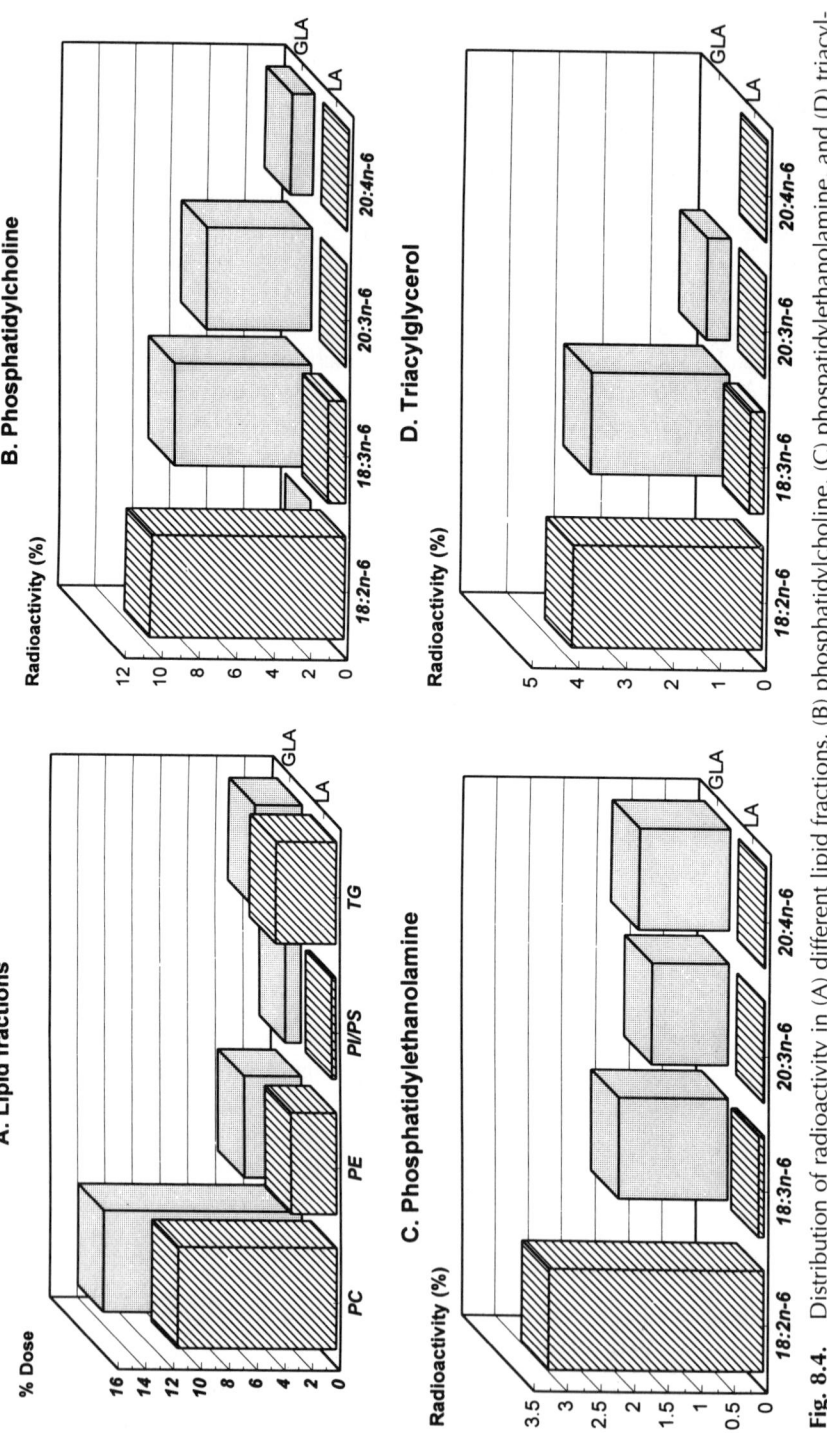

Fig. 8.4. Distribution of radioactivity in (A) different lipid fractions, (B) phosphatidylcholine, (C) phosphatidylethanolamine, and (D) triacylglycerol in rats orally gavaged with [1-^{14}C]18:2n-6 (LA, cross-hatched) and [1-^{14}C]18:3n-6 (GLA, shaded) (unpublished observation).

Similar results could be seen in rats maintained on LA- or GLA-supplemented diets for a longer period. Both LA and GLA feeding increased the levels of DGLA and AA (20). In the hamster, GLA feeding significantly increased the levels of DGLA, but only slightly increased the levels of AA in liver PL, because the D5-desaturase activity in hamsters is very low (19). In humans, both $\Delta 6$- and $\Delta 5$-desaturase activities are slower than in hamsters (19). As a result, the conversion rate of DGLA to AA is significantly lower in humans than in rats (1,21,22). It has been shown that excess LA intake [above the daily essential fatty acid (EFA) requirement] has no significant impact on the levels of GLA, DGLA, and AA in humans (4,23–26). On the other hand, dietary supplementation with GLA significantly increased the levels of DGLA (27), and to a lesser extent, AA (4) in plasma PL. Similar to humans, rabbits have lower $\Delta 5$-desaturase activity. Administration of DGLA had little effect on plasma AA in rabbits (21).

It should be noted that the levels of GLA in most animal tissues are extremely low, even after large quantities of exogenous GLA have been administered. This is because GLA is rapidly converted to DGLA by the elongase, which is not a rate-limiting step.

Factors Modulating *In Vivo* Metabolism of Linoleic and γ-Linolenic Acids

As mentioned early, the metabolisms of LA and GLA can be regulated by many nutritional and physiological factors (28). Frequently, several modulating factors can be present simultaneously and exert either synergistic or antagonistic effects more profound or less severe than would be expected from their independent effects. Some of these modulating factors will be discussed by others in this volume. The following presents only a few.

Bioavailability

Source. It has been suggested that the source of dietary GLA affects the formation of long-chain n-6 fatty acids and eicosanoids (29), whereas others have argued that the levels, but not the sources of dietary GLA modulate the conversion of GLA to DGLA and incorproation into tissue lipids (30).

Form. Fatty acids can be administered as natural or synthetic triglycerides, as free fatty acids, as phospholipids or as methyl or ethyl esters. In humans, it has been shown that the degree of absorption is affected significantly by the chemical form of long-chain PUFAs (31,32). Use of methyl esters is not recommended because of the formation of methanol and formaldehyde when the ester is metabolized.

Stereospecific Position. Distribution of fatty acids in the oil can also significantly modify the biological effects of fatty acids. Previously, it has been demonstrated that randomization of fatty acid distribution in natural peanut oil can significantly reduce its atherogenic effects (33,34). Distribution of GLA in TG differs among different sources (35), and this difference in stereospecific arrangement of GLA might affect its bioavailability. We have recently reported that GLA and LA located at different stereospecific positions were hydrolyzed differently when subjected to pancreatic lipase hydrolysis (36) (Fig. 8.5).

Enzyme Acitivities

Desaturase and Elongase. Hepatocytes (37–39), human endothelial cells (40), fibroblasts (41), and lymphocytes (42) can all desaturate and chain-elongate polyunsaturated fatty acids. Tissues other than liver do not sustain significant Δ6-desaturase activity (43). Kidney tissue cannot Δ6-desaturate LA to GLA, but can elongate GLA to DGLA, and to a smaller extent Δ5-desaturate DGLA to AA (44). Cardiac myocytes can take up both LA and GLA from the circulation, acylate or oxidize them, but do not desaturate or elongate these fatty acids (45). Platelets cannot desaturate LA to GLA (46), but can chain-elongate C_{18}- and C_{20}-polyunsaturated fatty acids (47). Chapkin and co-workers (13–15) have demonstrated that mouse peritoneal macrophages possess an active elongase capable of converting GLA to DGLA, but possess only modest Δ5-desaturase activities.

Esterification/Acylation. The enzyme which regulates the incorporation of fatty acids into PL is acyl-CoA:1-acyl-*sn*-glycero-3-phosphorylcholine acyltransferase (1-acyl-GPC-acyltransferase) (48). This enzyme is specific for long-chain n-6 fatty acids as the substrate. The *in vitro* rate studies (49–51) have shown that the activity of 1-acyl-GPC-acyltransferase [56 nmol/min/mg rat liver microsomal protein] for LA was 57-fold greater than that of Δ6-desaturase [0.98 nmol/(min·mg) microsomal

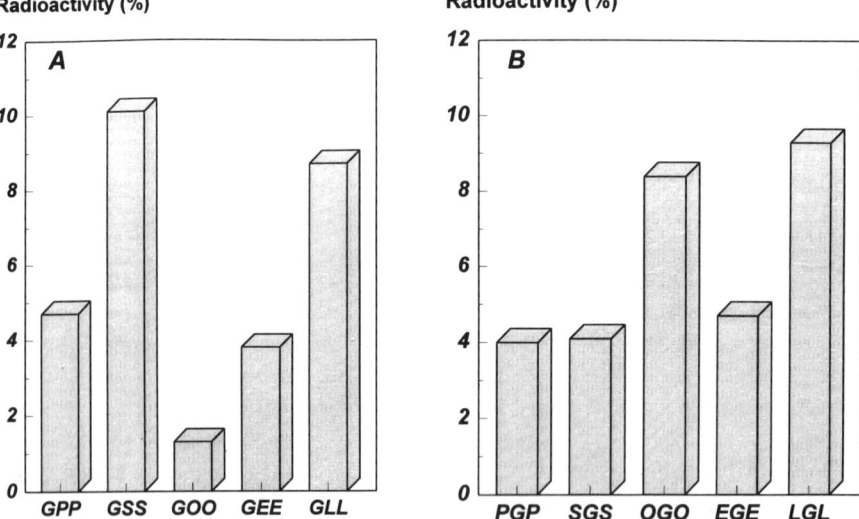

Fig. 8.5. Effect of stereospecific position of γ-linolenic acid at (A) *sn*-1/*sn*-3 and (B) *sn*-2 in triacylglycerols on the degree of hydrolysis. Abbreviations: G, γ-linolenic acid; P, palmitic acid; S, stearic acid; O, oleic acid; E, erucic acid; and L, linoleic acid. *Source:* Huang et al. (36).

protein] in EFA deficient rats (Fig. 8.6). These findings indicated that more of the administered LA was acylated to PC by 1-acyl-GPC-acyltransferase and less was available for Δ6-desaturation to form GLA. The *in vitro* rate studies have also shown that GLA is acylated more readily into PC [28 nmol/(min·mg) protein] than it is elongated to DGLA [4.43 nmol/(min·mg) protein in EFA deficient rat liver]. The acylation reaction was six times more common (49–51).

Oxidation. Leyton et al. (52) examined whole-body oxidation rates by measuring the extent of labeling in expired CO_2 over 24 h. They found that among the n-6 fatty acid family, increasing degree of desaturation and chain length resulted in a gradual reduction in the rate of fatty acid oxidation. Seven hours after administration, the rate of oxidation of GLA, DGLA, and AA was 27, 14, and 14%, respectively, of that observed for linoleic acid (Fig. 8.7).

Nutritional Effects

Essential Fatty Acid Deficiency. The metabolism of n-6 fatty acids by liver may be affected by the relative EFA concentration in different lipid pools (e.g., free acid, PL and TG). It is known that refeeding n-6 fatty acids following EFA deficiency increases their incorporation into PL fractions (53–55). Hassam et al. (56) have shown in suckling rats that [^{14}C]18:3n-6 and its metabolites were distributed evenly between PL and TG in liver, whereas most of the radioactivity in rats administered [^{3}H]18:2n-6 was recovered in the TG fraction. Similar results were also found in a preliminary study (unpublished data, Huang, Redden, Lin and Horrobin), in which the short-term

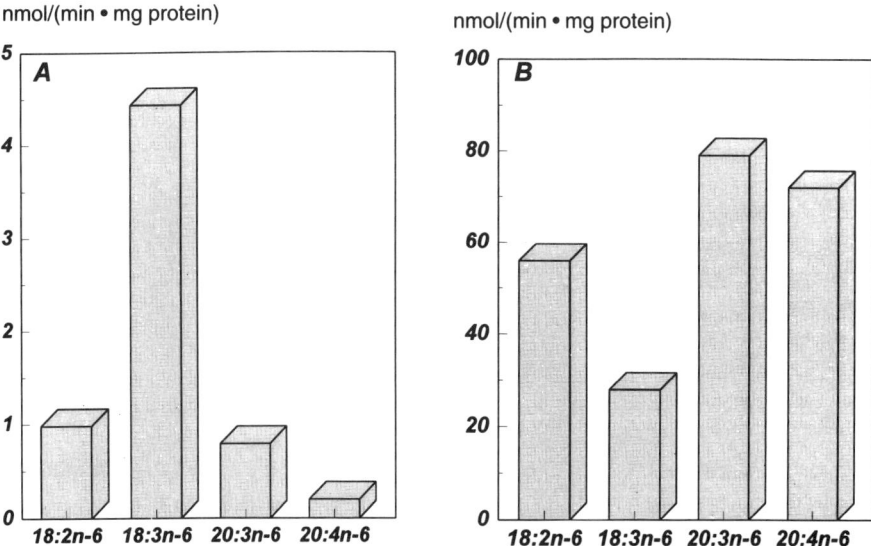

Fig. 8.6. *In vitro* activities of metabolic enzymes in rat liver microsomes. (A) Desaturase or elongase and (B) 1-acyl-*sn*-glycero-3-phosphorylcholine acyltransferase. *Sources:* Bernert and Sprecher (51) and Lands et al. (49).

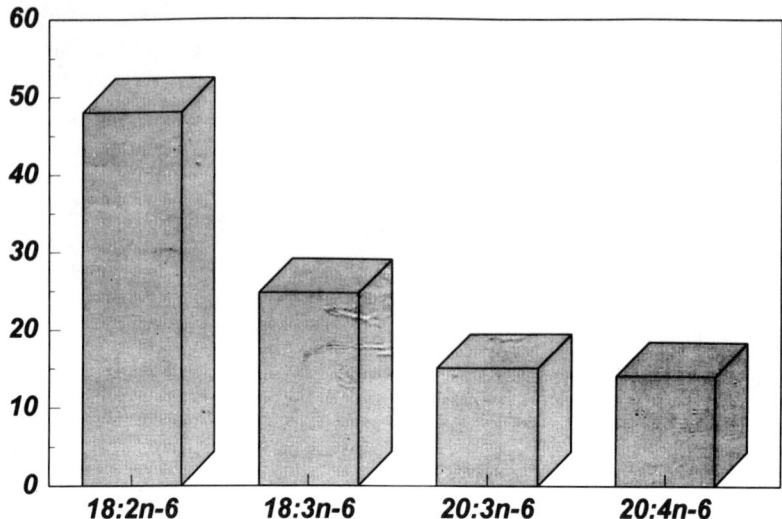

Fig. 8.7. *In vivo* oxidation rates of different n-6 fatty acids.
Source: Leyton et al. (52).

(8 h postadministration) metabolisms of [1-^{14}C]18:2n-6 and [1-^{14}C]18:3n-6 in growing rats previously fed an EFA-deficient diet for 9 wk were compared. In these animals, the majority of the radioactivity derived from [1-^{14}C]18:2n-6 and particularly from [1-^{14}C]18:3n-6 was associated with the liver PL fraction and to a lesser extent, the TG fraction (Fig. 8.4). In the PL fraction, some of the adminstered [1-^{14}C]18:3n-6 were elongated to DGLA and Δ5-desaturated to AA, but very little radioactivity in GLA metabolites was found in the TG fraction.

High Linoleic Acid Intake. There is ample evidence that high LA intake exerts an inhibitory effect on the rate-limiting activity of Δ6-desaturase and consequently the levels of metabolites of LA (28). Feeding a diet supplemented with sunflower seed oil for 22 wk resulted in an increase in linoleic acid and a marked decrease in arachidonic acid in mitochondrial membranes in marmoset monkeys (57). Intravenous administration of high levels of LA in parenteral lipid formulation reduced desaturation/elongation of essential fatty acids in PL in rats (58) and in newborn infants (59).

Dietary Cholesterol. It has previously been shown that dietary supplementation with cholesterol suppressed the conversion of LA to AA. In rats fed a GLA-rich diet, the addition of cholesterol in the diet increased the levels of DGLA whereas it decreased those of AA (60), and the AA/DGLA ratio (61) (Fig. 8.8). This is attributed to the inhibitory effect of dietary cholesterol on Δ6- and Δ5-desaturase activities (62,63). In guinea pigs, which have low D5D activity, feeding GLA-rich oil significantly increased the levels of DGLA and AA. The addition of cholesterol to the diet further elevated DGLA at the expense of AA (61) (Fig. 8.8).

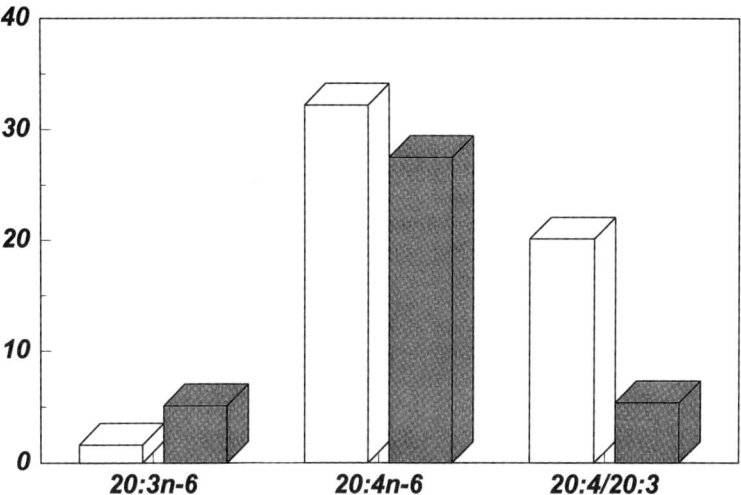

Fig. 8.8. Effect of dietary cholesterol on the proportions of 20:3n-6 and 20:4n-6, and the 20:4/20:3 ratios in rat liver phospholipids. *Source:* Huang et al. (60).

Fish Oil Supplementation. It is well established that fish oil or purified EPA and DHA suppress Δ6- and Δ5-desaturase activities (64–67). There is an inverse relationship between AA/DGLA ratios and EPA levels in rats fed GLA-rich oil and fish oil at various ratios (64). In developing mice, dietary supplementation with fish oil to the lactating dams increased the levels of DHA in brain and liver and was accompanied by a decrease in AA (68,69). The latter effect could be offset by partial replacement of LA with GLA, bypassing the suppressed Δ6 desaturase activity (Fig. 8.9).

Zinc Deficiency. Zinc is a cofactor for the desaturase activity. Zinc deficiency mimics many of the clinical features of essential fatty acid deficiency. Administration of GLA-rich oil as compared with LA-rich oil reversed most of the effects of zinc deficiency on plasma lipids (70) (Fig. 8.10).

Physiological and Pathological Factors

Diabetes. There is ample evidence that both Δ6- and Δ5-desaturase are impaired in experimental diabetes (71–74). Activities could be restored to normal levels by insulin treatment. Feeding a diet enriched with GLA raised the levels of GLA and DGLA in plasma phospholipids in the untreated diabetic rats (Fig. 8.11) and partially corrected the abnormal EFA metabolism in diabetic mice (75). In insulin-dependent diabetic patients, dietary supplementation with GLA (2 g/d) can also increase the incorporation of long-chain PUFA (76) and reduce diabetes-induced neuropathy (77).

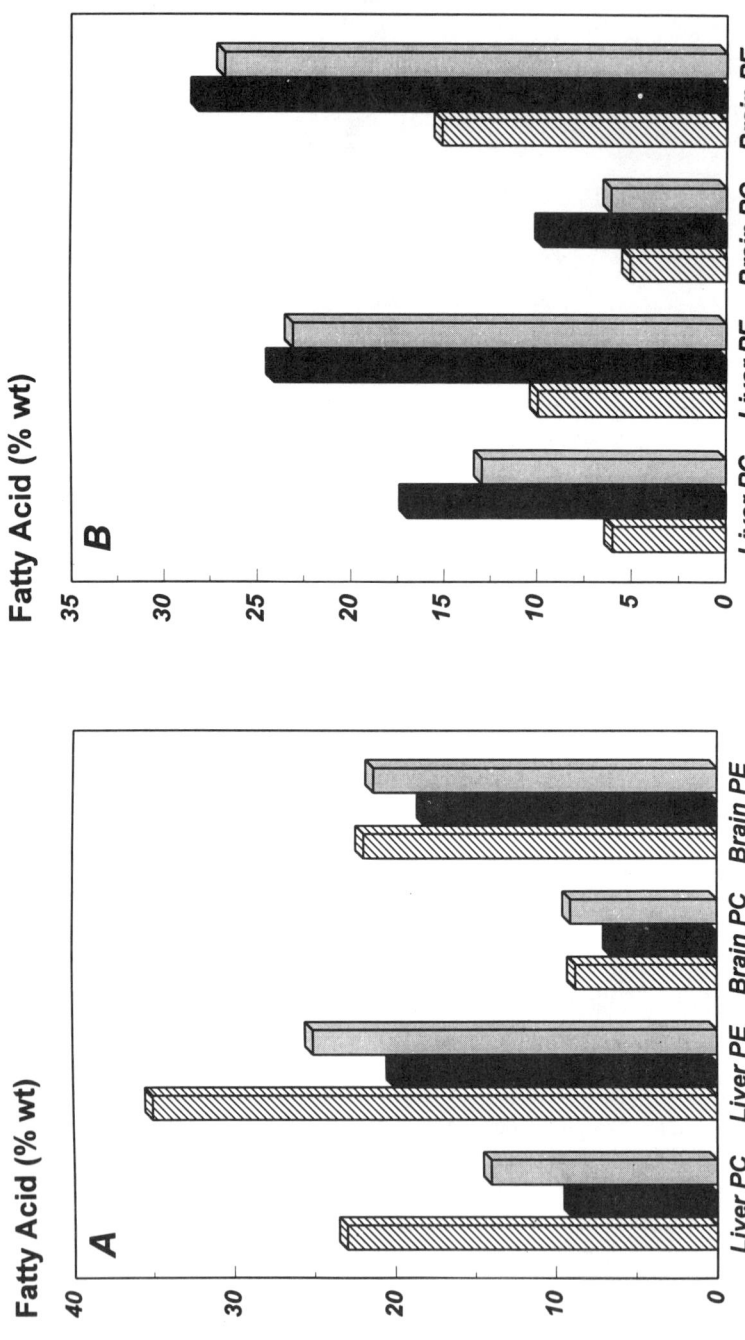

Fig. 8.9. Effect of maternal dietary fat (cross-hatched, control; ■, LA+fish oil; shaded, GLA + fish oil) on the levels of 20:4n-6 and 22:6n-3 in dam (A) and pup (B) liver and brain phosphatidylcholine (PC) and phosphatidylethanolamine (PE). *Source:* Wainwright et al. (68).

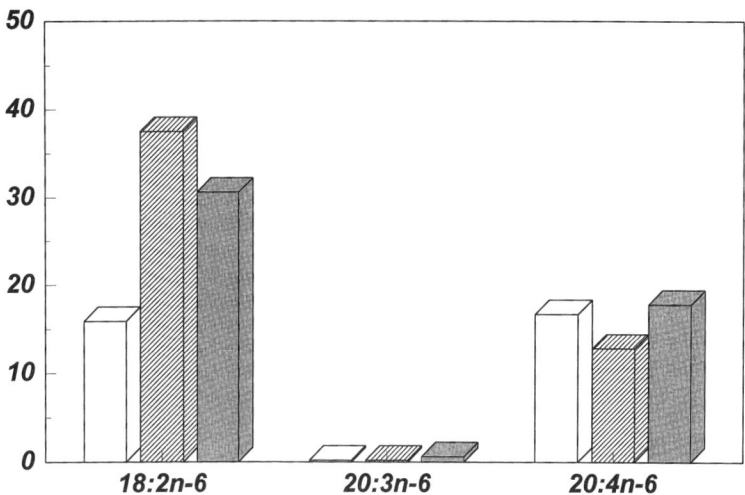

Fig. 8.10. Effect of zinc deficiency on levels of 18:2n-6, 20:3n-6 and 20:4n-6 in liver phospholipids of rats supplemented with linoleic acid (cross-hatched), γ-linolenic acid (shaded). *Source:* Huang et al. (70).

Chronic Alcohol Feeding. It has been demonstrated that chronic ethanol feeding reduced the levels of AA and other highly unsaturated fatty acids in liver PL in rats (78) and in pigs (79). The reduction was attributed to the selective inhibition of Δ6- and Δ5-desaturase activities. In golden Syrian hamsters, ethanol feeding led to

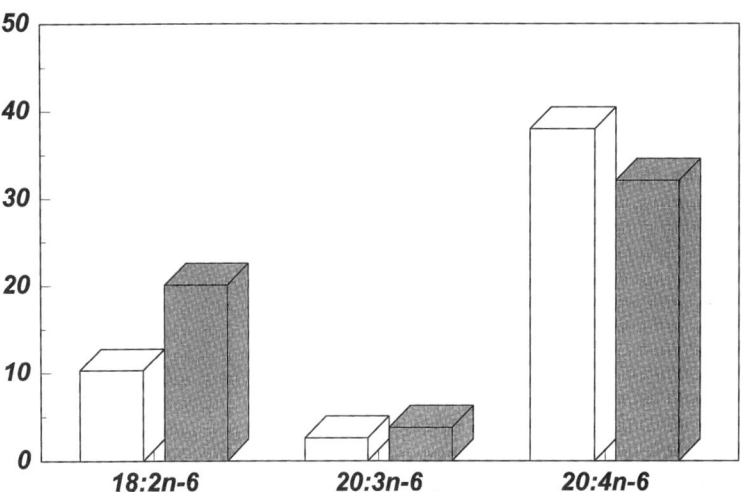

Fig. 8.11. Effect of diabeties on the levels of 18:2n-6, 20:3n-6 and 20:4n-6 in rat plasma phospholipids. (□) control; (shaded) diabetics. *Source:* Huang et al. (73).

an increase in DGLA with a concomitant decrease in AA in plasma and liver phospholipids (80) (Fig. 8.12).

Aging. The activity of Δ6-desaturase decreases during the aging process (81–83). Bourre et al. (84) showed in mice that Δ6-desaturase activity in brain decreases dramatically after birth, whereas liver activity increased for the first 7 d of life and then decreased progressively thereafter. Dietary supplementation with GLA partially reverses the abnormalities in fatty acid metabolism which accompany aging (81–83).

Non-Steroidal Anti-Inflammatory Drugs. Huang et al. (85,86) have shown that in aspirin-treated rats, the levels of all n-6 metabolites were decreased when LA was added in the diet. On the other hand, the levels of DGLA were increased in the treated rats fed a diet supplemented with GLA (Fig. 8.13). These findings demonstrate that aspirin suppresses the activities of Δ6- and Δ5-desaturase.

Stress. Brenner and his colleagues (87,88) showed that stress hormones such as catecholamines and glucocorticoids inhibit Δ6- and Δ5-desaturase activities. In rats fed a fat-free diet supplemented with 10% safflower oil (containing 79.5% 18:2n-6) and receiving daily injection of dexamethasone (1 mg/d) for 7 d, the proportions of LA and DGLA were increased, wherease those of other long-chain n-6 metabolites were reduced (Fig. 8.14).

Gender Difference. Gender difference affects desaturation and chain elongation of essential fatty acids in rat liver cells (89). Conversion of LA to long-chain n-6 polyun-

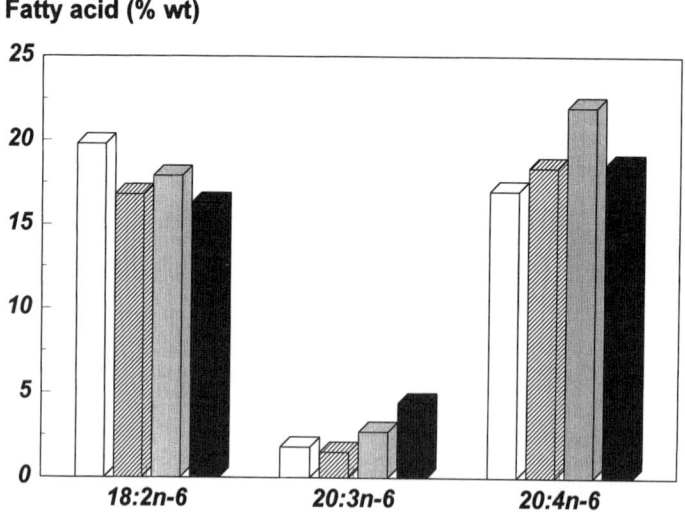

Fig. 8.12. Effect of chronic alcohol feeding on the levels of 18:2n-6, 20:3n-6, and 20:4n-6 in liver phospholipids of rats fed LA (□), LA + alcohol (cross-hatched), GLA (shaded), and GLA + alcohol (■). *Source:* Cunnane et al. (80).

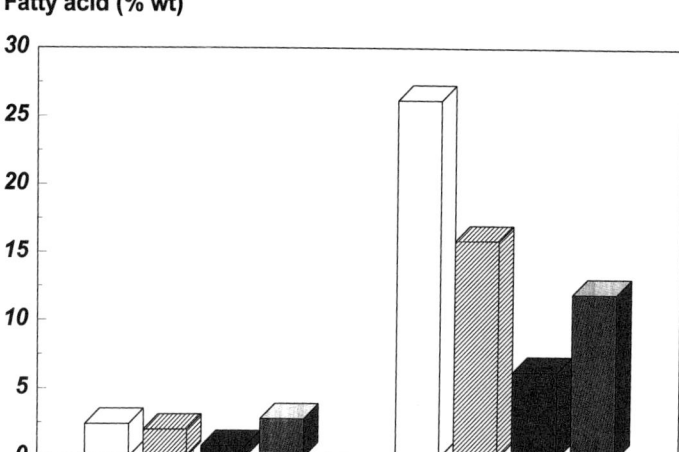

Fig. 8.13. Effect of aspirin administration on the levels of 20:3n-6 and 20:4n-6 in liver phospholipids in rats fed LA (□), LA + aspirin (cross-hatched), LA + fish oil + aspirin (■), and GLA + fish oil + aspirin (shaded). *Source:* Huang et al. (90).

saturated fatty acids was lower in the intact male than in the gonadectomized male fed a diet containing various levels of LA (90). Dietary supplementation with GLA increased the levels of DGLA more in male rats but increased the levels of AA more in the female rats (91). These findings suggest that the conversion of DGLA to AA was more active in female than in male rats (Fig. 8.15).

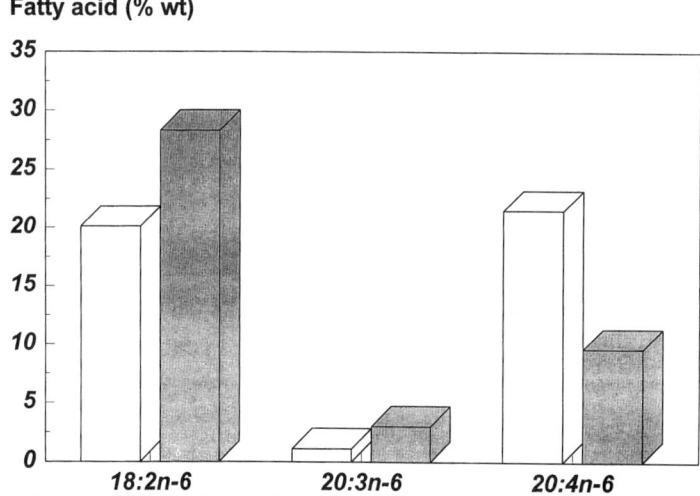

Fig. 8.14. Effect of dexamethasone administration on the levels of 18:2n-6, 20:3n-6, and 20:4n-6 in rat liver phospholipids. (□), nontreated, (shaded), treated. *Source:* Huang et al. (66).

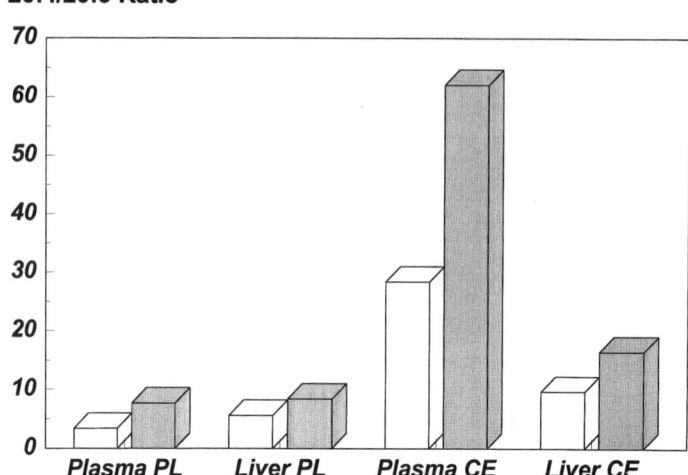

Fig. 8.15. Effect of gender on the 20:4/20:3 ratios in plasma and liver phospholipids and cholesteryl esters. (☐), male; (shaded), female. *Source:* Huang et al. (60).

Liver Injury. Biagi et al. (92) have reported that a significant decrease in D6D activity was observed in cirrhotic patients with no correlation with the etiology of the cirrhosis. It is not clear whether the liver disease caused the loss of enzyme activity, or the loss of enzyme activity led to the symptoms observed. Dietary supplementation with GLA (400 mg/d for 3 wk) resulted in an increase of GLA in cholesteryl esters and DGLA in both cholesteryl esters and PL in cirrhotic patients (93).

Summary

In view of evidence discussed above, major factors which are known to modulate the metabolic fate of LA and GLA may be grouped into 5 areas.

1. Balance Between Desaturation of LA to GLA and Acylation of LA to PL/TG. In the endoplasmic reticulum, competition occurs between acylation and desaturation. The rate of Δ6-desaturase which converts LA to GLA is significantly lower than that of acylation of LA to PL/TG. This may be further inhibited by many nutritional and physiological factors including high LA intake (28).

2. Balance Between the Elongation of GLA to DGLA and Desaturation of DGLA to AA, and Acylation of GLA and DGLA to PL (and to a lesser extent, TG). The *in vitro* rate studies have shown that GLA is acylated more readily to PC than it is elongated to DGLA (49–51). However, in rats administered radiolabeled GLA, significant proportions of the radioactivity were associated with DGLA (5.66% dose) and with AA (1.23% dose) in the PC fraction (unpublished observation). This suggests that the rates of metabolism (elongation and Δ5-desaturation) of GLA in this *in vivo* study were significantly faster than those in the *in vitro* studies (49–51). This may be due to the fact that an increase in elongation of GLA to DGLA, in conjunction with a reduction in Δ5-desaturation of DGLA to AA, leads to an accumulation of DGLA in the form of PL.

3. Opposite Responses of Δ6- and Δ5-Desaturases to the Same Modulating Factors.
EFA deficiency increases Δ6-desaturase activity, but depresses Δ5-desaturase activity. LA supplementation, on the other hand, depresses Δ6-desaturase activity but increases Δ5-desaturase activity (28,94). It is possible that feeding LA evokes an increase in the conversion of DGLA to AA.

4. Different Oxidation Rates. The *in vivo* oxidation rate of LA is greater than that of GLA. In comparison with C_{18} fatty acids, the oxidation rates of C_{20} fatty acids such as DGLA and AA are slow. This may result from their greater incorporation into PL than into TG (49). The C_{18} fatty acids are oxidized rapidly in mitochondria. However, the C_{20} fatty acids are first transported to peroxisomes where they are chain-shortened to C_{18} fatty acids (95). The released C_{18} fatty acids then enter the mitochondria for subsequent oxidation.

5. Role of Intestinal Cells. The cells of the small intestine have low Δ6- and Δ5-desaturase activity but high elongase activity (9). When GLA is supplemented in the diet, the absorbed GLA is elongated to DGLA in the cells of the intestine prior to release to plasma in the form of chylomicrons. Thus, the cells of the intestine may play an important role in raising the plasma levels of GLA and DGLA (4) (Fig. 8.16).

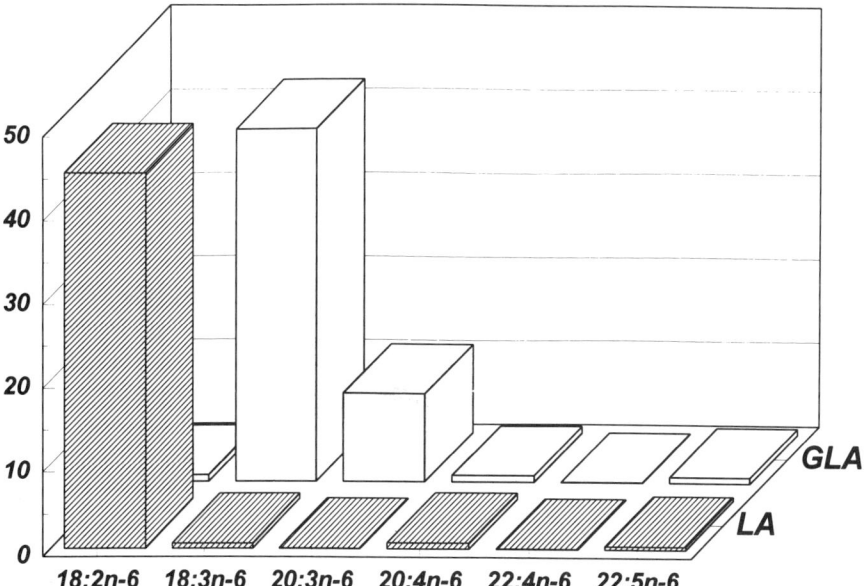

Fig. 8.16. The n-6 fatty acid composition of triacylglycerols secreted into the medium by Caco-2 cells incubated with linoleic acid (LA) or γ-linolenic acid (GLA). *Source:* Huang et al. (9).

References

1. Sprecher, H. Biochemistry of Essential Fatty Acids (1981) *Prog. Lipid Res. 20*, 13–22.
2. Blond, J.-P., Lamarchal, P., and Spielmann, D. Desaturation Comparée des Acides Linoléique et Dihomo-γ-Linolénique par des Homogénats de Foie Humain in Vitro (1981) *C.R. Acad. Sci. Paris 292*, 911–914.
3. Horrobin, D.F. Gamma-Linolenic Acid: An Intermediate in Essential Fatty Acid Metabolism with Potential as an Ethical Pharmaceutical and as a Food (1990) *Rev. Contemp. Pharmacother. 1*, 1–45.
4. Manku, M.S., Morse-Fisher, N., and Horrobin, D.F. Changes in Human Plasma Essential Fatty Acid Levels as a Result of Administration of Linoleic Acid and Gamma-Linolenic Acid (1988) *Eur. J. Clin. Nutr. 42*, 55–60.
5. Boberg, M., Vessby, B., and Selinus, I. Effect of Dietary Supplementation with n-6 and n-3 Long-Chain Polyunsaturated Fatty Acids on Serum Lipoproteins and Platelet Function in Hypertriglyceridemic Patients (1986) *Acta Med. Scand. 220*, 153–160.
6. Viikari, J., and Lethonen, A. Effect of Primrose Oil on Serum Lipids and Blood Pressure in Hyperlipidemic Subjects (1986) *Int. J. Clin. Pharm. Ther. Toxicol. 24*, 668–670.
7. Bourguignon, A., Jacotot, B., Lacroix, P., Maill, M., and Manus, A. Essai de l'Huile d'Onagre dans le Traitement de la Schizophrénie en Rapport avec un Déficit en Prostaglandine (1984) *L'Encéphale 10*, 241–244.
8. Howie, A., Huang, Y.-S., and Horrobin, D.F. Effects of Cholesterol on Viability and (n-6) Fatty Acid Metabolism in Cultured Human Monocyte-Like Cells (U937) (1992) *Biochem. Cell Biol. 70*, 643–649.
9. Huang, Y.-S., Liu, J.-W., Koba, K., and Anderson, S.N. Fatty Acid Metabolism in Undifferentiated and Differentiated Human Intestine Cell Line (Caco-2) (1995) *Mol. Cell Biochem. 151*, 121–130.
10. Cantrill, R.C., Huang, Y.-S., Ells, G.W., and Horrobin, D.F. Comparison of the Metabolism of α-Linolenic Acid and its Δ6 Desaturation Product, Stearidonic Acid, in Cultured NIH-3T3 Cells (1993) *Lipids 28*, 163–166.
11. Dunbar, L.M., and Bailey, J.M. Enzyme Deletions and Essential Fatty Acid Metabolism in Cultured Cells (1975) *J. Biol. Chem. 250*, 1152–1154.
12. Bailey, J.M. (1977) Lipid Metabolism in Cultured Cells. In: *Lipid Metabolism in Mammals,* Snyder, F., ed., Plenum Press, New York, pp. 352–364.
13. Chapkin, R.S., and Coble, K.J. Utilization of Gammalinolenic Acid by Mouse Peritoneal Macrophages (1991) *Biochim. Biophys. Acta 1085*, 365–370.
14. Chapkin, R.S., Miller, C.C., Somers, S.D., and Erickson, K.L. Utilization of Dihomo-γ-Linolenic Acid (8,11,14-eicosatrienoic acid) by Murine Peritoneal Macrophages (1988) *Biochim. Biophys. Acta 959*, 322–331.
15. Chapkin, R.S., Somers, S.D., and Erickson, K.L. Dietary Manipulation of Macrophage Phospholipid Classes: Selective Increase of Dihomogammalinolenic Acid (1988) *Lipids 23*, 766–770.
16. Horrobin, D.F., Huang, Y.-S., Cunnane, S.C., and Manku, M.S. Essential Fatty Acids in Plasma, Red Blood Cells and Liver Phospholipids in Common Laboratory Animals as Compared to Humans (1984) *Lipids 19*, 806–811.
17. Sinclair, A.J. Essential Fatty Acid Requirements of Different Species (1985) *Proc. Nutr. Soc. Aust. 10*, 41–48.

18. Rivers, J.P.W., Sinclair, A.J., and Crawford, M.A. Inability of the Cat to Desaturate Essential Fatty Acids. *Nature 258*, 171–173.
19. Ide, T., Sugano, M., Ishida, T., Niwa, M., Arima, M., and Morita, A. Effects of Gamma-Linolenic Acid on Fatty Acid Profiles and Eicosanoid Production of the Hamster (1987). *Nutr. Res. 7*, 1085–1092.
20. Engler, M.M., Karanian, J.W., and Salem, N. Jr. Influence of Dietary Polyunsaturated Fatty Acids on Aortic and Platelet Fatty Acid Composition in the Rat (1991) *Nutr. Res. 11*, 753–763.
21. Stone, K.J., Willis, A.L., Hart, M., Kirtland, S.J., Kernoff, P.B.A., and McNicol, G.P. The Metabolism of Dihomo-γ-linolenic Acid in Man (1979) *Lipids 14*, 174–180.
22. El Boustani, S., Descomps, B., Monnier, L., Warnant, J., Mendy, F., and Crastes de Paulet, A. *In Vivo* Conversion of Dihomo-gamma Linolenic Acid into Arachidonic Acid in Man (1986) *Prog. Lipid Res. 25*, 67–72.
23. Gibson, R.A. The Effect of Dietary Supplementation with Evening Primrose Oil in Hyperactive Children (1985) *Proc. Nutr. Soc. Aust. 10*, 196.
24. Horrobin, D.F., Ells, K.M., Morse-Fisher, N., and Manku, M.S. The Effects of Evening Primrose Oil, Safflower Oil and Paraffin on Plasma Fatty Acid Levels in Humans: Choice of an Appropriate Placebo for Clinical Studies on Primrose Oil (1991) *Prostaglandins Leukotrienes Essen. Fatty Acids 42*, 245–249.
25. Lasserre, M., Mendy, F., and Spielman, D. Effects of Different Dietary Intakes of Essential Fatty Acids on 20:3n-6 and 20:4n-6 Serum Levels in Human Adults (1985) *Lipids 20*, 227–233.
26. Dayton, S., Hashimoto, S., and Dixon, W. Composition of Lipids in Human Serum and Adipose Tissue During Prolonged Feeding of a Diet High in Unsaturated Fat (1966) *J. Lipid Res. 7*, 103–111.
27. Richard, J.-L., Martin, C., Maille, M., Mendy, F., Delplanque, B., and Jacotot, B. Effects of Dietary Intake of Gamma-Linolenic Acid on Blood Lipids and Phospholipid Fatty Acids in Healthy Human Subjects (1990) *J. Clin. Biochem. Nutr. 8*, 75–84.
28. Brenner, R.R. Nutritional and Hormonal Factors Influencing Desaturation of Essential Fatty Acids (1981) *Prog. Lipid Res. 20*, 41–48.
29. Jenkins, D.K., Mitchell, J.C., Manku, M.S., and Horrobin, D.F. Effects of Different Sources of Gamma-Linolenic Acid on the Formation of Essential Fatty Acid and Prostanoid Metabolites (1988) *Med. Sci. Res. 16*, 525–526.
30. Raederstorff, D., and Moser,U. Borage or Primrose Oil Added to Standardized Diets Are Equivalent Sources for γ-Linolenic Acid in Rats (1992) *Lipids 27*, 1018–1023.
31. El Boustani, S., Colette, C., Mannier, L., Descomps, B., Crastes de Paulet, A., and Mendy, F. Enteral Absorption in Man of Eicosapentaenoic Acid in Different Chemical Forms (1987) *Lipids 22*, 711–714.
32. Lawson, L.D., and Hughes, B.G. Human Absorption of Fish Oil Fatty Acids as Triacylglycerols, Free Acids or Ethyl Esters (1988) *Biochem. Biophys. Res. Commun. 152*, 328–335.
33. Kritchevsky, D. Effects of Triglyceride Structure on Lipid Metabolism (1988) *Nutr. Rev. 46*, 171–181.
34. Myher, J.J., Marai, L., and Kuksis, A. Acylglycerol Structure of Peanut Oils of Different Atherogenic Potential (1977) *Lipids 12*, 775–785.

35. Lawson, L.D., and Hughes, B.G. Triacylglycerol Structure of Plant and Fungal Oils Containing γ-Linolenic Acid (1988) *Lipids 23*, 313–317.
36. Huang, Y.-S., Redden, P.R., Lin, X., and Horrobin, D.F. In vitro Hydrolysis of Synthetic or Natural γ-Linolenic Acid-Containing Triacylglycerols (1995) *J. Am. Oil Chem. Soc. 72*, 625–631.
37. Hagve, T.A., and Christophersen, B.O. Linolenic Acid Desaturation and Chain Elongation and Rapid Turnover of Phospholipid n-3 Fatty Acids in Isolated Liver Cells (1983) *Biochim. Biophys. Acta 753*, 339–349.
38. Hagve, T.A., and Christophersen, B.O. Effect of Dietary Fats on Arachidonic Acid and Eicosapentaenoic Acid Biosynthesis and Conversion to C_{22} Fatty Acids in Isolated Rat Liver Cells (1984) *Biochim. Biophys. Acta 796*, 205–217.
39. Voss, A.C., and Sprecher, H. Regulation of the Metabolism of Linoleic Acid to Arachidonic Acid in Rat Hepatocytes (1988) *Lipids 23*, 660–665.
40. Rosenthal, M.D., and Whitehurst, M.C. Selective Effects of Isomeric *cis* and *trans* Fatty Acids on Fatty Acyl Delta-9 and Delta-6 Desaturation by Human Skin Fibroblasts (1983) *Biochim. Biophys. Acta 753*, 450–459.
41. Rosenthal, M.D., and Whitehurst, M.C. Fatty Acyl Delta-6 Desaturation Activity of Cultured Human Endothelial Cells: Modulation by Fetal Bovine Serum (1983) *Biochim. Biophys. Acta 750*, 490–496.
42. Hagve, T.A., Christophersen, B.O., Høie, K., and Johansen, Y. Effect of a Low Fat Diet on Essential Fatty Acid Metabolism in Healthy Human Subjects (1986) *Scand. J. Clin. Lab. Invest. 46 (Suppl. 184)*, 61–66.
43. Zevenberger, J.L. (1986) in *Enzymes of Lipid Metabolism II*, L. Freysz et al., eds., Plenum Publishing Corporation, New York, NY, pp. 647–649.
44. Huang, Y.-S., Cantrill, R.C., DeMarco, a., Campbell, L., Lin, X., Horrobin, D.F., and Mills, D.E. Differences in the Metabolism of 18:2n-6 and 18:3n-6 by the Liver and Kidney May Explain the Anti-Hypertensive Effect of 18:3n-6 (1994) *Biochem. Med. Metab. Biol. 51*, 27–34.
45. Hagve, T.-A., and Sprecher, H. Metabolism of Long-Chain Polyunsaturated Fatty Acids in Isolated Cardiac Myocytes (1989) *Biochim. Biophys. Acta 1001*, 338–344.
46. Needleman, S.W., Spector, A.A., and Hoak, J.C. Enrichment of Human Platelet Phospholipods with Linoleic Acid Diminishes Thromboxane Release (1982) *Prostaglandins 24*, 607–622.
47. Weiner, T.W., and Sprecher, H. 22-Carbon Polyenoic Acids. Incorporation into Platelet Phospholipids and the Synthesis of These Acids from 20-Carbon Polyenoic Acid Precursors by Intact Platelets (1985) *J. Biol. Chem. 260*, 6032–6038.
48. Lands, W.E.M., and Crawford, C.G. (1976) in *The Enzymes of Biological Membranes* A. Martonosi, ed., Plenum Press, New York, vol. 2, pp. 3–20.
49. Lands, W.E.M., Inoue, M., Sugiura, Y., and Okuyama, H. Selective Incorporation of Polyunsaturated Fatty Acids into Phosphatidylcholine by Rat Liver Microsomes (1982) *J. Biol. Chem. 257*, 14968–14972.
50. Sprecher, H., Voss, A.C., Careaga, M., and Hadjiagapiou, C. Inter-Relationships Between Polyunsaturated Fatty Acid and Membrane Lipid Synthesis (1987) in *Polyunsaturated Fatty Acids and Eicosanoids*, Lands, W.E.M., ed., American Oil Chemists' Society, Champaign, IL, pp. 154–168.

51. Bernert, J.T., and Sprecher, H. Studies to Determine the Role Rates of Chain Elongation and Desaturation Play in Regulating the Unsaturated Fatty Acid Composition of Rat Liver Lipids (1975) *Biochim. Biophys. Acta 398,* 354–363.
52. Leyton, J., Drury, P.J., and Crawford, M.A. Differential Oxidation of Saturated and Unsaturated Fatty Acids *in Vivo* in the Rat (1987) *Br. J. Nutr. 57,* 383–393.
53. Becker, W., and Månsson, J.E. Incorporation of ^{14}C into Tissue Lipids after Oral Administration of 1-^{14}C-Linoleic Acid in Rats Fed Different Levels of Essential Fatty Acids (1985) *J. Nutr. 115,* 1248–1258.
54. Mercuri, O., and DeTomas, M.E. Early Steps on the *in Vivo* Incorporation of 1-^{14}C-Linoleic Acid into Liver Lipids from Normal and Essential Fatty Acid-Deficient Rats (1971) *Lipids 6,* 858–859.
55. Hassam, A.G., Rivers, J.P., and Crawford, M.A. Metabolism of Gamma-Linolenic Acid in Essential Fatty Acid Deficient Rats (1977) *J. Nutr. 107,* 519–524.
56. Hassam, A.G., Sinclair, A.J., and Crawford, M.A. The Incorporation of Orally Fed Radioactive γ-Linolenic Acid and Linoleic Acid into the Liver and Brain Lipids of Suckling Rats (1975) *Lipids 10,* 417–420.
57. McMurchie, E.J., Gibson, R.A., Charnock, J.S., and McIntosh, G.H. Mitochondrial Membrane Fatty Acid Composition in the Marmoset Monkey Following Dietary Lipid Supplementation (1986) *Lipids 21,* 315–323.
58. Innis, S.M. Effect of TPN with Linoleic Acid Rich Emulsions on Tissue ω-6 and ω-3 Fatty Acids in the Rat (1986) *Lipids 21,* 132–138.
59. Martizez, M., and Ballabriga, A. Effects of Parenteral Nutrition with High Doses of Linoleate on the Developing Human Liver and Brain (1987) *Lipids 22,* 31–33.
60. Huang, Y.-S., Manku, M.S., and Horrobin, D.F. The Effects of Dietary Cholesterol on Blood and Liver Polyunsaturated Fatty Acids and Plasma Cholesterol in Rats Fed Various Types of Fatty Acid Diet (1984) *Lipids 19,* 664–672.
61. Huang, Y.-S., and Horrobin, D.F. Effect of Dietary Cholesterol and Polyunsaturated Fatty Acids in Plasma and Liver Lipids in Guinea Pigs (1987) *Ann. Nutr. Metab. 31,* 18–28.
62. Garg, M.L., Snoswell, A.M., and Sabine, J.R. Influence of Dietary Cholesterol on Desaturase Enzymes of Rat Liver Microsomes (1986) *Prog. Lipid Res. 21,* 639–644.
63. Leikin, A.I., and Brenner, R.R. Cholesterol-Induced Microsomal Changes Modulate Desaturase Activities (1987) *Biochim. Biophys. Acta 922,* 294–303.
64. Nassar, B.A., Huang, Y.-S., Manku, M.S., Das, U.N., Morse, N., and Horrobin, D.F. The Influence of Dietary Manipulation with n-3 and n-6 Fatty Acids on Liver and Plasma Phospholipid Fatty Acid in Rats (1986) *Lipids 21,* 652–656.
65. Brenner, R.R., and Peluffo, R.O. Inhibitory Effect of Docosa-4,7,10,13,16,19-hexaenoic Acid upon the Oxidative Desaturation of Linoleic into γ-Linolenic Acid and of γ-Linolenic Acid into Octadeca-6,9,12,15-tetraenoic acid (1967) *Biochim. Biophys. Acta 137,* 184–186.
66. Huang, Y.-S., Nassar, B.A., and Horrobin, D.F. Changes of Plasma Lipids and Long-Chain n-3 and n-6 Fatty Acids in Plasma, Liver, Heart and Kidney Phospholipids of Rats Fed Variable Levels of Fish Oil with or without Cholesterol Supplementation (1986) *Biochim. Biophys. Acta 879,* 22–27.
67. Grønn, M., Christensen, E., Hagve, T.A., and Christophersen, B.O. Effects of Dietary Purified Eicosapentaenoic Acid (20:5(n-3)) and Docosahexaenoic Acid (22:6(n-3)) on

Fatty Acid Desaturation and Oxidation in Isolated Rat Liver Cells (1992) *Biochim. Biophys. Acta 1125*, 35–43.

68. Wainwright, P.E., Huang, Y.-S., Bulman-Fleming, B., Dalby, D., Mills, D.E., Redden, P., and MuCutcheon, D. The Effects of Dietary n-3/n-6 Ratio on Brain Development in the Mouse: A Dose Response Study with Long-Chain n-3 Fatty Acids (1992) *Lipids 27*, 98–103.

69. Huang, Y.-S., Wainwright, P.E., Redden, P.E., Mills, D.E., Bulman-Fleming, B., and Horrobin, D.F. Effect of Maternal Dietary Fats with Variable n-3/n-6 Ratios on Tissue Fatty Acid Composition in Suckling Mice (1992) *Lipids 27*, 104–110.

70. Huang, Y.-S., Cunnane, S.C., Horrobin, D.F., and Davignon, J. Most Biological Effects of Zinc Deficiency Corrected by γ-Linolenic Acid (18:3ω-6) but Not by Linoleic Acid (18:2ω-6) (1982) *Atherosclerosis 41*, 193–207.

71. Mercuri, O., Peluffo, R.O., and Brenner, R.R. Depression of Microsomal Desaturation of Linoleic to Gamma-Linolenic Acid in the Alloxan Diabetic Rat (1966) *Biochim. Biophys. Acta 116*, 407–411.

72. Faas, F.H., and Carter, W.J. Altered Fatty Acid Desaturation and Microsomal Fatty Acid Composition in Streptozotocin Diabetic Rat (1980) *Lipids 15*, 953–961.

73. Huang, Y.-S., Fujii, K., Takahashi, R., Mitchell, J., and Horrobin, D.F. Effect of Diabetes on the Metabolism of n-3 and n-6 Fatty Acids in Rats (1985) *IRCS Med. Sci. 13*, 1145–1146.

74. Mimouni, V., and Poisson, J.-P. Altered Desaturase Activities and Fatty Acid Composition in Liver Microsomes of Spontaneously Diabetic Wistar BB Rat (1992) *Biochim. Biophys. Acta 1123*, 296–302.

75. Cunnane, S.C., Manku, M.S., and Horrobin, D.F. Abnormal Essential Fatty Acid Composition of Tissue Lipids in Genetically Diabetic Mice is Partially Corrected by Dietary Linoleic and Gamma-Linolenic Acids (1985) *Br. J. Nutr. 53*, 449–458.

76. Chaintreuil, J., Monnier, L., Colette, C., Crastes de Paulet, P., Orsetti, A., Spielmann, D., Mendy, F., and Crastes de Paulet, A. Effects of Dietary γ-Linolenate Supplementation on Serum Lipids and Platelet Function in Insulin-Dependent Diabetic Patients (1983) *Human Nutr. Clin. Nutr. 38C*, 121–130.

77. Jamal, G.A., Carmichael, H.A., and Weir, A.I. Gamma-Linolenic Acid in Diabetic Neuropathy (1986) *Lancet i*, 1098.

78. Nervi, A.M., Peluffo, R.O., Brenner, R.R., and Leikin, A.I. Effect of Ethanol Administration on Fatty Acid Desaturation (1980) *Lipids 15*, 263–268.

79. Nakamura, M.T., Tan, A.B., Villanueva, J., Halsted, C.H., and Phinney, S.D. Selective Reduction of $\Delta 6$ and $\Delta 5$ Desaturase Activities but Not $\Delta 9$ Desaturase in Micropigs Chronically Fed Ethanol (1994) *J. Clin. Invest. 93*, 450–454.

80. Cunnane, S.C., Huang, Y.-S., Manku, M.S., and Horrobin, D.F. Influence of Different Dietary Fatty Acid Sources on Erythrocyte Lipids and Plasma and Liver Essential Fatty Acids in Hamsters Fed Ethanol (1986) *Ann. Nutr. Metab. 30*, 81–86.

81. Bordoni, A., Biagi, P.L., Turchetto, E., and Hrelia, S. Aging Influences on Delta-6-Desaturase Activity and Fatty Acid Composition of Rat Liver Microsomes (1988) *Biochem. Int. 17*, 1001–1009.

82. Hrelia, S., Bordoni, A., Celadon, M., Turchetto, E., Biagi P.L., and Rossi, C.A. Age-Related Changes in Linoleate and Alpha-Linolenate Desaturation by Rat Liver Microsomes (1989) *Biochem. Biophys. Res. Commun. 163*, 348–355.

83. Biagi, P.L., Bordoni, A., Hrelia, S., Celadon, M., and Horrobin, D.F. γ-Linolenic Acid Dietary Supplementation Can Reverse the Aging Influence on Rat Liver Microsome Δ^6-Desaturase Activity (1991) *Biochim. Biophys. Acta 1083,* 187–192.
84. Bourre, J.-M., Piciotti, M., and Dumont, O. Δ6-Desaturase in Brain and Liver During Development and Aging (1990) *Lipids 25,* 354–356.
85. Huang, Y.-S., Drummond, R., and Horrobin, D.F. Protective Effect of Gamma-Linolenic Acid on Aspirin-Induced Gastric Hemorrhage in Rats (1987) *Digestion 36,* 36–41.
86. Huang, Y.-S., Watanabe, Y., Horrobin, D.F., and Simmon, V. Fatty Acid Changes in Liver Choline and Ethanolamine Glycerophospholipids in Aspirin Treated Rats Fed Linoleate, Gamma-linolenate and Fish Oil (1989) *Clin. Physiol. Biochem. 7,* 79–86.
87. de Goméz Dumm, I.N.T., de Alaniz, M.J.T., and Brenner, R.R. Effect of Epinephrine on the Oxidative Desaturation of Fatty Acids in the Rat (1976) *J. Lipid Res. 17,* 616–621.
88. de Goméz Dumm, I.N.T., de Alaniz, M.J.T., and Brenner, R.R. Effect of Glucocorticoids on the Oxidative Desaturation of Fatty Acids by Rat Liver Microsomes (1979) *J. Lipid Res. 20,* 834–839.
89. Hagve, T.A., and Christophersen, B.O. Sex-Related Differences in Desaturation and Chain Elongation of Essential Fatty Acids Studied in Isolated Rat Hepatocytes (1987) *Biochim. Biophys. Acta 920,* 149–154.
90. Huang, Y.-S., and Horrobin, D.F., Watanabe, Y., Bartlett, M.E., and Simmons, V. Effects of Dietary Linoleic Acid on Growth and Liver Phospholipid Fatty Acid Composition in Intact and Gonadectomized Rats (1990) *Biochem. Arch. 6,* 47–54.
91. Huang, Y.-S., and Horrobin, D.F. Sex Differences in n-3 and n-6 Fatty Acid Metabolism in EFA-Depleted Fats (1987) *Proc. Soc. Exp. Biol. Med. 185,* 291–296.
92. Biagi, P.L., Hrelia, S., Stefanini, G.F., Zunarelli, P., and Bordoni, A. Delta-6-Desaturase Activity of Human Liver Microsomes from Patients with Different Types of Liver Injury (1990) *Prostaglandins Leukotrienes Essent. Fatty Acids 39,* 39–42.
93. Paccalin, J., Delhaye, N., Bernard, M., Lacomere, R.P., Spielmann, D., Piganeau, P., and Mendy, F. Étude des Acides Gras au Niveau des Esters de Cholesterol et des Pholsholides Circulant chez des Sujets Cirrhotiques et Variation sous l'Effet d'une Supplémentation en Acide Gamma-Linolénique (1982) *Cah. Nutr. Diét. 17,* 211–214.
94. Jeffcoat, R., and James, A.T. Interrelationship Between the Dietary Regulation of Fatty Acid Synthesis and the Fatty Acyl-CoA Desaturases (1977) *Lipids 12,* 469–474.
95. Lazarow, P.B., and de Duve, C. A Fatty Acyl-CoA Oxidizing System in Rat Liver Peroxisomes: Enhancement by Clofibrate, a Hypolipidemic Drug (1976) *Proc. Natl. Acad. Sci. U.S.A. 73,* 2043–2046.

Chapter 9

γ-Linolenic Acid and Immune Function

Dayong Wu and Simin Nikbin Meydani

Jean Mayer USDA HNRCA at Tufts University, Boston, MA 02111

Introduction

There are two groups of essential fatty acids (EFAs), (n-6) and (n-3) EFAs. Linoleic acid (LA, 18:2 n-6)) and α-linolenic acid (ALA, 18:3 n-3) are the parent fatty acids of the (n-6) and (n-3) EFAs, respectively. Other members of the (n-6) and (n-3) families can be derived (through desaturation and elongation) from their parent EFAs and thus are called derived EFAs. It is commonly believed that both pathways involving (n-6) and (n-3) EFA metabolism share the same enzymes (Fig 9.1). In the (n-6) family, LA can be converted to γ-linolenic acid (GLA) by action of Δ6-desaturase and further to dihomo-γ-linolenic acid (DGLA), the precursor of 1-series prostaglandins (PGs) and 3-series leukotrienes (LTs), by elongase. DGLA can be also converted by Δ5-desaturase to arachidonic acid (AA) which is the precursor of 2-series PGs and 4-series LTs. Δ6-Desaturase is the rate-limiting factor in the (n-6) EFA metabolism cascade (1,2), and it is influenced by changes in metabolic and endocrine regulation as well as by the progression of certain diseases. For example, Δ6 desaturase activity has been demonstrated to be increased by insulin and inhibited by epinephrine, cortisol, thyroxin, glucagon, saturated fat and aging (3–5). Decreased levels of GLA are reported in patients with inflammatory diseases (6–8). GLA supplementation has been used to by-pass Δ6-desaturase and to increase levels of GLA and other derived EFAs, in particular 20-carbon precursors of eicosanoids in phospholipids. GLA in substantial amounts is found naturally in plant oils such as evening primrose oil (9%), borage oil (23%) and black currant seed oil (18%). These oils are commonly used in most studies as the sources of GLA.

Abnormal essential fatty acid metabolism including that of eicosanoid production has been implicated in the impairment of the immune function and pathogeneses of inflammatory, autoimmune, and neoplastic diseases. This has led investigators to use fatty acid modulation as a way to improve immune response and decrease pathogenesis of diseases. This review will summarize studies related to the effect of GLA and cell-mediated immune responses as well as to some immune-related diseases.

Immune Function

Immune cells, especially lymphocytes, have a high content of polyunsaturated fatty acids (PUFAs) in their membrane phospholipids. Numerous studies have shown

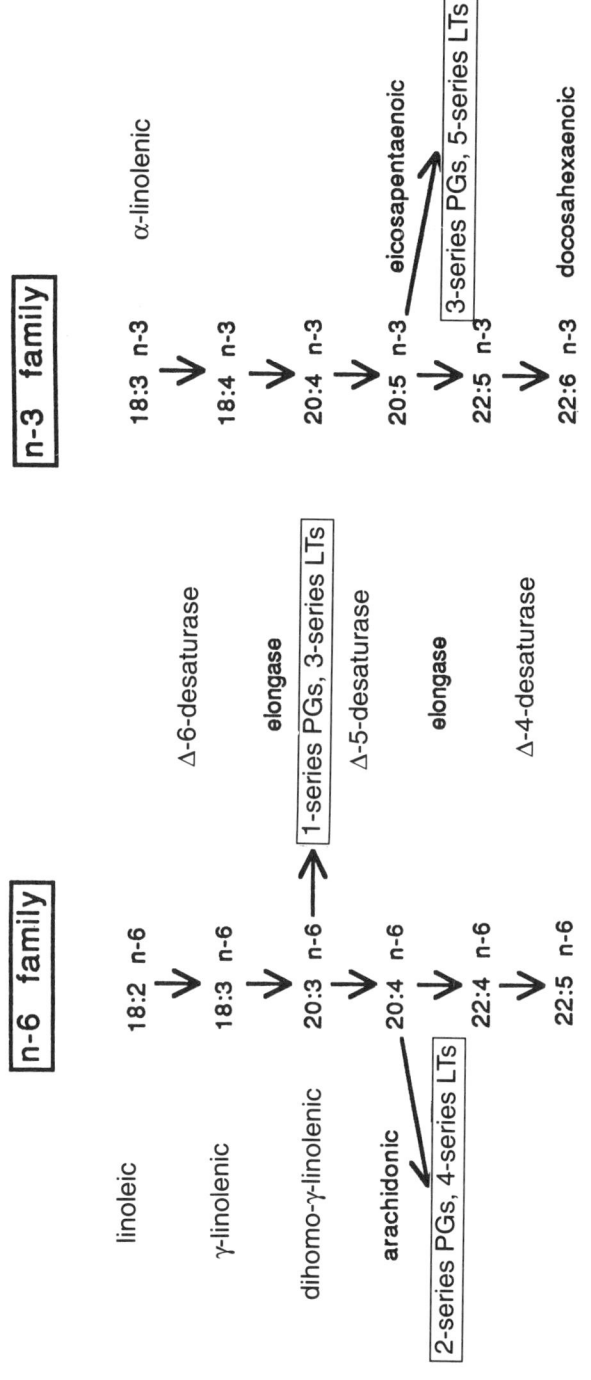

Fig. 9.1. Metabolic pathways of essential fatty acids.

that dietary fats can influence the fatty acid composition of membrane phospholipids. These fatty acid alterations contribute to the changes in immune function through alteration of the biophysical properties of membranes (such as membrane fluidity) and enzyme activity as well as through affecting the availability of the fatty acid precursors of immune-regulating eicosanoids. In recent years, increasing dietary intake of individual (n-6) and (n-3) PUFAs has been shown to cause quantitative and qualitative changes in the immune response of animals and humans. GLA is an intermediate precursor of both the 1- and 2-series PGs and 3- and 4-series LTs. Previous studies have shown that an increase in GLA consumption decreases PGE_2 levels while increasing PGE_1 levels (9–11). PGE_2 has been shown, for the most part, to have a suppressive effect on cell-mediated immunity including lymphocyte proliferation and the production of T cell growth factor interleukin-2 (IL-2) (12,13). Thus, increasing the intake of GLA can be expected to influence immune function. Few studies, however, have focused on the effect of GLA on immune function.

In Vitro *Studies*

Devi and Das examined the *in vitro* effect of several PUFAs on normal human lymphocytes and abnormal human lymphocytes (leukemic cell line Molt-4) (14). They observed that all of the PUFAs tested (LA, ALA, GLA, AA, eicosapentaenoic acid [EPA, 20:5 n-3] and docosahexaenoic acid [DHA, 22:6 n-3]) inhibited proliferation of both human lymphocytes and Molt-4 cells in a dose-dependent manner with GLA being the most inhibitory. It is interesting to note that all of the PUFAs reduced IL-2 production in the normal lymphocytes but elevated IL-2 levels in Molt-4 cells. The authors attributed the inhibition of cell proliferation by PUFAs to increased free radical generation and lipid peroxidation (measured as nitroblue tetrazolium and thiobarbituric acid reactive substances, respectively). However, this conclusion can not explain why GLA, instead of EPA or DHA, which are more oxidizable, was the most suppressive to lymphocyte proliferation. Unfortunately, the authors did not examine PUFAs other than GLA for their effect on free radical production and lipid peroxidation. In a recent study, Madhavi et al. (15) confirmed inhibition of lymphocyte proliferation by PUFAs including GLA. They further demonstrated that the inhibitors of cyclooxygenase or lipoxygenase did not reverse the inhibitory effect of PUFAs on lymphocyte proliferation. However, vitamin E and superoxide dismutase completely reversed the PUFA-induced inhibition. These findings suggest that PUFA-induced suppression of lymphocyte proliferation is a free radical-dependent process. GLA is the immediate precursor of DGLA. Increased consumption of GLA increases the level of DGLA. Santoli and Zurier (16) reported that the addition of DGLA to human peripheral blood mononuclear cells (PBMC) inhibited IL-2 production in a dose-dependent manner. Indomethacin, a cyclooxygenase inhibitor that has been shown to decrease PGE_2 and increase IL-2 production, had no effect on the capacity of DGLA to suppress IL-2 production. This indicates that a cyclooxygenase pathway-independent mechanism contributes to DGLA-induced inhibition of IL-2 production.

In Vivo Studies

Nerad et al. (10) reported that dietary supplementation with GLA altered both *in vivo* and *in vitro* indices of cell-mediated immune response. In this double-blind prospective trial, the healthy young volunteers consumed 7.5 g/d of either olive oil/coconut oil (CNO) or borage seed oil (providing 2 g GLA) for 12 wk. After 8 and 12 wk of supplementation, phytohemagglutinin- (PHA, T cell mitogen) stimulated lymphocyte proliferation was suppressed in the GLA group and had not returned to baseline levels by wk 32 (after 20 wk of washout). Decreased lymphocyte proliferation was also seen in the CNO group but only after 32 wk (washout). However, there was a significant increase in IL-2 production in both groups after 12 and 32 wk. The PGE_1 level was not changed in either group. PHA-stimulated PGE_2 production was lower after consumption of GLA for 8 and 12 wk and went back to baseline levels after the washout period. A significant increase in IL-1-induced IL-1β and tumor necrosis factor (TNF) production was also observed. *In vivo* cell-mediated immune function was evaluated in this study as a delayed-type hypersensitivity (DTH) skin test using multitest CMI. The results showed unchanged antigen scores (number of positive antigen responses) in both groups but an increased cumulative score (total diameter of induration) in the GLA-supplemented group.

In a study conducted by Taki et al. (17), DGLA emulsion was intravenously injected into mice. After 1 h, DGLA concentrations in the total phospholipid fraction of spleen cells were increased, and at the same time DTH response was greatly suppressed. These paradoxical *in vitro* and *in vivo* results might reflect the different impact of GLA on different types of cells present *in vivo* and not under *in vitro* conditions as well as other experimental conditions such as species of animal and the level and duration of GLA supplementation.

It is well documented that aging is associated with a decline in immune function. Age-related decrease in Δ6-desaturase activity and its contribution to age-associated cellular dysfunction has been reported (5). Because cell-mediated immune response is decreased and PGE_2 production is increased in the aged, we are currently conducting a double-blind, placebo-controlled study to investigate the effect of GLA supplementation on the immune response of elderly human subjects. Subjects are assigned to either a placebo group or blackcurrant seed oil (BCO) group. Each subject is supplemented with 4.5 g soybean oil (SBO) or BCO (containing 15–19% GLA) per day for 2 mo. Several indices of *in vitro* and *in vivo* immune response will be compared before and after supplementation. The results of this study are currently being analyzed and will be reported later.

Immune-Related Diseases

Eicosanoids, including PGs and LTs, are oxygenated metabolites of PUFAs via cyclooxygenase and lipoxygenase pathways, respectively. Many studies have shown eicosanoids to be mediators of inflammation (18). This has led to the hypothesis that manipulation of PUFA status might modulate eicosanoid metabolism and, in turn, regulate inflammation and the course of inflammatory diseases. Studies using animal models of acute and chronic inflammation as well as limited human studies have provided preliminary evidence to support this hypothesis.

Animal Models of Inflammation

In a rat model of acute inflammation developed by injection of monosodium urate (MSU), Tate et al. (9) found that feeding diets enriched (15% fat) with borage seed oil (23% GLA) for 24 d reduced the total volume, leukocytes count, lysosomal enzyme activity, and protein concentration in air pouch exudates. They obtained similar results using a chronic inflammation model developed by injection of complete Freund's adjuvant. In addition, PGE_2 and LTB_4 concentrations in the exudates were reduced. The same group has demonstrated that in an acute inflammation of rat air pouch induced by MSU, supplementation with 25% fat as primrose oil (8% GLA) for 24 d suppressed the cellular phase but not the fluid phase (exudate volume and protein concentration) of inflammation (19). In another study, this group used 25% fat as blackcurrant seed oil (BCO, containing 19% GLA and 14% ALA) (20). Both cellular and fluid phases of air pouch inflammation induced by MSU were suppressed in rats fed BCO for 24 d compared with those fed normal chow or diets enriched with safflower oil. Topical administration of GLA (1% as eye drop) was shown to inhibit leukocyte infiltration, edema and neovascularization in an experimentally provoked inflammatory keratitis in rabbits (21).

Rheumatoid Arthritis

Rheumatoid arthritis (RA) is an inflammatory disease of the joints characterized by both acute and chronic inflammation. Eicosanoids and cytokines such as IL-1 have been implicated in the pathogenesis of the disease. The effects of this disease can usually be alleviated by administering corticosteroids and non-steroidal antiinflammatory drugs (NSAIDs), but detrimental effects of these drugs have often caused more problems than the disease itself. Medical researchers have been searching for alternate treatments to reduce the need for NSAIDs. Dietary lipids, because of their modulatory effect on eicosanoids, have been considered as one such alternative. A number of studies have focused on GLA as a potentially effective treatment for RA. Clinically important reductions in the signs and symptoms of disease activity in RA patients have been observed after a daily supplementation of 1.4 g GLA (in the form of borage seed oil) for 24 wk (22). In another 6-mo study, the RA patients taking 6 g evening primrose oil per day showed a mild improvement (23). Belch et al. (24) reported that 15-mo administration of evening primrose oil to RA patients resulted in a significant improvement in subjective measures of the disease. Furthermore, by 12 mo, the patients significantly reduced their NSAID intake without adversely affecting the clinical symptoms of the disease. There was, however, no improvement in objective measures of the disease. Lack of an effect of GLA on objective measures of the disease was also reported by Hansen et al. (25).

Inflammatory Skin Disorders

Patients with atopic eczema have been shown to have higher levels of LA and lower levels of its metabolites especially GLA (6–8), indicating impaired Δ6-desaturase activity. The (n-3) EFAs appear to be similarly affected because eczema patients show an elevation of ALA and a decrease in its long-chain metabolites (6). In a number of clinical trials, GLA supplementation produced significant improvement in itching and antihistamine use, as well as gradual improvement in erythema, excoriations and lichenification (26–28). Dietary supplementation with GLA increased epidermal levels of GLA, DGLA, 15-hydroxy-eicosatrienoic acid, and PGE (29).

Multiple Sclerosis

Multiple sclerosis (MS) is a chronic disabling neurological disease with no recognized treatment. The favored hypothesis for the etiology of MS is that the immune system in susceptible individuals fails to eliminate chronic virus infection in the central nervous system, resulting in the development of an autoimmune response directed toward myelin. Studies have indicated a link between abnormal EFA metabolism and altered lymphocyte function in the development of MS (30,31). GLA supplementation in some studies was shown to cause modest clinical improvement in patients with MS (32–34). Others, however, reported no benefit from GLA supplementation for these patients (35).

Cancer

Studies related to the anti-tumor properties of GLA have been conducted by a number of laboratories. Horrobin was the first to suggest a possible link between cancer and GLA content (36). Malignant cells have been found to be deficient in Δ6 desaturase and, consequently, deficient in GLA. GLA was shown to inhibit or kill many tumor cells without harming normal cells (37–39). The anti-tumor properties of GLA are believed to be the result of a direct effect of GLA on tumor cells by increasing the formation of free radicals and peroxides which are toxic to the cells. Others, however, have proposed the possibility that, apart from having a direct effect on cancer cells, GLA may enhance the ability of the host to resist cancer development by modulating immune response. The specific tumorocidal activity of mouse peritoneal macrophages was shown to be dependent in part on appropriate levels of GLA (40). An increase in GLA level in the macrophages was responsible for the increase in lymphokine activation of macrophages (40,41).

Infection

There have been a limited number of reports regarding the possible effect of GLA in protection of the body from infection-related injury. Elevated levels of AA and its metabolites (2-series PGs) have been found in endotoxemia (42). Furthermore, PGE_1 has been shown to be protective in models of endotoxic shock (43). GLA may shift PG production towards 1-series PGs and away from 2-series PGs and is, therefore, expected to attenuate endotoxic shock. Based on this hypothesis, Hirschberg et al. (44) intravenously administered black currant seed oil emulsion (20% GLA) to a guinea pig model of endotoxic shock. No improvement in resistance to the development of endotoxic shock was observed despite the higher levels of GLA and DGLA as well as the higher ratio of DGLA/AA in plasma phospholipids. Considering that the animals were fed GLA for only 3 d and no eicosanoids were measured, more work is required to determine if GLA is effective in reducing pathogenesis of endotoxic shock.

Mechanism of γ-Linolenic Acid Effect

The mechanism by which GLA exerts its effects on immune response and immune-related diseases is still not completely understood. As an immediate EFA metabolite after the rate-limiting step $\Delta 6$ desaturase, GLA tends to be most affected in its metabolism by a variety of factors that influence $\Delta 6$ desaturase. For example, an abnormal fatty acid profile was found in patients with atopic illness. In these cases of atopy, elevated levels of LA and ALA and reduced levels of their metabolites have been demonstrated, which suggests an impairment in desaturation of LA and ALA by $\Delta 6$ desaturase (6–8,45). This might explain the finding that supplementation with (n-6) and (n-3) EFA metabolites in the form of plant (borage, evening primrose and black currant seed) oils and fish oil has been shown to improve the status of some inflammatory diseases. The change in GLA content will have an effect on subsequent metabolites of (n-6) EFAs, especially DGLA and AA, the substrates for synthesis of eicosanoids. Previous studies showed that GLA supplementation increases GLA and DGLA, resulting in an increased DGLA/AA ratio (9,46,47). DGLA can be metabolized by cyclooxygenase to PGE_1. PGE_1 has been reported to affect several aspects of immune and inflammatory response (48) such as reducing histamine level in atopic dermatitis (49,50), promoting T lymphocyte maturation and function (51,52), stimulating suppressor T cells (53) and inhibiting B cell responses (54). It has, therefore, been suggested that a deficit in PGE_1 would lead to defective T lymphocyte function with increased susceptibility both to infections and to autoimmune diseases (30). On the other hand, DGLA cannot be converted to proinflammatory LTs by 5-lipoxygenase. Rather, it inhibits LTB_4 formation and is also simultaneously converted to the 15-lipoxygenase product 15-hydroxy eicosatrienoic acid which has anti-inflammatory potential (29,55). When GLA was observed to suppress adjuvant-induced inflammation in rat air pouch, the levels of LTB_4 and PGE_2 were reduced (9). Furthermore, a recent study showed that women with regular menstrual cycles have a suppressed endometrial PGE_2 and $PGF_{2\alpha}$ synthesis following dietary GLA supplementation and suggested a direct competition between GLA and AA for incorporation into membrane phospholipids (56). These changes in eicosanoid production could, in turn, lead to modified production of the proinflammatory cytokines such as IL-1 and TNF (57,58).

Some studies have shown a significant benefit from reducing proinflammatory cytokines in the treatment of inflammatory diseases (59). In a clinical trial conducted by Byars et al. (60), preliminary results indicated that the levels of IL-1 and IL-6 secreted from the monocytes of RA patients appeared to be higher than those of healthy volunteers. In this study, BCO supplementation slightly reduced IL-1 production. However, in another study reported by Nerad et al. (61), interleukin but not endotoxin or Staphylococcus epidermidis-induced IL-1 and TNF production was increased after dietary supplementation with GLA for 12 wk. They also demonstrated that the increased production of IL-1 and TNF was accompanied by an increase in spontaneous PGE_2 production and a decrease in mitogen-stimulated PGE_2 production (61).

The few reports available in the literature on the effect of GLA on cell-mediated immunity are controversial. The *in vitro* studies have shown GLA to be as suppressive for lymphocyte proliferation as other PUFAs. This inhibitory effect has been attributed to increased production of free radicals by GLA rather than a change in eicosanoid production. The *in vivo* studies have indicated that there is an increase in cytokine production and DTH, an effect which might be related to decreased production of PGE_2, an eicosanoid with a suppressive effect on cell-mediated immunity, by GLA. Some of the effect of GLA on cell-mediated immunity might also be related to increased PGE_1 production. In a previous study (unpublished), we found that adding PGE_1 to human PBMC *in vitro* at 1×10^{-8} and 1×10^{-7} M was less effective than PGE_2 in inhibiting lymphocyte proliferation (30.6 and 43.9% *vs.* 48.5 and 69.4% inhibition, respectively).

Conclusions

Mechanistically, it is feasible to suggest that GLA supplementation could modulate immune and inflammatory responses and related diseases. However, to date, the few published studies have produced controversial results. Further investigation is required to confirm the biological effect of increased GLA consumption on immune and inflammatory responses in animal models as well as in humans.

Acknowledgments

The authors' work was funded in part with Federal funds from the U.S. Department of Agriculture, Agricultural Research Service under contract number 53-K06-01 and a grant from Nestle, Inc. The contents of this publication do not necessarily reflect the views or policies of the U.S. Department of Agriculture, nor does mention of trade names, commercial products, or organizations imply endorsement by the U.S. government.

References

1. Brenner, R.R., De Tomas, M.E., and Peluffo, R.O. Effect of Polyunsaturated Fatty Acids on the Desaturation in Vitro of Linoleic to γ-Linolenic Acid (1965) *Biochim. Biophys. Acta 106*, 640–642.
2. Marcel, Y.L., Christiansen, K., and Holman, R.T. The Preferred Metabolic Pathway from Linoleic Acid to Arachidonic Acid *in Vitro* (1968) *Biochim. Biophys. Acta 164*, 25–34.
3. de Goméz Dumm, I.N.T., de Alianiz, J.T., and Brenner, R.R. Effect of Epinephrine on the Oxidative Desaturation of Fatty Acids in the Rat (1976) *J. Lipid Res. 17*, 616–621.

4. de Goméz Dumm, I.N.T., de Alianiz, J.T., and Brenner, R.R. Effect of Glucocorticoids on the Oxidative Desaturation of Fatty Acids by Rat Liver Microsomes (1976) *J. Lipid Res. 20,* 834–839.
5. Hrelia, S., Bordoni, A., Celadon, M., Turchetto, E., Biagi, P.L., and Rossi, C.A. Age-related Changes in Linoleate and α-Linolenate Desaturation by Rat Liver Microsomes (1989) *Biochem. Biophys. Res. Commun. 163,* 348–355.
6. Manku, M.S., Horrobin, D.F., Morse, N.L., Wright, S., and Burton, J.L. Essential Fatty Acids in the Plasma Phospholipids of Patients with Atopic Eczema (1984) *Br. J. Dermatol. 110,* 643–648.
7. Morse, P.F., Horrobin, D.F., Manku, M.S., Stewart, J.C.M., Allen, R., Littlewood, S., Wright, S., Burton, J., Gould, D.J., Holt, P.J., Jansen, C.T., Mattila, L., Weigel, W., Dettke, T.H., Wexler, D., Guenther, L., Bordoni, A., and Patrizi, A. Metaanalysis of Placebo-Controlled Studies of the Efficacy of Epogam in the Treatment of Atopic Eczema. Relationship Between Plasma Essential Fatty Acid Changes and Clinical Response (1989) *Br. J. Dermatol. 121,* 75–90.
8. Lindskov, R., and Holmer, G. Polyunsaturated Fatty Acids in Plasma, Red Blood Cells and Mononuclear Cell Phospholipids of Patients with Atopic Dermatitis (1992) *Allergy 47,* 517–521.
9. Tate, G., Mandell, B.F., Laposata, M., Ohliger, D., Baker, D.G., Schumacher, H.R., and Zurier, R.B. Suppression of Acute and Chronic Inflammation by Dietary Gamma Linolenic Acid (1989) *J. Rheumatol. 16,* 729–733.
10. Nerad, J.L., Meydani, S.N., and Dinarello, C.A. Dietary Supplementation with Gamma-Linolenic Acid (GLA) and Parameters of Cell-Mediated Immunity (1991) *Cytokine 3,* 513.
11. Fan, Y.-Y., and Chapkin, R.S. Mouse Peritoneal Macrophage Prostaglandin E Synthesis Is Altered by Dietary γ-Linolenic Acid (1992) *J. Nutr. 122,* 1600–1606.
12. Goodwin, J.S., and Webb, D.R. Regulation of the Immune Response by Prostaglandins (1977) *Clin. Immunol. Immunopathol. 15,* 106–122.
13. Rappaport, R.S., and Dodge, G.R. Prostaglandin E Inhibits the Production of Human Interleukin 2 (1982) *J. Exp. Med. 155,* 943–948.
14. Devi, M.A., and Das, N.P. Antiproliferative Effect of Polyunsaturated Fatty Acids and Interleukin-2 on Normal and Abnormal Human Lymphocytes (1994) *Experientia 50,* 489–492.
15. Madhavi, N., Das, U.N., Prabha, P.S., Kumar, G.S., Koratkar, R., and Sagar, P.S. Suppression of Human T-cell Growth *in Vitro* by *cis*-unsaturated Fatty Acids: Relationship to Free Radicals and Lipid Peroxidation (1994) *Prostaglandins Leukotrienes Essen. Fatty Acids 51,* 33–40.
16. Santoli, D., and Zurier, R.B. Prostaglandin E Precursor Fatty Acids Inhibit Human IL-2 Production by a Prostaglandin E-independent Mechanism (1989) *J. Immunol. 143,* 1303–1309.
17. Taki, H., Nakamura, N., Hamazaki, T., and Kobayashi, M. Intravenous Injection of Tridihomo-γ-linolenoyl-glycerol into Mice and Its Effects on Delayed-Type Hypersensitivity (1993) *Lipids 28,* 873–876.
18. Williams, T.J., and Peck, M.J. Role of Prostaglandins in Inflammation (1977) *Nature 270,* 530–532.
19. Tate, G., Mandell, B.F., Karmali, R.A., Laposata, M., Baker, D.G., Schumacher, H.R., and Zurier, R.B. Suppression of Monosodium Urate Crystal-Induced Acute Inflammation by Diets Enriched with Gamma-Linolenic Acid and Eisosapentaenoic Acid (1988) *Arthritis Rheum. 31,* 1543–1551.

20. Tate, G., and Zurier, R.B. Suppression of Monosodium Urate Crystal-Induced Inflammation by Black Currant Seed Oil (1994) *Agents Actions 43*, 35–38.
21. Verbey, N.L.J., van Haeringen, N.J., and de Jong, P.T. V.M. Modulation of Immunogenic Keratitis in Rabbits by Topical Administration of Polyunsaturated Fatty Acids (1988) *Curr. Eye Res. 7*, 549–556.
22. Leventhal, L.J., Boyce, E.G., and Zurier, R.B. Treatment of Rheumatoid Arthritis with γ-Linolenic Acid (1993) *Ann. Intern. Med. 119*, 867–873.
23. Brzeski, M., Madhok, R., and Capell, H.A. Evening Primrose Oil in Patients with Rheumatoid Arthritis and Side-Effects of Non-Steroidal Anti-Inflammatory Drugs (1991) *Br. J. Rheumatol. 30*, 370–372.
24. Belch, J.J.F., Ansell, D., Madhok, R., O'Dowd, A., and Sturrock, R.D. Effects of Altering Dietary Essential Fatty Acids on Requirements for Non-steroidal Anti-Inflammatory Drugs in Patients with Rheumatoid Arthritis: A Double Blind Placebo Controlled Study (1988) *Ann. Rheum. Dis. 47*, 96–104.
25. Hansen, T.M., Lerche, A., Kassis, A., Lorenzen, V., and Sondergaard, J. Treatment of Rheumatoid Arthritis with Prostaglandin E_1 Precursors *cis*-Linoleic Acid and γ-Linolenic Acid (1983) *Scand. J. Rheumatol. 12*, 85–88.
26. Fiocchi, A., Sala, M., Signoroni, P., Banderali, G., Agostoni, C., and Riva, E. The Efficacy and Safety of γ-Linolenic Acid in the Treatment of Infantile Atopic Dermatitis (1994) *J. Int. Med. Res. 22*, 2~32.
27. Bordoni, A. Biagi, P.L., Masi, M., Ricci, G., Fanelli, C., Patrizi, A., and Ceccolini, E. Evening Primrose Oil in the Treatment of Children with Atopic Eczema (1988) *Drugs Exp. Clin. Res. 14*, 291–297.
28. Moa, S.-K., Leena, M., Jansen, C.T., and Uotila, P. Evening Primrose Oil in the Treatment of Atopic Eczema: Effect on Clinical Status, Plasma Phospholipid Fatty Acids and Circulating Blood Prostaglandins (1987) *Br. J. Dermatol. 117*, 11–19.
29. Miller, C.C. and Ziboh, V.A. γ-Linolenic Acid-enriched Diet Alters Cutaneous Eicosanoids (1988) *Biochem. Biophys. Res. Commun. 154*, 967–974.
30. Horrobin, D.F. Multiple Sclerosis: The Rational Basis for Treatment with Colchicine and Evening Primrose Oil (1979) *Med. Hypotheses 5*, 365–378.
31. Bates, D. Lipids and Multiple Sclerosis (1989) *Biochem. Soc. Trans. 17*, 289–291.
32. Meyer-Rieneckerk, H.J., Jenssen, H.L., Kohler, H., Field, E.J., and Shenion, B.K. Effect of γ-Linolenate on Multiple Sclerosis (1976) *Lancet ii*, 966.
33. Field, E.J. Gamma-Linolenate in Multiple Sclerosis (1978) *Lancet I*, 780.
34. Field, E.J., and Joyce, G. Effect of Prolonged Ingestion of Gamma-Linolenate by Multiple Sclerosis Patients (1978) *Eur. Neurol. 17*, 67–76.
35. Bates, D., Fawcett, P.R.W., Shaw, D.A., and Weightman, D. Polyunsaturated Fatty Acids in Treatment of Acute Remitting Multiple Sclerosis (1978) *Br. Med. J. 2*, 1390–1391.
36. Horrobin, D.F. The Reversibility of Cancer: The Relevance of Cyclic Amp, Calcium, Essential Fatty Acids and Prostaglandin E_1 (1980) *Med. Hypotheses 6*, 469–486.
37. Dippenaar, N., Booyens, J., Fabbri, D., Engelbrecht, P., and Katzeff, I.E. The Reversibility of Cancer: Evidence That Malignancy in Human Hepatoma Cells Is Gamma-Linolenic Acid Deficiency Dependent (1982) *S. Afr. Med. J. 62*, 683–685.
38. Booyens, J., Dippenaar, N., Fabbri, D., Engelbrecht, P., and Katzeff, I.E. The Effect of Gamma-Linolenic Acid on the Growth of Human Osteogenic Sarcoma and Oesophageal Carcinoma Cells in Culture (1984) *S. Afr. Med. J. 65*, 240–242.

39. Begin, M.E., Das, U.N., Ells, G., and Horrobin, D.F. Selective Killing of Human Cancer Cells by Polyunsaturated Fatty Acids (1985) *Prostaglandins Leukotrienes Med. 19*, 177–186.
40. Schlager, S.I., Madden, L.D., and Meltzer, M.S. Role of Macrophage Lipids in Regulating Tumorocidal Activity (1983) *Cell Immunol. 77*, 52–68.
41. Schlager, S.I., Meltzer, M.S., Bara, S., and Mamula, M.J. Role of Macrophage Lipids in Regulating Tumorocidal Activity (1983) *Cell. Immunol. 80*, 10–19.
42. Collier, J.G., Herman, A.G., and Vane, J.R. Appearance of Prostaglandins in the Renal Venous Blood of Dogs in Response to Acute Systemic Hypotension Produced by Bleeding or Endotoxin (1973) *J. Physiol. 230*, 19–20.
43. Raflo, G.T., Wangensteen, S.L., Glenn, T.M., and Lefer, A.M. Mechanism of the Protective Effects of Prostaglandin E_1 and $F_{2\alpha}$ in Canine Endotoxin Shock (1973) *Eur. J. Pharmacol. 24*, 86–95.
44. Hirschberg, Y., Shackelford, A., Mascioli, E.A., Babayan, V.K., Bistrian, B.R., and Blackburn, G.l. The Response to Endotoxin in Guinea Pigs After Intravenous Black Currant Seed Oils (1990) *Lipids 25*, 491–496.
45. Galland, L. Increased Requirements for Essential Fatty Acids in Atopic Individuals: A Review with Clinical Descriptions (1986) *J. Am. Coll. Nutr. 5*, 213–228.
46. Chapkin, R.S., and Coble, K.J. Utilization of γ-linolenic Acid by Mouse Peritoneal Macrophages (1991) *Biochim. Biophys. Acta 1085*, 365–370.
47. Karlstad, M.D., DeMichele, S.J., Leathem, W.D., and Peterson, M.B. Effect of Intravenous Lipid Emulsions Enriched with γ-Linolenic Acid on Plasma n-6 Fatty Acids and Prostaglandin Biosynthesis after Burn and Endotoxin Injury in Rats (1993) *Crit. Care Med. 21*, 1740–1749.
48. Samuelsson, B., Goldyne, M., Granstrom, E., Hamberg, M., Hammastrom, S., and Malmsten, C. Prostaglandins and Thromboxanes (1978) *Ann. Rev. Biochem. 47*, 997–1029.
49. Ruzicka, T., and Ring, J. Enhanced Releasability of Prostaglandin E_2 and Leukotrienes B_4 and C_4 from Leukocytes of Patients with Atopic Eczema (1987) *Acta Derm. Venereol. 67*, 469–475.
50. von der Helm, D., Ring, J., and Dorsch, W. Comparison of Histamine Release and Prostaglandin E_2 Production of Human Basophils in Atopic and Normal Individuals (1987) *Arch. Dermatol. Res. 279*, 536–542.
51. Zurier, R.B., Sayadoff, D.M., Torrey, S.B. and Rothfield, N.F. Prostaglandin E Treatment of NZB/NZW Mice. I. Prolonged Survival of Female Mice (1977) *Arthritis Rheum. 20*, 723–728.
52. Horrobin, D.F., Manku, M.S., Oka, M., Morgan, R.O., Cunnane, S.C., Ally, A.I., Ghayur, T., Schweitzer, M., and Karmali, R.A. The Nutritional Regulation of T-Lymphocyte Function (1979) *Med. Hypotheses 5*, 969–985.
53. Pillay, D.J., and Pope, B.I. Requirement of Prostaglandin E_1 (PGE_2) for the Secretion of Suppressor Cell Inducer Factors by Spleen Cells of Tumor-Bearing Mice (1986) *Int. J. Immunopharmacol. 8*, 221–226.
54. Ohsugi, Y., and Gershwin, M.E. Inhibition by Various Antiarthritic Agents of Murine Splenic B Cell Colony Formation (1984) *Immunopharmacology 7*, 1–7.
55. Iverson, L., Fogh, K., Bojesen, G., and Kragballe, K. Linoleic Acid and Dihomo-γ-Linolenic Acid Inhibit Leukotriene B_4 Formation and Stimulate the Formation of Their 15-Lipoxygenase Products by Human Neutrophils *in Vitro*. Evidence of Formation of Antiinflammatory Compounds (1991) *Agents Actions 33*, 286–291.

56. Graham, J., Franks, S., and Bonney, R.C. *In Vivo* and *in Vitro* Effects of Gamma-linolenic Acid and Eicosapentaenoic Acid on Prostaglandin Production and Arachidonic Acid Uptake by Human Endometrium (1994) *Prostaglandins Leukotrienes Essen. Fatty Acids 50,* 321–329.
57. Watson, J., Madhok, R., Wijelath, E., Capell, H.A., Gillespie, J., Smith, J., and Byars, M.L. Mechanism of Action of Polyunsaturated Fatty Acids in Rheumatoid Arthritis (1990) *Biochem. Soc. Trans. 18,* 284–285.
58. Enders, S., Ghorbani, R., Kelley, V.E., Georgilis, K., Lonnemann, G., van der Meer, J.W.M., Cannon, J.G., Rogers, T.S., Klempner, M.S., Weber, P.C., Schaefer, E.J., Wolff, S.M., and Dinarello, C.A. The Effect of Dietary Supplementation with n-3 Polyunsaturated Fatty Acids on the Synthesis of Interleukin-1 and Tumor Necrosis Factor by Mononuclear Cells (1989) *N. Engl. J. Med. 320,* 265–271.
59. Feldmann, M., Brennan, F.M., Chantry, D., Haworth, C., Turner, M., Abney, E., Buchan, G., Barrett, K., Barkley, D., Chu, A., Field, M., and Maini, R.N. Cytokine Production in the Rheumatoid Joint: Implications for Treatment (1990) *Annals Rheum. Dis. 49,* 480–486.
60. Byars, M.L., Watson, J., and McGill, P.E. Blackcurrant Seed Oil as a Source of Polyunsaturated Fatty Acids in the Treatment of Inflammatory Disease (1992) *Biochem. Soc. Trans. 20,* 139S.
61. Nerad, J.L., Meydani, S.N., and Dinarello, C.A. Dietary Supplementation with Gamma-Linolenic Acid (GLA) and Synthesis of IL-l and TNF by Peripheral Blood Mononuclear Cells (PBMC) (1991) *Cytokine 3,* 513.

Chapter 10

The Biological/Nutritional Significance of γ-Linolenic Acid in the Epidermis: Metabolism and Generation of Potent Biological Modulators

V.A. Ziboh

Department of Dermatology, University of California, Davis, Davis, CA 95616

Historical Perspective

γ-Linolenic acid (GLA, 18:3n-6) is a Δ6-desaturase product of linoleic acid (LA, 18:2n-6). An increasing number of reports have appeared which indicate that dietary constituents containing this polyunsaturated fatty acid are capable of influencing cellular eicosanoid biosynthesis. For instance, orally administered evening primrose oil (EPO) containing LA and GLA was reported to increase tissue levels of 1-series prostaglandins (PGs) and to suppress chronic inflammation (1,2). A notable feature of GLA in the epidermis is its *in vivo* elongation to dihomo-γ-linolenic acid (DGLA, 20:3n-6), followed by the latter's oxidative metabolism via either the cyclooxygenase pathway to prostaglandins of the 1-series (PGE_1), or the lipoxygenase pathway into mainly the hydroxy fatty acids. PGE_1 has been reported to exert anti-inflammatory effects in a variety of *in vitro* and *in vivo* systems. For instance, it has been reported to suppress the inflammations of adjuvant arthritis (3) and immune complex vasculitis in rats (4). Taken together, the generation of PGE_1 and its suppression of inflammatory reactions seem consistent with an *in vivo* regulatory role for GLA-containing diets.

The Biological Significance of γ-Linolenic Acid in the Epidermis

The excitement generated by reports of clinical improvement of patients with atopic eczema after oral administration of primrose oil (5,6) signalled a possible role for GLA-containing oil in cutaneous biology. To evolve clear biochemical mechanisms for this dietary PUFA, we embarked on a progressive series of studies to delineate whether a relationship exists between the dietary intake of three vegetable oils: (i) safflower oil (containing predominantly 18:2n-6), (ii) primrose oil (containing 18:2n-6 and 18:3n-6), and (iii) borage oil (also containing predominantly 18:2n-6 and 18:3n-6), and the generation of oxidative metabolites of GLA with anti-inflammatory properties.

As a first step in the elucidation of these biochemical events, we investigated *in vitro*, whether LA was desaturated into GLA. Our findings revealed that both guinea pig and human epidermal preparations lacked the capability to transform LA to GLA, suggesting a lack of Δ6-desaturase. Next, we investigated the *in vitro* metabolism of GLA by guinea pig and human epidermal enzyme preparations. The incubation of

18:3n-6 plus manonyl CoA revealed the elongation of GLA into DGLA (7,8). In a follow-up study, we explored whether DGLA can be desaturated to arachidonic acids (AA). Our findings revealed the inability of human epidermal preparations to desaturate the biosynthesized DGLA into arachidonic acid (AA, 20:4n-6), indicating a negligible amount or absence of Δ5-desaturase in this tissue (8). These findings underscore that the arachidonic acid found principally esterified to epidermal membrane phospholipids is not biosynthesized locally from tissue LA, but rather is biosynthesized and transported to skin epidermis from systemic sources, possibly by the liver.

We next tested the hypothesis that, because epidermal enzymes can elongate GLA into DGLA, but lack the Δ5-desaturase to transform the DGLA into AA, dietary intake of a high GLA-containing oil should result first in the *in vivo* accumulation of DGLA in epidermal phospholipids. We suggest that the elevated tissue level of DGLA should enhance the metabolism of DGLA via both the cyclooxygenase and the lipooxygenase pathways, thereby generating potent biological metabolites.

Metabolism of DGLA via the Cyclooxygenase Pathway

To test the preceding hypothesis, we explored the *in vitro* metabolic products of DGLA. Specifically, the incubation of guinea pig epidermal high-speed particulate (microsomal) enzyme preparation with ^{14}C-labeled DGLA ([1-^{14}C]20:3n-6), revealed the formation of prostaglandin E_1 (^{14}C-PGE$_1$) as shown in Fig. 10.1. Minor metabolites include ^{14}C-PGF$_\alpha$ and other unidentified products.

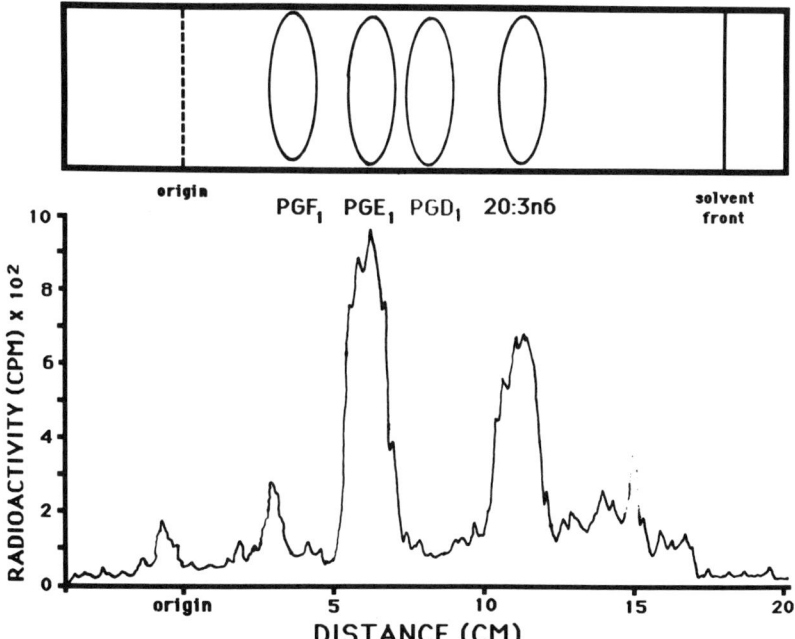

Fig. 10.1. Argentation TLC radiochromatogram of epidermal microsomal metabolites of [l-^{14}C] 20:3n-6.

Metabolism of GLA via the Lipoxygenase Pathway

In separate experiments, the incubation of epidermal high-speed supernatant (cytosolic) with ^{14}C-labeled DGLA, [1-^{14}C]20:3n-6, and fractionation of the extracted metabolites on high performance liquid chromatography (HPLC) revealed the formation of a major radioactive metabolite, 15-hydroxy-8,11,13-eicosatrienoic acid (15-OH-20:3n-6), as shown in Fig. 10.2. The HPLC metabolite was confirmed further by GLC-Mass Spectrometry. Taken together, the subcellular epidermal enzyme preparations possess the capacities *in vitro* to transform DGLA into a cyclooxygenase product prostaglandin E_1 (PGE_1) and a 15-lipoxygenase product (15-OH-20:3n-6) or 15-HETrE.

Anti-Inflammatory Potential of the Dihomo-γ-Linolenic Metabolites

To test the anti-inflammatory potential of the 15-lipoxygenase metabolite of DGLA (15-HETrE), a cellular model generating proinflammatory metabolites from AA was used. First, we tested *in vitro* the effects of varying concentrations of 15HETrE on Ca^{++} ionophore-activated rat basophilic leukemia (RBL-1) cell line which elaborates 5-lipoxygenase activity. Metabolites derived from this lipoxygenase pathway,

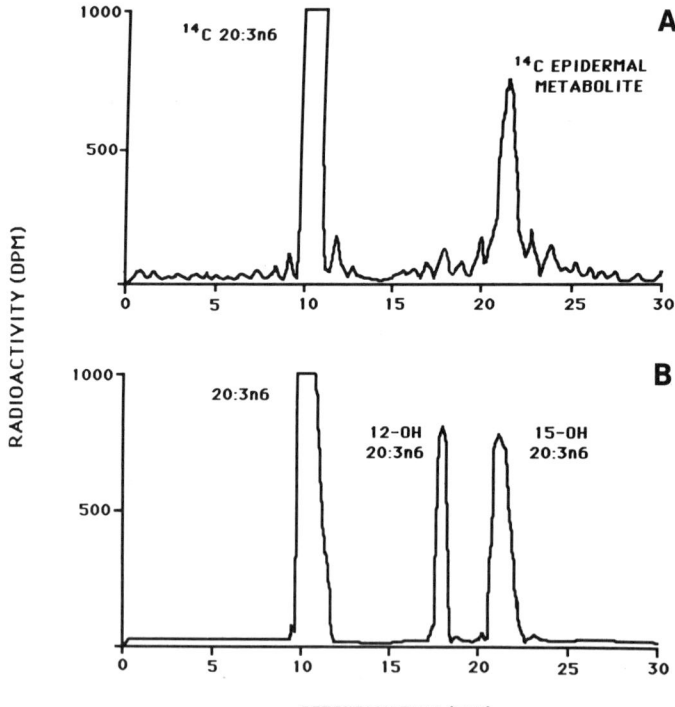

Fig. 10.2. Normal phase HPLC chromatograms of: (A) metabolism of ^{14}C.20:3n-6 by epidermal cytosolic extract and (B) authentic reference standards.

particularly leukotriene B_4 (LTB_4), are known to induce hyperproliferation in epidermal tissues and keratinocytes (9) as well as cutaneous inflammatory reactions (10–12).

In vitro *Inhibition of 5-Lipoxygenase Activity by 15-HETrE*

The incubation of 15-HETrE derived from DGLA with supernatant enzyme preparations from RBL cells used as the LTB_4-generating system resulted in a dose-dependent inhibition of LTB_4 formation. A similar incubation with 15-HETE derived from AA also revealed a dose-dependent inhibition of LTB_4 formation. The results in Fig. 10.3 show the dose-dependent inhibitory effects of 15-HETrE and 15-HETE (0–50 µM) on the ability of RBL-1 enzyme preparations to convert [1-^{14}C]20:4n-6 to [^{14}C]LTB_4.

Effect of Dietary Intake of GLA-Enriched Oils in Experimental Animals

The demonstration *in vitro* that epidermal preparations have the capacity to transform GLA/DGLA into the cyclooxygenase product PGE_1 and the 15-lipoxygenase product, 15-HETrE (both inhibitors of the generation of proinflammatory metabolites from arachidonic acid) suggests that dietary supplementation with a GLA-enriched oil could lead to local elongation of GLA to DGLA. The accumulated DGLA could then undergo oxidative metabolism to PGE_1 and 15-HETrE. Should this occur *in vivo*, it should be possible to identify both metabolites in the excised epidermis after a GLA-supplemented diet.

Generation of Epidermal Hydroxy Fatty Acids. In our first dietary protocol, guinea pig diets were supplemented with safflower oil (SFO, containing <0.5% GLA) and borage oil (BO, containing 25% GLA) for 8 wk. The epidermis from these two

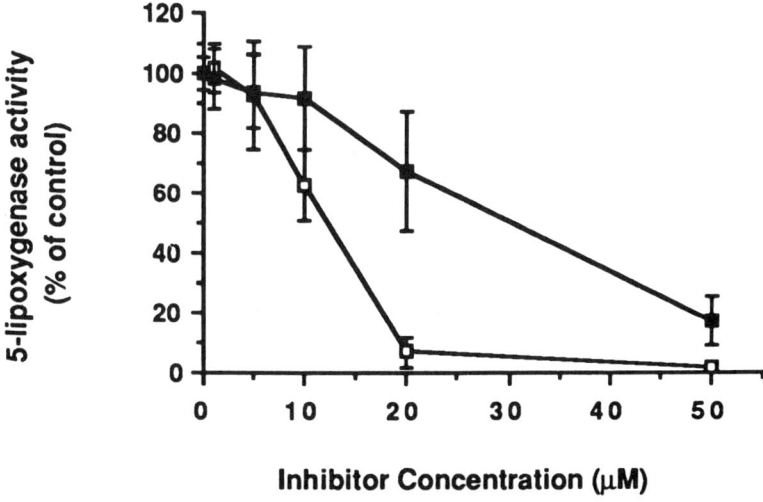

Fig. 10.3. The effects of epidermal 15-HETrE (□) and 15-HETE (■) on RBL-I 5 lipoxygenase activity.

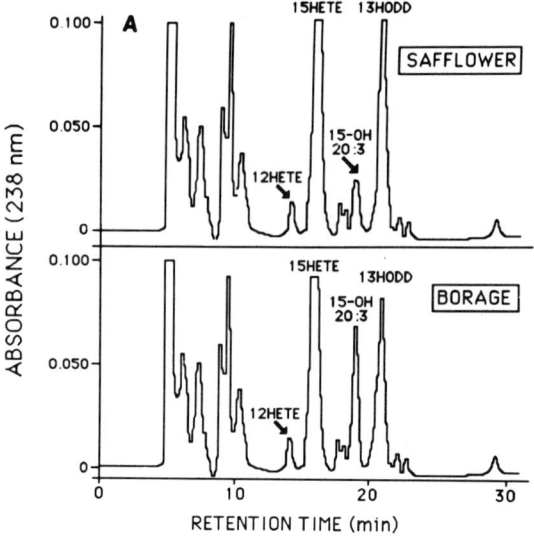

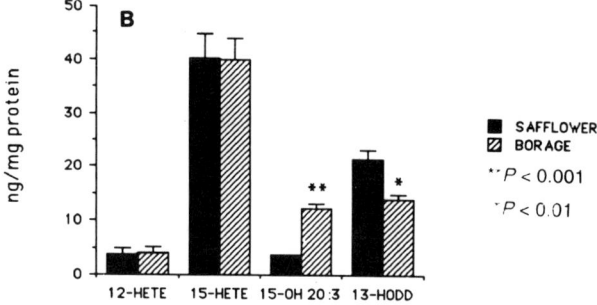

Fig. 10.4. Effect of GLA-enriched diets on the generation of epidermal monohydroxy fatty acids.

groups of animals were excised after the study and analyzed for: (1) tissue levels of monohydroxy fatty acids and (2) epidermal levels of prostaglandins. A comparison of the hydroxy fatty acid contents of the epidermis from the BO- and SFO-fed guinea pigs is shown in Fig. 10.4A and B.

Extracts of the epidermis from the two groups of animals revealed no significant differences in arachidonic acid-derived monohydroxy fatty acids such as 12-HETE and 15-HETE. In contrast, the epidermis of the BO-fed animals revealed a significant increase in the DGLA-derived monohydroxy fatty acid (15 HETrE) ($P < 0.001$), indicating *in vivo* metabolism of DGLA into 15-HETrE by epidermal 15-lipoxygenase.

Generation of Epidermal Cyclooxygenase Products. A comparison of the epidermal prostaglandins from the BO- and SFO-fed guinea pigs is shown in Fig. 10.5A and B. The epidermis of the BO-fed animals showed significant tissue elevation of the major

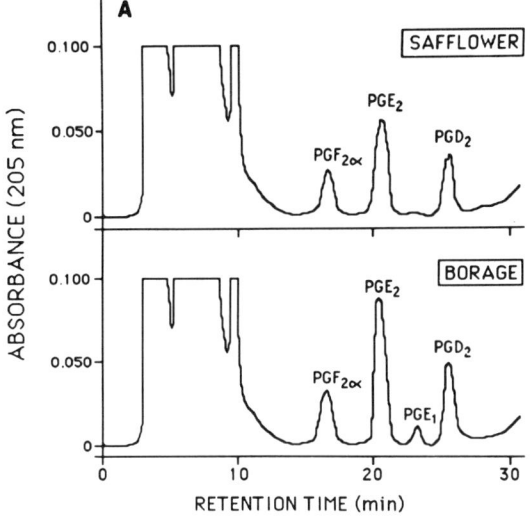

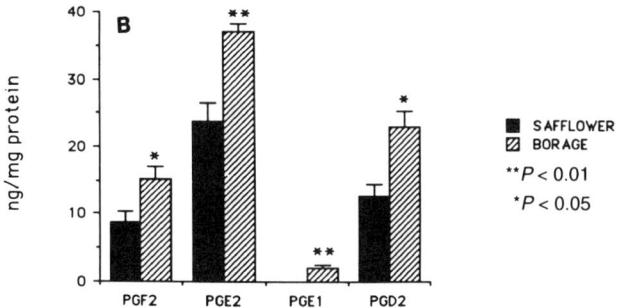

Fig. 10.5. Effect of GLA-enriched diet on the generation of cyclooxygenase products.

arachidonic acid-derived prostaglandins: $PGF_{2\alpha}$ ($P < 0.05$), PGE_2 ($P < 0.01$), and PGD_2 ($P < 0.05$). Interestingly, $PGF_{2\alpha}$ (a prostanoid with reported antiinflammatory properties) was increased significantly. Of particular interest as shown in Fig. 10.5B is the significant tissue elevation in the amount of DGLA-derived PGE_1 ($P < 0.005$) by BO-fed animals, indicating the metabolism of DGLA into PGE_1 via the cyclooxygenase pathway. This PGE_1 (with reported antiinflammatory properties) was not detectable in the epidermis of control SFO-fed animals.

Effect of Dietary Supplementation with GLA-Enriched Oil in Humans: Modulation of Leukotriene B_4 Generation by GLA-Rich Polymorphonuclear Cells

To determine whether the dietary effects of the intake of GLA-enriched oil observed in experimental animals was also possible in humans, we examined the effects of the dietary intake on the ability of human polymorphonuclear cells (PMNs) to generate LTB_4. Normal human volunteers with approval by the Human Research and Ethical Committee of the University of California, Davis were assigned to two dietary groups. Specifically, our protocol included two groups initially placed on a 2-wk baseline period on olive oil to normalize the *in vivo* basal levels of fatty acids. After the baseline period, 60 mL of heparinized blood was taken from each participant. The PMNs were isolated, employing a standard Hypaque-Ficoll gradient centrifugation, dextran sedimentation and hypotonic lysis (13). The isolated PMNs were used to determine the baseline fatty acid profile in the PMNs of both groups. Then the participants (six per group) were randomly assigned to continue for an additional 6 wk either as controls taking control capsules of olive oil (equivalent to 0.55 g) or as the GLA-supplemented group, taking capsules of GLA-enriched borage oil (BO) (equivalent to 1.5 g GLA/d). At the end of the study, 60 mL of blood was obtained from each participant, and PMNs were isolated as described above and

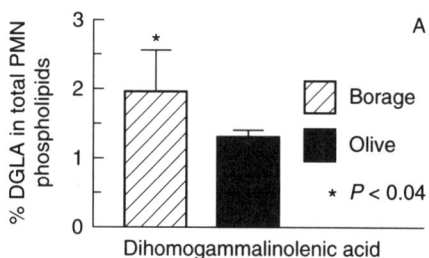

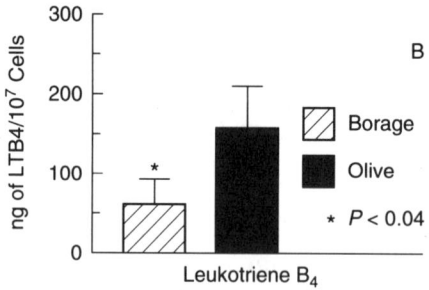

Fig. 10.6. The effect of dietary GLA-enriched oil on Ca^{2+}-ionophore-induced PMN generation of LTB_4.

assessed for cellular concentrations of PMN phospholipid GLA, DGLA and for PMN induced-generation of LTB_4.

The data shown in Fig. 10.6 (A and B) summarize data from the two dietary groups on olive oil and GLA-containing borage oil. Fig. 10.6A indicates a marked increase in cellular accumulation of DGLA in PMN phospholipids of the BO-fed group when compared with the control olive oil-fed group. Interestingly, the effect of ingested GLA-fortified capsules resulted in the inhibition of Ca^{++} ionophore-induced PMN generation of LTB_4 (Fig. 10.6B). Thus, these results indicate that the *in vivo* elevation of DGLA in PMN phospholipids derived from dietary GLA inhibits the Ca^{++} ionophore-induced PMN generation of LTB_4. This finding suggests that 15-HETrE (the 15-lipoxygenase metabolite of DGLA) generated by PMN *in vivo* may play a role in the *in vivo* suppression of PMN generation of proinflammatory LTB_4 in the BO-fed group.

A speculative scenario of the possible modulatory effects of the constituent fatty acids and metabolites from dietary LA- and GLA-enriched oils, their putative generation of metabolites *in vivo*, and the resultant effects of these metabolites on the generation of proinflammatory leukotrienes from AA is shown in Fig. 10.7.

The pathway labeled (A) in Fig. 10.7 illustrates the metabolic transformations from dietary intake of LA-enriched safflower oil which results on the one

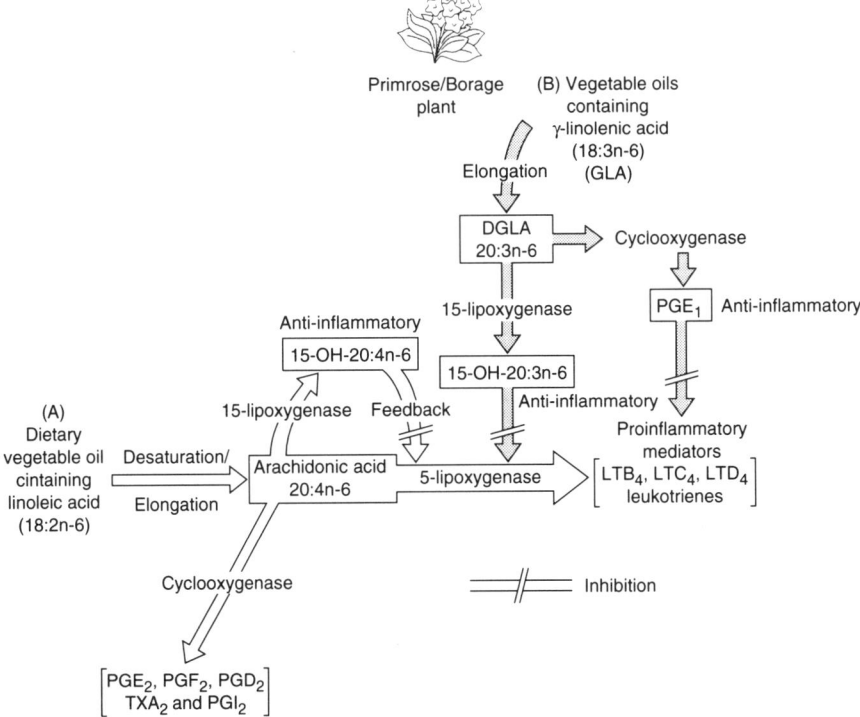

Fig. 10.7. A speculative scenario of *in vivo* modulatory effects of dietary GLA-enriched oils on AA generation of LTB_4, C_4, and D_4.

hand in the generation of 15-HETE via the 15-lipoxygenase of pathway and, on the other hand, in the generation of the proinflammatory leukotrienes by PMNs via the 5-lipoxygenase pathway. The pathway labeled (B) represents the epidermal transformation of dietary GLA-enriched oils (primrose oil and/or borage oil) into DGLA and the tissue generation of 15-HETrE (via 15-lipoxygenase pathway) as well as PGE_1 (via the cyclooxygenase pathway). It is therefore reasonable to speculate that the metabolites from the pathway labeled (B) can inhibit the *in vivo* generation of local cellular proinflammatory leukotrienes LTB_4, C_4, and D_4 from AA. These possibilities imply that the dietary intake of highly purified vegetable oils containing sufficient amounts of GLA (because cellular/tissue concentrations are pivotal) may offer an alternative or an adjunct therapeutic modality for alleviating inflammatory disorders.

Involvement of Monohydroxy Fatty Acids in Cutaneous Signal Transduction Processes

We next explored whether the notable biological effects of the various monohydroxy fatty acids in the epidermis occur via the signal transduction pathway. As a first step, we demonstrated that a diet supplemented with SFO (linoleic acid-enriched oil) resulted in epidermal elevation of 13-hydroxyoctadecadienoic acid (13-HODE), a 15-lipoxygenase metabolite of linoleic acid. This finding indicated that LA was metabolized into 13-HODE *in vivo*. Furthermore, we demonstrated that 13-HODE can display an antiproliferative activity in this tissue (14). More recently, we have shown that 13-HODE is incorporated into epidermal phosphatidyl 4,5-bisphosphate (PtdIns4,5-P2) and is subsequently released as a novel putative 13-HODE-containing diacylglycerol (13-HODE-DAG) by epidermal phospholipase C (15). The putative 13-HODE-DAG was shown to selectively inhibit the activity of PKC-β isozyme, while exerting negligible effect on the PKC-α isozyme (16). Interestingly, an increase in PKC-β was shown to parallel epidermal hyperproliferation. This selective inhibitory effect of 13-HODE-DAG on epidermal-β PKC isozyme activity suggests that 13-HODE-containing DAG seemingly can modulate epidermal PKC activity and hyperproliferation. A speculative scenario of the effect of dietary linoleic acid-enriched SFO on the cutaneous elevation of 13-HODE, the generation of putative 13-HODE-DAG and its downregulation of PKC-β is illustrated in Fig. 10.8.

Excited about the findings of putative 13-HODE-DAG and because 15-HETrE is a potent anti-inflammatory monohydroxy fatty acid *in vitro*, we investigated whether 15-HETrE is similarly metabolized by epidermis. In a preliminary study, the intralesional injection of 15-HETrE into human psoriatic lesion (plaque) revealed its selective incorporation into phospholipids (particularly, the inositol phospholipids). This initial observation in human epidermis prompted further explorations using guinea pigs as a model. Our preliminary data revealed that 15-HETrE is incorporated into phosphatidylinositol 4,5-bisphosphate (PtdIns-4,5P_2) and that phospholipase C catalysis of PtdIns-containing 15-HETrE yielded a putative 15-HETrE-containing DAG (15-HETrE-DAG). The possibility that the novel

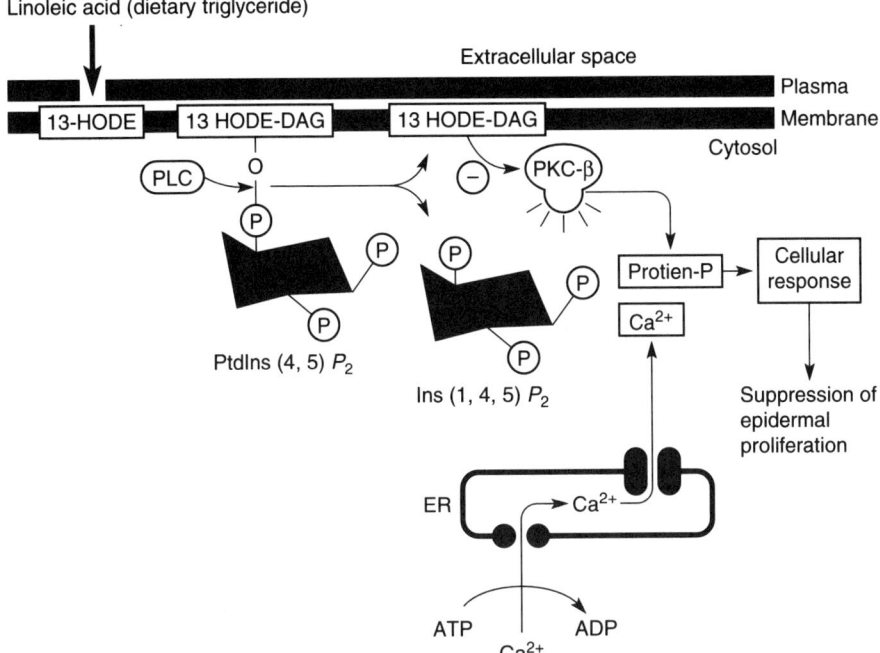

Fig. 10.8. Speculative scenario of dietary linoleic acid and the cutaneous generation of putative 13-HODE-DAG.

15-HETrE substituted diacylglycerol may exert its biological functions via the modulation of protein kinase C remains to be determined.

Acknowledgments

The author thanks Linda Starr for preparation of the manuscript. Some of the studies referenced in this review were supported in part by Research Grant AM30679 from the National Institutes of Health of the United States Public Health Service.

References

1. Kunkel, S.L., Ogawa, H., Ward, P.A., and Zurier, R.B. Suppression of Chronic Inflammation by Evening Primrose Oil (1981) *Prog. Lipid Res. 20,* 885–888.
2. Zurier, R.B. Use of Prostaglandins and Evening Primrose Oil (Efamol) in Experimental Models of Inflammation (1982). in Horrobin, D.F., ed., *Clinical Uses of Essential Fatty Acids,* Eden Press, Montreal, pp. 113–124.
3. Zurier, R.B., and Quagliata, F. Effect of Prostaglandin E_1 on Adjuvant Arthritis (1971) *Nature 234,* 304–305.
4. Kunkel, S.L., Thrall, R.S., Kunkel, R.G., Mccormick, J.R., Ward, P.A., and Zurier, R.B. Suppression of Immune Complex Vasculitis in Rats by Prostaglandins (1979) *J. Clin. Invest. 64,* 1525–1529.

5. Lovell, C.R., Burton, J.L., and Horrobin, D.F. Treatment of Atopic Eczema with Evening Primrose Oil (1981) *Lancet i,* 278.
6. Wright, S., and Burton, J.L. Oral Evening Primrose-seed Oil Improves Atopic Eczema (1982) *Lancet ii,* 1120–1122.
7. Chapkin, R.S., and Ziboh, V.A. Inability of Skin Enzyme Preparations to Biosynthesize Arachidonic Acid from Linoleic Acid (1984) *Biochem. Biophys. Res. Commun. 124,* 784–792.
8. Chapkin, R.S., Ziboh, V.A., Marcelo, C.L., and Voorhees, J.J. Metabolism of Essential Fatty Acids by Human Epidermal Enzyme Preparations: Evidence of Chain Elongation (1986) *J. Lipid Res. 27,* 945–954.
9. Kragballe, K., Desjarlais, L., and Voorhees, J.J. Leukotrienes B_4, C_4, and D_4 Stimulate DNA Synthesis in Cultured Human Epidermal Keratinocytes (1985) *Br. J. Dermatol. 113,* 43–52.
10. Soter, N.A., Lewis, R.A., Corey, E.J., and Austen, K.F. Local Effects of Synthetic Leukotrienes (LTC_4, LTD_4, LTE_4, LTB_4) in Human Skin (1983) *J. Invest. Dermatol. 80,* 115–118.
11. Camp, R., Jones, R.R., Brain S., Woollard, P., Greaves, M. Production of Intraepidermal Microabscesses by Topical Application of Leukotriene B_4 (1984) *J. Invest. Dermatol. 82,* 202–204.
12. Dowd, P.M., Black, A.K., Woollard P.M., Camp, R.D., and Graves, M.W. Cutaneous Responses to 12-Hydroxy-5,8,10,14-eicosatetraenoic Acid (12-HETE) (1985) *J. Invest. Dermatol. 84,* 537–541.
13. Fletcher, M.P., and Seligmann, B.E. Monitoring Human Neutrophil Granule Secretion by Flow Cytometry: Secretion and Membrane Potential Changes Assessed by Light Scatter and a Fluorescent Probe of Membrane Potential (1985) *J. Leukol. Biol. 37,* 431–447.
14. Miller, C.C., and Ziboh, V.A. Induction of Epidermal Hyperproliferation by Topical n-3 Polyunsaturated Fatty Acids on Guinea Pig Skin Linked to Decreased Levels of 13-Hydroxyoctadecadienoic Acid (13-HODE) (1990) *J. Invest. Dermatol. 94,* 353–358.
15. Cho, Y., and Ziboh, V.A. Incorporation of 13-Hydroxyoctadecadienoic Acid (13-HODE) into Epidemal Ceramides and Phospholipids: Phospholipase Catalyzed Release of Novel 13-HODE-containing Diacylglycerol (1994) *J. Lipid Res. 35,* 255–262.
16. Cho, Y., and Ziboh, V.A. Expression of Protein Kinase C Isozymes in Guinea Pig Epidermis: Selective Inhibition of PKC-β Activity by 13-Hydroxyoctadecadienoic Acid Containing Diacylglycerol (1994) *J. Lipid Res. 35,* 913–921.

Chapter 11

γ-Linolenic Acid, Inflammation, Immune Responses, and Rheumatoid Arthritis

Robert B. Zurier, Pamela DeLuca, and Deborah Rothman

University of Massachusetts Medical Center, 55 Lake Avenue North, Worcester, MA 01655-0335

Essential fatty acids (EFA) are "essential" not only because of their physiological importance, but because they must be derived directly or in partially elaborated form from the diet. Thus, these acids may be classified as vitamins (indeed they were once called vitamin F). Two groups of fatty acids are essential to the body: the ω-6 (n-6) series derived from linoleic acid (18:2 n-6), and the ω-3 (n-3) series derived from α-linolenic acid (18:3 n-3). Fatty acids provide energy, are an integral part of cell membranes, and certain ones are precursors for prostaglandins (PG), thromboxanes (TX), and leukotrienes (LT), collectively termed eicosanoids. Abundant experimental evidence supports the view that eicosanoids participate in the development and regulation of immunological and inflammatory responses (1). Because rheumatoid arthritis (RA) is characterized by inflammation, disordered immune regulation, and tissue injury, there is much interest in the role of eicosanoids in the regulation of host defense in RA patients. Because the detrimental effects of therapy for RA may be more difficult to manage than the disease itself, there is a need for new, safe approaches to the treatment of these patients.

Generation of a unique eicosanoid profile with different biological effects by administration of fatty acid precursors other than arachidonic acid (AA, 20:4n-6) is one approach under investigation. Although changes in eicosanoid production due to alteration of fatty acid intake formed the basis of the initial hypothesis for the anti-inflammatory effects of this type of treatment, it is likely that the precursor fatty acids themselves alter immune responses. The n-3 fatty acids eicosapentaenoic acid (EPA; 20:5n-3) and docosahexaenoic (DHA; 22:6n-3), prominent in fish oil lipids, inhibit formation of cyclooxygenase and lipoxygenase products derived from AA (2,3). Diets enriched in fish oil reduce the generation of platelet-activating factor by peripheral blood monocytes (4), and reduce production of interleukin-1 (IL-1) and tumor necrosis factor (TNF) by stimulated peripheral blood mononuclear cells (5). Fish oil supplements have therefore been used with modest success to suppress inflammation in experimental animal models (6,7) and in patients with RA (8,9).

Evidence obtained from experiments *in vitro* and *in vivo* suggests that other novel fatty acids may be safe and effective anti-inflammatory and immunomodulatory agents. For example, certain botanical lipids, notably those extracted from seeds of the evening primrose and borage plants, contain relatively large amounts of γ-linolenic acid (GLA; 18:3 n-6) which can be converted rapidly to dihomo-γ-linolenic acid (DGLA; 20:3 n-6), the fatty acid precursor of the monoenoic PGE_1, an eicosanoid with anti-inflammatory and immunoregulating properties (10–12). These properties include suppression of diverse T lymphocyte functions such as proliferation, cytotoxicity, and interleukin-2 (IL-2) production. PGE_1 also suppresses polymorphonuclear leucocyte and monocyte activation.

It is now known that PGE_1, PGE_2, and PGI_2 have separate receptors on cells (13). Although the biologic activities of corresponding members of the monoenoic (PGE_1) and dienoic (PGE_2) prostaglandins are in many cases qualitatively similar, in other respects they differ markedly. For example, PGE_1 inhibits aggregation of human platelets *in vitro* whereas PGE_2 does not influence this activity (14). Also, PGE_1 is much more effective than PGE_2 in increasing concentrations of cyclic AMP in human synovial cells in culture and in suppressing synovial cell proliferation (15,16). In addition, PGE_1 relaxes and PGE_2 contracts guinea pig tracheal muscle. More striking are the antagonistic effects of PGE_1 (vasodilate) and PGE_2 (vasoconstrict) on bovine coronary and human chorionic plate arteries (17,18). In fact, PGE_1 prevents PGE_2-induced constriction of chorionic plate arteries. Many effects of PGE_1 *in vitro* are seen at concentrations of 10^{-9}–10^{-13} M (19).

An approach to PGE_1 therapy, first suggested by Willis (20), is provision of PGE_1 precursors such as GLA or DGLA. The extremely short half-life of natural prostaglandins allows moment to moment regulation of cell function in response to external stimuli and internal messengers. Therefore, enrichment of cells with DGLA should enable PGE_1 production to be increased as needed without overriding the physiological controls which modulate rapid changes in its synthesis and degradation.

DGLA competes with arachidonate for oxidative enzymes, thereby reducing production of cyclooxygenase products derived from arachidonate. In addition, DGLA cannot be converted to inflammatory LT by 5-lipoxygenase. Instead, it is converted to 15-hydroxy-DGLA, which can inhibit 5-lipoxygenase activity (21). GLA enrichment of diet suppresses acute and chronic inflammation as well as joint tissue injury in several experimental animal models (22,23). In animals treated with evening primrose or borage seed oils, cells from inflammatory exudate are enriched in GLA and DGLA, exudate PGE_2 and LTB_4 concentrations are reduced, and leucocyte effector functions (chemotaxis, lysosomal enzyme release) are suppressed. Enrichment with DGLA of synovial cells in culture leads to a marked reduction in PGE_2 synthesis, a substantial increase in PGE_1 production, and reduction of IL-1 induced synovial cell proliferation (16). The addition of AA (which increases PGE_2 substantially) or of EPA to cultures does not modify synovial cell proliferation. The antiproliferative effect of DGLA is prevented by indomethacin. GLA administration to normal volunteers increases monocyte production of PGE_1 and reduces production of LTB_4 (24). Pullman-Mooar et al. (25) observed that the ratio of DGLA to AA in circulating mononuclear cells increased significantly in both healthy subjects and

RA patients given 1.1 g/d GLA for 12 wk. The DGLA/AA ratio reflects the potential capacity of DGLA to compete with arachidonic acid for oxidative enzymes. LTB_4, LTC_4, and total PGE production by stimulated peripheral blood monocytes were also reduced. Thus, botanical lipids have anti-inflammatory actions due to their ability to reduce synthesis of those oxygenation products of AA which are potent mediators of inflammation.

In addition to their role as eicosanoid precursors, fatty acids are of major importance in maintaining cell membrane structure and are key determinants of the behavior of membrane-bound enzymes and receptors (26). Fatty acids can exert these functions directly and therefore may themselves be important regulators of immune responses. DGLA suppresses IL-2 production by human PBMC *in vitro*, suppresses proliferation of IL-2-dependent human T lymphocytes, and reduces expression of activation markers on T lymphocytes directly, in a manner which is independent of its conversion to an eicosanoid (27,28). In addition, DGLA, AA, and EPA all suppress long-term growth of T lymphocytes harvested from synovial tissue and fluid obtained from RA patients (29). These observations indicate that fatty acids can modulate immune responses by acting directly on T cells and suggest that alteration of cellular fatty acids may be a worthwhile approach to the control of inflammation.

Treatment of Rheumatoid Arthritis with γ-Linolenic Acid

In one of the first efforts to treat RA with GLA, 20 patients were given 432 mg/d GLA in evening primrose oil for 3 mo (30). Several days before the study began, patients stopped treatment with anti-inflammatory drugs. GLA treatment did not influence disease activity or plasma or urine concentrations of PGE_1. However, because disease activity remained stable despite the absence of other medication, it is possible the GLA did have a small therapeutic effect. The results might have been more impressive if a higher dose of GLA had been given for a longer period of time.

In a subsequent double-blind placebo-controlled trial of 49 RA patients (31), both GLA alone (540 mg/d) and GLA with EPA (450mg/d GLA and 240 mg/d EPA) were studied. Patients remained on a stable nonsteroidal anti-inflammatory drug (NSAID) dose for the first 3 mo of a 15-mo study. Thereafter, they were instructed to decrease or stop the NSAID if it could be done without exacerbation of symptoms. Although objective improvement was not seen in either treatment group, over 90% of patients in each treatment group (GLA alone and GLA with EPA) felt subjective improvement in their condition at 12 mo. Also, 73% of patients on GLA alone and 80% on GLA plus EPA, compared with 33% of patients given placebo, were able to reduce or stop NSAID by 12 mo.

Based on these promising results, Brzeski et al. (32) did a 6-mo study of 40 patients with RA who had evidence (endoscopic, radiographic, or clinical symptoms) suggestive of upper gastrointestinal lesions, presumably due to NSAID use. The aim of the study was to determine whether patients given GLA would experience enough improvement in joint symptoms to allow reduction of the NSAID dose. Patients were given either 6 g/d of evening primrose oil (540 mg/d GLA) or 6 g/d of olive oil. Morning stiffness was reduced significantly at both 3 and 6 mo in the GLA-treated group, and a reduction in pain and articular index was seen at 6 mo in patients given olive oil. However, only 23% of the patients in the GLA group and 18% of patients in the olive oil group were able to reduce their NSAID dose. Although patients in this study had more severe RA than patients in the earlier study cited above (31), none were treated with second-line drugs. Beneficial effects of olive oil on RA have been reported (33). Therefore, olive oil can no longer be considered an inert placebo. Also, individual variations in levels of $\Delta 5$ desaturase may alter the response to GLA. It is generally believed that humans have low levels of this enzyme, and hence limited conversion of DGLA to arachidonic acid. However, a small but significant increase in serum arachidonic acid was reported in one group of RA patients who took 1.8 g/d GLA for 3 mo (34). Reduced plasma PGE_2 in these patients was associated with a good therapeutic response to GLA.

In a study designed to evaluate the effects of GLA administration on *in vitro* biochemical responses, Pullman-Mooar et al. (25) noted clinical improvement in RA patients who were given 1.1 g/d GLA in borage seed oil for 3 months in an open manner. Sleep patterns, joint scores, duration of morning stiffness, and the patients' overall assessment of disease activity all improved.

More recently, GLA treatment of RA was evaluated in a 24-wk, randomized, double-blind, placebo-controlled (cottonseed oil) trial (35). Only patients with RA on stable NSAID and/or low corticosteroid doses (less than 10 mg/d prednisone or equivalent) were allowed to participate. Treatment with GLA (1.4 g/d in borage seed oil; 4 capsules three times daily) resulted in clinically important reductions in signs and symptoms of disease activity. In contrast, patients given placebo exhibited no change or worsening of disease. GLA reduced the number of tender joints by 36%, the tender joint score by 45%, swollen joint count by 28%, and the swollen joint score by 41%, whereas the placebo group did not demonstrate significant improvement in any measure. Overall clinical responses (greater than 25% improvement in four measures) were also significantly better in the treatment group. Platelet counts were reduced significantly in the GLA group but erythrocyte sedimentation rate did not change appreciably in either group. A second controlled trial of GLA treatment of 56 RA patients is being done at the University of Massachusetts Medical Center. The GLA dose has been increased to 2.4 g/d; the higher dose of GLA appears to be well tolerated. Although compliance does not appear to be a major problem in clinical trials of RA in general, and in these studies with GLA in particular, long-term ingestion of 8–12 capsules daily is a concern. Compliance in these studies was monitored by capsule counts. In some patients, plasma fatty acid analyses were done, and concentrations of DGLA as high as 40 μg/mL were achieved. It is possible that further experience with GLA therapy will allow lower maintenance doses of GLA to be used, in the manner of treatment with gold salts.

Another source of GLA that has been studied in the treatment of RA is black currant seed oil (BCO). In addition to GLA, BCO contains α-linolenic acid which can be metabolized to EPA, an eicosanoid precursor that can compete with arachidonate for oxidative enzymes. Fish oil, also rich in EPA, enhances the antiinflammatory effect of GLA in animal models (36). BCO suppresses inflammation in rats

(37), and it reduced joint pain and swelling in a small placebo-controlled clinical trial of RA patients with active synovitis (38).

Few adverse effects of plant seed oil administration have been observed. Stool softening, belching, and an occasional feeling of abdominal bloating have been reported. Nonetheless, potential adverse effects cannot be dismissed. Experience teaches that the longer a given therapy is used, the greater the incidence of adverse effects. Administration of long-chain polyunsaturated fatty acids increases the likelihood of lipid peroxidation with its associated toxic effects on cells. It is not known whether an increased requirement for an antioxidant (such as vitamins E and C) accompanies increased intake of long-chain unsaturated fatty acids. Our own *in vitro* studies (Baker et al., unpublished) indicate no increase in lipid peroxidation after addition of DGLA to human cells. Because these novel fatty acids can reduce inflammation and affect immunocytes, the question arises whether they can compromise the immune system. Susceptibility to infection has not been observed but must be considered. Another concern (39) of prolonged GLA administration is the potential for slow accumulation of tissue arachidonic acid. Adverse effects of increased arachidonate levels might be more pronounced after GLA treatment is stopped, when DGLA production would no longer be increased. We have not observed increased arachidonate in plasma, leucocytes, or platelets from RA patients on GLA for 6- to 12-mo periods.

GLA appears to be a safe and useful therapy for treatment of RA patients. A minimum dose of 1.4 g/d GLA for at least 3 mon appears to be necessary before the full effectiveness of GLA therapy can be expected. It is possible that the addition of GLA to other drugs may prove to be the most effective way to use this agent.

The potential ability of particular fatty acids to regulate cell activation, immune responses, and inflammation is exciting to consider at the clinical, cellular, and molecular levels. A better understanding of how fatty acids modulate the function of cells involved in host defense might lead to development of new, benign treatment for diseases characterized by acute and chronic inflammation.

Acknowledgments

The work was supported in part by National Institutes of Health grants RO-1 AR38501 and T32-AR07572, and Food and Drug Administration grant FD-R-000756. The manuscript was typed by Mrs. Carol Mader.

References

1. Goodwin, J.S., and Ceuppens, J. The Regulation of Immune Responses by Prostaglandins (1983) *J. Clin. Immunol. 3*, 295–308.
2. Needleman, P., Raz, A., Minkes, M.S., Ferrendelli, J.A., and Sprecher, H. Trienoic Prostaglandins: Prostacyclin and Thromboxane Biosynthesis and Unique Biological Properties (1979) *Proc. Natl. Acad. Sci. U.S.A 76*, 944–950.
3. Lee, T.H., Hoover, R.L., Williams, J.D., Sperling, R.I., Ravelese, J., Spur, B.W., Robinson, D.R., Corey, E.J., Lewis, R.A., and Austen, K.E. Effect of Dietary Enrichment

with Eicosapentaenoic and Docosahexaenoic Acids on in Vitro Neutrophil and Monocyte Leukotriene Generation and Neutrophil Function (1986) *N. Engl. J. Med. 312,* 1217–1224.

4. Sperling, R.I., Weinblatt, M., Robin, J.L., Ravalese, J., Hoover, R.L., House, F., Coblyn, J.S., Fraser, P.A., Spur, B.W., Robinson, D.R., Lewis, R.A., and Austen, K.E. Effects of Dietary Supplementation with Marine Fish Oil on Leukocyte Lipid Mediator Generation and Function in Rheumatoid Arthritis (1987) *Arthritis Rheum. 30,* 988–997.

5. Endres, S., Ghorbani, R., Kelly, V.E., Georgilis, K., Lonnemann, G., VanderMeer, J.W.M., Cannon, J.G., Rogers, T.S., Klempner, M.S., Weber, P.C., Schaefer, E.J., Wolff, S.M., and Dinarello, C.A. The Effect of Dietary Supplementation with n-3 Polyunsaturated Fatty Acids on the Synthesis of Interleukin-1 and Tumor Necrosis Factor by Mononuclear Cells (1989) *N. Engl. J. Med. 320,* 265–271.

6. Prickett, J.D., Robinson, D.R., and Steinberg, A.D. Dietary Enrichment with the Polyunsaturated Fatty Acid Eicosapentaenoic Acid Prevents Proteinuria and Prolongs Survival in NZB × NZW F_1 Mice (1981) *J. Clin. Invest. 68,* 556–567.

7. Leslie, C.A., Gonnerman, W.A., Ullman, M.D., Hayes, K.C., Franzblau, C., and Cathcart, E.S. Dietary Fish Oil Modulates Macrophage Fatty Acids and Decreases Arthritis Susceptibility in Mice (1985) *J. Exp. Med. 162,* 1336–1349.

8. Kremer, J.M., Jubiz, W., Michalek, A., Rynes, R.I., Bartholomew, L.E., Bigaouette, J., Timchalk, M., Beeler, D., and Lininger, L. Fish–Oil Fatty Acid Supplementation in Active Rheumatoid Arthritis (1987) *Ann. Int. Med. 106,* 497–504.

9. Cleland, L.G., French, J.K., Betts, W.H., Murphy, G.A., and Elliott, M.J. Clinical and Biochemical Effects of Dietary Fish Oil Supplements in Rheumatoid Arthritis (1988) *J. Rheumatol. 15,* 1471–1475.

10. Fantone, J.C., Kunkel, S.L., Ward, P.A., and Zurier, R.B. Suppression by Prostaglandin E_1 of Vascular Permeability Induced by Vasoactive Inflammatory Mediators (1980) *J. Immunol. 125,* 2591–2600.

11. Kunkel, S.L., Thrall, R.S., Kunkel, R.G., McCormack, J.R., Ward, P.A., and Zurier, R.B. Suppression of Immune Complex Vasculitis by Prostaglandins (1979) *J. Clin. Invest. 64,* 1525–1535.

12. Zurier, R.B. Prostaglandin E_1: Is It Useful? (1990) *J. Rheumatol. 17,* 1439–1441, (editorial).

13. Datta-Roy, A.K., Colman, R.W., and Sinha, A.K. Prostaglandin E_1 and E_2 Receptors of Human Erythrocyte Membrane (1983) *J. Cell Biol. 97,* 403–404.

14. Kloeze, J. Relationship Between Chemical Structure and Platelet Aggregation Activity of Prostaglandins (1969) *Biochim. Biophys. Acta 187,* 285–292.

15. Newcombe, D.S., Coisek, C.P., Ishikawa, Y., and Fahey, J.V. Human Synoviocytes: Activation and Desensitization by Prostaglandins and L-epinephrine (1975) *Proc. Natl. Acad. Sci. U.S.A. 72,* 3124–3128.

16. Baker, D.G., Krakauer, K.A., Tate, G.A., Laposata, M., and Zurier, R.B. Suppression of Human Synovial Cell Proliferation by Dihomo-γ-Linolenic Acid (1989) *Arthritis Rheum. 32,* 1273–1281.

17. Suzuki, T., Nakanishi, H., and Makahata, N. Antagonism Between Prostaglandin E_1 and PGE_2 in Bovine Coronary Arteries (1982) *Fukushima J. Med. Sci. 29,* 1–11.

18. Kitson, G.E., and Pipkin, F.B. Effects of Interactions of Prostaglandins E_1 and E_2 on Human Chorionic Plate Arteries (1981) *Am. J. Obstet. Gynecol. 140,* 683–692.

19. Manevich, E.M., Lakin, K.M., Archakov, A.I., Li, V.S., Molotkovskyu, J.G., Bezuglov, V.V., and Bergelson, L.D. Influence of Cholesterol and Prostaglandin E_1 on the Molecular

Organization of Phospholipids in the Erythrocyte Membrane. A Fluorescent Polarization Study with Lipid Specific Probes (1985) *Biochim. Biophys. Acta 815,* 455–460.
20. Willis, A.L. Nutritional and Pharmacological Factors in Eicosanoid Biology (1981) *Nutr. Rev.,* 289–300.
21. Ziboh, V.A., and Chapikin, R.S. Biologic Significance of Polyunsaturated Fatty Acids in the Skin (1987) *Arch. Dermatol. 123,* 1686–1690.
22. Tate, G., Mandell, B.F., Karmali, R.A., Laposata, M., Baker, D.G., Schumacher. H.R., and Zurier, R.B. Suppression of Monosodium Urate Crystal-induced Acute Inflammation by Diets Enriched with Gamma-linolenic Acid and Eicosapentaenoic Acid (1988) *Arthritis Rheum. 31,* 1543–1551.
23. Tate, G., Mandell, B.F., Laposata, M., Ohliger, D., Baker, D.G., Schumacher, H.R., and Zurier, R.B. Suppression of Acute and Chronic Inflammation by Dietary Gamma Linolenic Acid (1989) *J. Rheumatol. 16,* 1729–1736.
24. Callegari, P., and Zurier, R.B. Botanical Lipids: Potential Role in Modulation of Immunologic Responses and Inflammatory Reactions (1991) *Rheum. Dis. Clin. N. Amer. 17,* 415–425.
25. Pullman-Mooar, S., Laposata, M., Lem, D., Holman, R.T., Leventhal, L.J., DeMarco, D.M., and Zurier, R.B. Alterations of the Cellular Fatty Acid Profile and the Production of Eicosanoids in Human Monocytes by Gamma-linolenic Acid (1990) *Arthritis Rheum. 33,* 1526–1533.
26. McMurchie, E.J. Dietary Lipids and the Regulation of Membrane Fluidity and Function (1988) in *Physiological Regulation of Membrane Fluidity,* Alan R. Liss, Inc., New York, pp. 189–237.
27. Santoli, D., and Zurier, R.B. Prostaglandin E Precursor Fatty Acids Inhibit Human IL-2 Production by a PGE-Independent Mechanism (1989) *J. Immunol. 143,* 1303–1309.
28. Santoli, D., Phillips, P.D., Colt, T.L., and Zurier, R.B. Suppression of Interleukin 2-Dependent Human T Cell Growth by E-series Prostaglandins (PGE) and Their Precursor Fatty Acids: Evidence for a PGE-Independent Mechanism of Inhibition by the Fatty Acids (1990) *J. Clin. Invest. 85,* 424–432.
29. DeMarco, D.M., Santoli, D., and Zurier, R.B. Effects of Fatty Acids on Proliferation and Activation of Human Synovial Compartment Lymphocytes (1994) *J. Leuk. Biol. 56,* 612–615.
30. Mörk-Hansen, T., Lerche, A., Kassis, V., Lorenzen, I., and Sondergaard, J. Treatment of Rheumatoid Arthritis with Prostaglandin E_1 Precursors *cis*-Linoleic Acid and γ-Linolenic Acid (1983) *Scand. J. Rheumatol. 12,* 85–88.
31. Belch, J.J.F., Ansell, D., Madhok, A.R., O Dowd, A., and Sturrock R.D. Effects of Altering Dietary Essential Fatty Acids on Requirements for Non-steroidal Anti-Inflammatory Drugs in Patients with Rheumatoid Arthritis: A Double Blind Placebo Controlled Study (1988) *Ann. Rheum. Dis. 47,* 96–104.
32. Brzeski, M., Madhok, R., and Capell, H.A. Evening Primrose Oil in Patients with Rheumatoid Arthritis and Side-effects of Non-Steroidal Antiinflammatory Drugs (1991) *Br. J. Rheum. 30,* 370–372.
33. Darlington, L.G., and Ramsey, N.W. Olive Oil for Rheumatoid Patients? (1987) *Br. J. Rheum. 26 (Suppl.),* 215.
34. Jantti, J., Nikkari, T., and Solakivi, T. Evening Primrose Oil in Rheumatoid Arthritis: Changes in Serum Lipids and Fatty Acids (1989) *Ann. Rheum. Dis. 48,* 124–127.

35. Leventhal, L.J., Boyce, E.G., and Zurier, R.B. Treatment of Rheumatoid Arthritis with Gammalinolenic Acid (1993) *Ann. Int. Med. 119*, 867–873.
36. Tate, G.A., Mandell, B.F., Karmali, R.A., Laposata, M., Baker, D.G., Schumacher, H.R., and Zurier, R.B. Suppression of Monosodium Urate Crystal-induced Inflammation by Diets Enriched with Gamma-linolenic Acid and Eicosapentaenoic Acid (1988) *Arthritis Rheum. 31*, 1543–1551.
37. Tate, G.A., and Zurier, R.B. Suppression of Monosodium Urate Crystal-induced Inflammation by Black Currant Seed Oil (1994) *Agents and Actions 43*, 35–38.
38. Leventhal, L.J., Boyce, E.G., and Zurier, R.B. Treatment of Rheumatoid Arthritis with Black Currant Seed Oil (1994) *Br. J. Rheumatol. 33*, 847–852.
39. Phinney, S. Potential Risk of Prolonged Gamma-linolenic Use (1994) *Ann. Int. Med. 120*, 692.

Chapter 12

The Anti-Inflammatory Role of γ-Linolenic and Eicosapentaenoic Acids in Acute Lung Injury

Michael D. Karlstad,[a] John D. Palombo,[b] Michael J. Murray,[c] and Stephen J. DeMichele[d]

[a]Department of Anesthesiology, Graduate School of Medicine, University of Tennessee Medical Center, Knoxville, TN 37920-6999

[b]New England Deaconess Hospital, Harvard Medical School, Boston, MA 02215

[c]Department of Anesthesiology and Critical Care Service, Mayo Clinic and Mayo Foundation, Rochester, MN 55905

[d]Ross Products Division, Abbott Laboratories, Columbus, OH 43215

Introduction

Proinflammatory eicosanoids are thought to play a central role in the development of systemic inflammatory response syndrome, septic shock, acute lung injury (ALI), and adult respiratory distress syndrome (ARDS). Important advances in the understanding of lung injury as an inflammatory disease have resulted in a shift of emphasis from supportive to anti-inflammatory therapy. We will review in this chapter the results of three animal studies (1–3) that show that nutritional intervention with diets containing fish and borage oil rapidly modulates the phospholipid fatty acid composition of inflammatory cell membranes, reduces the synthesis of important proinflammatory eicosanoids of lung injury, attenuates endotoxin-induced increases in pulmonary microvascular protein permeability, and improves cardiopulmonary hemodynamics and respiratory gas exchange in models of ALI. We have attributed these beneficial anti-inflammatory effects of nutritional therapy, in large part, to eicosapentaenoic acid (EPA, 20:5n-3) and γ-linolenic acid (GLA, 18:3n-6), the fatty acids present at high levels in fish and borage oil, respectively, and to modulation of the synthesis of 1-, 2-, and 3-series prostaglandins (PGs) and 4- and 5-series leukotrienes (LTs) by cells of the inflammatory process.

Rationale for the Provision of Eicosapentaenoic Acid in Inflammatory Disorders

Experimental and clinical studies have shown that the host's immune response can be modulated by nutritional intervention with diets enriched with fish oil containing EPA and docosahexaenoic (DHA, 22:6n-3) acids. EPA, DHA, and other n-3 polyunsaturated fatty acids (PUFAs) displace arachidonic acid (AA, 20:4n-6) from cell membrane phospholipids (4). AA, a membrane polyunsaturated fatty acid derived from dietary linoleic acid (LA, 18:2n-6), has a central role in the proinflammatory effects of activated macrophages. Trauma and sepsis activate phospholipase A_2 and promote the cleavage of AA from the phospholipid pools of macrophages (5–7). AA may then be oxidized by cyclooxygenase and lipoxygenase to form eicosanoids that enhance platelet aggregation, immunosuppression, and leukosequestration. AA has been identified as a primary intracellular activator of macrophage NADPH oxidase, which elicits the respiratory burst reaction (8,9). Oxygen radicals generated during the respiratory burst from alveolar macrophages (AMϕ) promote membrane lipid peroxidation, potentiating damage to type II pneumocytes that generate surfactant (10). The persistent and uncontrolled release of AA-derived inflammatory mediators and reactive oxygen species causes lung inflammation, edema, and alveolar collapse. These clinical signs are hallmark features that characterize ARDS (6,11,12). Thus, therapeutic modalities that limit the availability and/or release of AA from AMϕ phospholipids may prove beneficial to critically ill patients at risk of developing ARDS.

Activated macrophages from animals fed n-3 fatty acid-enriched diets form reduced amounts of proinflammatory PGs and LTs relative to control animals given a standard diet containing n-6 (i.e., LA) PUFAs (13,14). EPA competes with AA for binding sites on cyclooxygenase and lipoxygenase, thereby serving as the progenitor of trienoic eicosanoids which exhibit reduced inflammatory, chemotactic and vasoactive properties relative to the dienoic series derived from AA (Fig. 12.1).

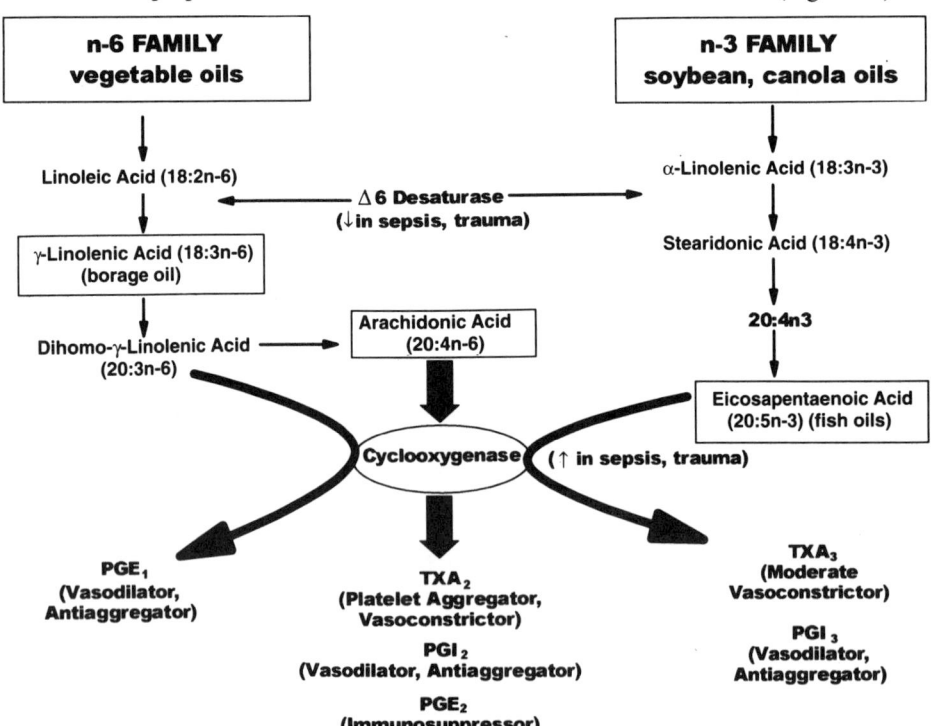

Fig. 12.1. Metabolic pathways for conversion of dietary polyunsaturated fatty acids to eicosanoids by the alveolar macrophage.

Other putative benefits derived from dietary intervention with n-3 PUFA include reduced formation of tumor necrosis factor α (TNF-α) and interleukin 1β by mononuclear cells (13,15). Neutrophil chemotaxis also appears to be attenuated in association with n-3 PUFA supplementation (16). It has been shown that oral supplementation with n-3-enriched diets reduced pulmonary leukosequestration and improved arterial oxygen pressure (PaO$_2$), lung morphology and survival in animals challenged with endotoxin (17,18) or live *Escherichia coli* (19) relative to animals pretreated with an LA-enriched diet. Improved lung function in the animals pretreated with the diets containing n-3 PUFAs was directly associated with decreased concentrations of plasma AA-derived eicosanoids.

Rationale for the Provision of γ-Linolenic Acid in Inflammatory Disorders

A common misconception exists that LA is rapidly converted to its desaturated and elongated intermediates, GLA, dihomo-γ-linolenic acid (DGLA, 20:3n-6), and AA and that there is a simple and direct relationship between LA intake and 2-series PG production. The conversion of LA to GLA in tissues is incomplete (4–20%) and may not occur when the enzyme Δ6-desaturase is absent or inactivated (20–22). GLA may become essential in pathological situations, such as stress, major surgical and medical disorders, diabetes, cancer, premature birth, and aging, in which Δ6-desaturase is thought to be deficient (20,23,24). A chronic imbalance between the essential fatty acid metabolites GLA, DGLA, AA, and EPA and their derivatives (1-, 2-, and 3-series PGs) has been proposed to be one contributing factor in the etiology of many serious diseases (inflammatory disorders, cardiovascular disorders, menstrual cycle disorders, and malignancy).

The oil extracted from the seeds of borage plant seeds contains relatively high concentrations of GLA (20–25%) as compared with black currant (15–20%) and evening primrose (8–10%) seed oils (25). GLA as a nutritional supplement is considered to be responsible for the apparent effectiveness of treatment of a variety of diseases including premenstrual syndrome and atopic eczema (20,21,26). GLA is elongated to DGLA which competes with AA for cyclooxygenase binding sites and serves as the precursor of the monoenoic PGs, e.g., PGE$_1$, which have anti-inflammatory properties (Fig. 12.1) (26). The biologic responses of PGE$_1$ include vasodilatation and suppression of leukocyte effector functions, e.g., chemotaxis and lysosomal enzyme release (26,27). DGLA can be converted to a 15-hydroperoxy derivative which inhibits conversion of AA to the undesirable 4-series LTs (26). In a recent clinical study, continuous enteral administration of a GLA-enriched high fat (45.7% of kcal) diet to critically injured patients for 3 wk promoted DGLA incorporation into red cell phospholipids without increasing AA (28). Short-term intravenous infusion of a parenteral diet enriched with GLA to endotoxemic rats with a 30% surface area scald burn increased plasma DGLA and modulated plasma ratios of dienoic eicosanoids relative to injured rats receiving an isocaloric quantity of LA-enriched diet (29). Peritoneal macrophages from mice fed a borage oil-enriched diet had greater incorporation of DGLA into the phospholipid fraction and yielded significantly higher amounts of PGE_1 *in vitro* after zymosan stimulation compared with control mice given a corn oil (i.e., LA-enriched) diet (30). Both GLA and DGLA supplements suppress acute and chronic inflammation as well as joint tissue injury in several experimental animal models (27,31–33). In animals treated with borage oil, cells from inflammatory exudate are enriched in GLA and DGLA, exudate PGE_2 and LTB_4 concentrations are reduced (27,31,32) and leukocyte effector functions (chemotaxis, lysosomal enzyme release) are suppressed (33). Thus GLA should have anti-inflammatory actions analogous to those of the more extensively studied n-3 fatty acids due to its capacity to reduce synthesis of AA-derived proinflammatory mediators.

Rationale for the Combination of Eicosapentaenoic and γ-Linolenic Acids in Acute Lung Injury

Gram-negative sepsis and endotoxemia initiate inflammatory responses that have been implicated in the pathogenesis of ARDS (34). The clinical treatment of critically ill patients with ARDS is usually supportive, consisting primarily of fluid resuscitation for circulatory support and mechanical ventilation to improve arterial oxygenation. However, current treatment modalities are associated with a mortality rate greater than 50% (35) and have not addressed the role of proinflammatory mediators in the pathogenesis of ARDS. High fat, low carbohydrate enteral diets have been designed to reduce minute ventilation and ventilatory demand by lowering CO_2 production in ventilator-dependent patients. However, the lipids found in these formulations may not be suitable for patients at risk of or exhibiting signs of ARDS because they are typically rich in LA, the metabolic precursor of AA and the proinflammatory 2-series PGs and 4-series LTs. These eicosanoids, along with various cytokines (interleukin-1 [IL-1], TNF-α, IL-6, and IL-8), complement (C5a), and platelet-activating factor, are important mediators of inflammation of the lung. The remainder of this chapter will review our research findings on the effects of enteral nutrition with both fish and borage oil on the modulation of 1-, 2-, and 3-series PGs and 4- and 5-series LTs in animal models of ALI and endotoxemia.

Study I. Attenuation of Cardiopulmonary Dysfunction with GLA and EPA in a Pig Model of Acute Lung Injury

The use of diets containing high levels of fat in patients with respiratory distress has led to an increased interest in understanding the role of fatty acids in lung physiology. It has been shown that the lungs play a major role in eicosanoid metabolism. Metabolites of AA, thromboxane A_2 (TXA_2), and LTB_4 have potent effects on bronchial and vascular smooth muscle by promoting bronchoconstriction (36) and pulmonary arteriolar vasoconstriction (37), and by increasing microvascular permeability (38). Reduction in the production of these proinflammatory agents has been associated with improved outcome in clinical (39) and animal studies (40). Dietary supplementation with n-3 fatty acids from fish oil can alter the production of proinflammatory eicosanoids produced from n-6 fatty acids. The n-3 fatty acids, EPA and DHA from fish oil, compete with AA in several ways. They inhibit Δ5-desaturase activity and thereby reduce the conversion of dietary LA to AA (22). EPA and DHA also competitively displace LA and AA from tissue phospholipid pools, thereby reducing the availability of AA for eicosanoid production (2-series PGs, 4-series LTs). When EPA is substituted for AA, the resulting PGs and LTs are markedly less chemotactic, vasoconstrictive and proinflammatory than their AA counterparts. The net effect of substituting n-3 fatty acids for n-6 fatty acids is a change in the eicosanoid balance which then strongly favors an anti-inflammatory and vasodilatory state. To assess this, we examined the physiologic effects of diets containing fish and borage oils in a porcine model of endotoxin-induced ALI. An unanesthetized pig model was selected because of its physiologic and metabolic similarities to humans.

Methods

Approval to conduct this study was granted by the Animal Care and Use Committee of Mayo Clinic. Thirty-six, 15–25 kg castrated male pigs (sus scrofa: mixed breeds) were initially randomized into three groups of 12 pigs each and were fed eucaloric (175 kcal/kg per day) and isonitrogenous enteral diets for eight days containing either LA, EPA, or a combination of EPA and GLA; Diets A, B, and C, respectively. Diets provided 16.7% of calories from protein, 28.1% of calories from carbohydrate, and 55.1% of calories from lipid: Diet A, corn oil; Diet B, fish oil; Diet C, fish and borage oils. Diets B and C had nearly identical levels of medium-chain triglycerides and fish oil. To maintain a similar n-6 to n-3 fatty acid ratio between the two diets, LA was replaced with GLA in Diet C. All diets were formulated and supplied by Ross Products Division, Abbott Laboratories, Columbus, OH (Table 12.1).

On the 8th day, after the daily diet had been consumed, the animals were fasted. Eighteen hours later the unanesthetized animal was placed in a standing harness. A pulmonary artery catheter was inserted via the previously placed femoral venous introducer into the pulmonary artery for hemodynamic and cardiac output measurements. Systemic arterial, pulmonary arterial, right atrial, and pulmonary capillary wedge pressures, electrocardiogram and cardiac output were monitored continuously. Cardiac output was measured by a thermodilution technique utilizing

TABLE 12.1 Fatty Acid Composition of Experimental Enteral Diets

Fatty Acid (%)	Diet A Corn Oil	Diet B Fish Oil	Diet C Fish and Borage Oil
18:2n-6	58.9	22.5	16.7
18:3n-6	0	0.08	4.7
18:3n-3	1.1	5.2	3.7
20:5n-3	0	5.4	5.7
22:6n-3	0	2.4	2.5
n-6/n-3 Ratio	53.5	1.6	1.6

an American Edwards cardiac output computer. Normal saline was infused in all animals at a rate of 60 mL/h. After a brief stabilization period (1 h), baseline measures were obtained.

ALI was induced with a 0.1 mg/kg intravenous bolus of *E. coli* endotoxin (lipopolysaccharide from *E. coli* serotype 055:B5; Sigma Chemical, St Louis, MO) with continuous intravenous infusion of endotoxin at 0.075 mg/(kg·h) for 4 h. Only normal saline was infused into pigs randomized to the control group. Hemodynamic and blood gas measurements were repeated at 20 min, 1, 2, and 4 h postinfusion. Blood was drawn for TXB_2 and platelet phospholipid fatty acid analyses using RIA and gas chromatography, respectively. Results observed for the saline control animals did not alter the conclusions associated with data gathered on the endotoxin-treated pigs. Thus, to minimize redundancy, only those findings from the endotoxin-challenged animals are presented. Saline data are presented to qualify noteworthy effects seen in the endotoxemic pigs.

Results and Discussion

Our model of porcine ALI was chosen to assess the potential therapeutic benefits of a GLA-supplemented diet on hemodynamic and pulmonary dysfunction and its effects on vasoactive eicosanoids. The intravenous infusion of endotoxin in pigs has been used in many studies to provide an experimental model of ALI (18,41–44). *E. coli* endotoxin has been shown to initiate an inflammatory cascade, both by a direct effect on neutrophils as well as on microvascular endothelium, with accumulation of inflammatory cells in the microcirculation, interstitium, and the air spaces of the lung (45–47). Intravenous infusion of *E. coli* endotoxin produces pulmonary arterial hypertension, increases in pulmonary vascular resistance (PVR), bronchoconstriction, hypoxemia, shock and pulmonary edema (48–50). Many of the pathophysiologic features of ALI, mimicked in animal models, have been attributed to the effects of eicosanoids and in particular TXA_2 (51,52). These cyclooxygenase and lipoxygenase metabolites of AA stimulate aggregation of both platelets and neutrophils, constriction of both the vasculature and airways and may also cause increased permeability (36–38). Thus, these mediators may all contribute to the development of pulmonary hypertension, hypoxemia, and increased airway resistance observed during ALI.

In this study, important physiologic differences were found in pigs supplemented with GLA during endotoxemia. Pigs prefed a corn oil-supplemented diet for 8 d displayed the classical physiological indices of septic shock. However, nutritional intervention with either Diet B or C resulted in a significant attenuation of the early increase in PVR (Fig. 12.2), and an attenuation of the decrease in PaO_2 (Fig. 12.3), cardiac index (Fig. 12.4), and oxygen delivery (Fig. 12.5). These attenuations were diminished in the late phase response to endotoxin (2 to 4 h after endotoxin infusion) in pigs given Diet B (fish oil) only. These observations are consistent with those from previous studies that showed that the short-term consumption of a diet supplemented with n-3 fatty acids attenuated the early phase of pulmonary dysfunction associated with the administration of endotoxin (18,19). Pigs given Diet C (EPA + GLA), however, maintained the attenuation in hemo-

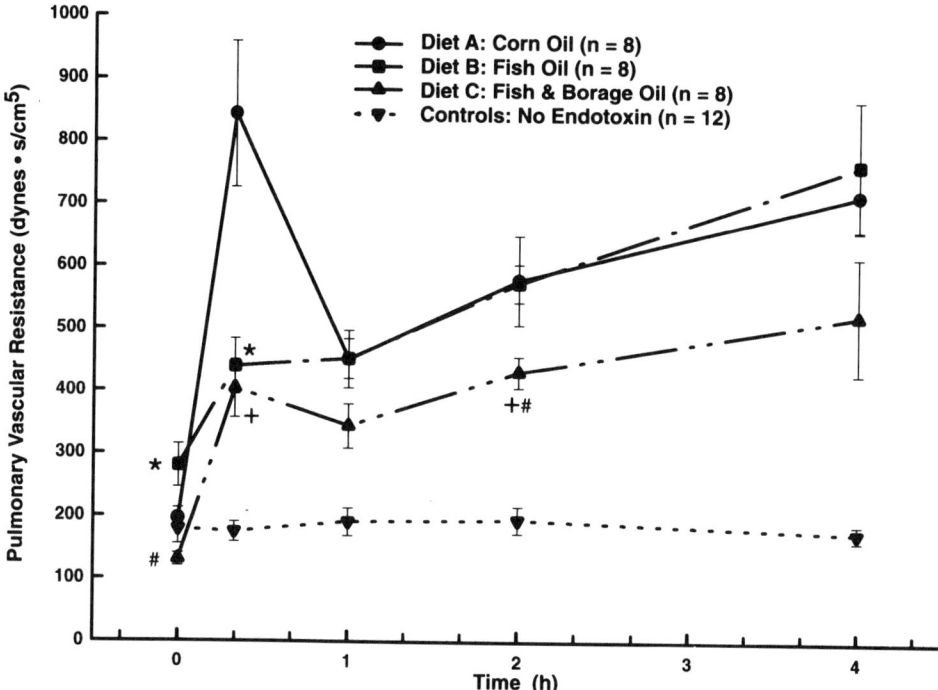

Fig. 12.2. Pulmonary vascular resistance was measured before and after endotoxin infusion in pigs fed enteral diets for 8 d containing either corn oil (Diet A), fish oil (Diet B), or a combination of fish and borage oils (Diet C). Pooled control pigs were infused with normal saline. $+P < 0.05$, Diet C compared with Diet A; $*P < 0.05$, Diet B compared with Diet A; $\#P < 0.05$, Diet B compared with Diet C.

dynamic deterioration and improvement in oxygenation throughout the 4-h study period. This was evident by sustained improvements in PVR, cardiac index, and oxygen delivery.

Another important finding in this study was that short-term dietary supplementation of EPA and EPA + GLA significantly decreased the release of the AA metabolite, TXB_2, in response to endotoxin. At 4 h (Fig. 12.6), TXB_2 showed a 20-fold increase over baseline in group A, while groups B and C had significant attenuation of the increase in levels compared with baseline. These decreased TXB_2 levels may explain in part the hemodynamic benefits observed in pigs prefed Diets B or C. The sustained metabolic benefits seen with Diet C may also be contributed from synthesis of the vasodilatory PGE_1. Although we did not measure PGE_1 levels in this study, we speculate that the GLA in Diet C was elongated to DGLA with little desaturation to AA, thus potentially augmenting the synthesis of monoenoic PGs. Diets B and C increased the ratio of DGLA to AA by two- to three-fold in platelet phospholipids, and this may provide additional means to alter the generation of vasoactive AA-derived eicosanoids.

Short-term feeding for 8 d prior to endotoxin infusions had an impact on the composition of platelet phospholipid fatty acids. A 50% reduction in the n-6/n-3 ratio was observed in groups B and C compared with group A (Table 12.2). This was the result of a five-fold increase in EPA and a two-fold increase in DHA, whereas a

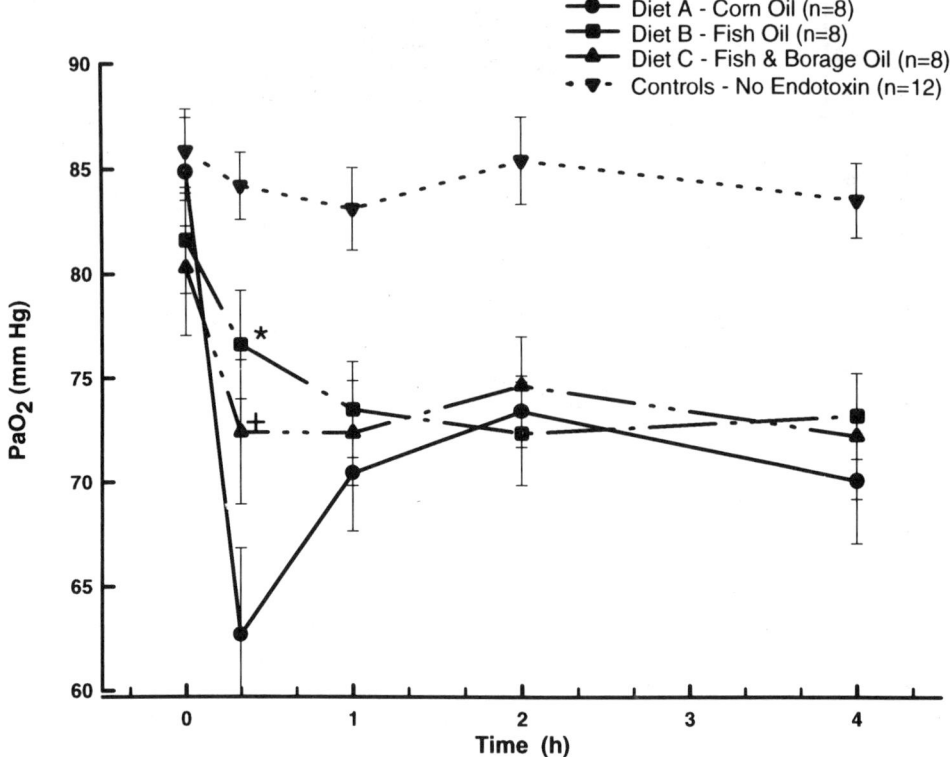

Fig. 12.3. PaO_2, arterial oxygen pressure, was measured before and after endotoxin infusion in pigs fed enteral diets for 8 d containing either corn oil (Diet A), fish oil (Diet B), or a combination of fish and borage oils (Diet C). Pooled control pigs were infused with normal saline. $+P = 0.06$, Diet C compared with Diet A; $*P < 0.05$, Diet B compared with Diet A.

significant decrease occurred in both LA and AA. GLA and DGLA were significantly elevated in pigs receiving Diet C only. These findings are viewed as physiologically important. Endotoxin is known to stimulate the release of eicosanoids from platelets (53) and platelets, in turn, are involved in the pathogenesis of ALI (54). Other evidence suggests that EPA suppresses the formation of eicosanoids via a direct inhibitory effect on cyclooxygenase (55). Our results confirm this in that both TXB_2 and 6-keto-$PGF_{1\alpha}$ (stable metabolite of prostacyclin, PGI2) levels (data not shown) were markedly decreased in pigs prefed Diet B or C.

Several reports have demonstrated the benefit of prophylactic administration of novel cyclooxygenase or selective thromboxane inhibitors in the treatment of sepsis-induced ALI (43,56–59). Such agents block the formation and activity of vasoactive metabolites of AA and thereby attenuate the hemodynamic consequences of sepsis-induced lung injury. We hypothesize that with a decrease in the amount of vasoactive eicosanoids, the GLA-supplemented pigs had an improved physiologic response to endotoxin compared with the other two groups.

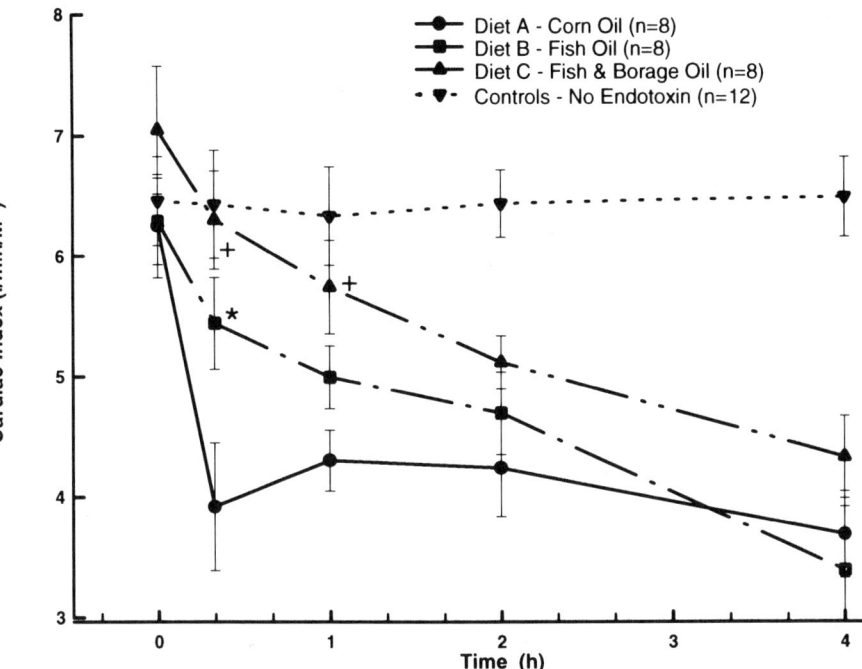

Fig. 12.4. Cardiac index was measured before and after endotoxin infusion in pigs fed enteral diets for 8 d containing either corn oil (Diet A), fish oil (Diet B), or a combination of fish and borage oil (Diet C). Pooled control pigs were infused with normal saline. $+P < 0.05$, Diet C compared with Diet A; $*P < 0.05$, Diet B compared with Diet A.

Dietary supplementation with GLA should increase PGE_1 and other monoenoic eicosanoids. The substitution of n-3 fatty acids for n-6 fatty acids should increase the formation of trienoic eicosanoids. Therefore, the combination of GLA and EPA will foster a change in the eicosanoid balance to strongly favor an anti-inflammatory, vasodilatory state.

This study demonstrated that short-term feeding (8 d) of diets containing EPA and EPA and GLA attenuated the early phase of cardiopulmonary dysfunction following endotoxin-induced lung injury. Although pigs prefed Diet B containing EPA showed a diminished early phase response to endotoxin, the late phase response was identical to that observed in the group fed Diet A. The supplementation of GLA in the diet significantly diminished both the early and late phase responses to endotoxin infusion by a sustained decrease in PVR while minimizing the decrease in cardiac index and arterial oxygen saturation.

In conclusion, enteral diets enriched with EPA from fish oil and GLA from borage oil improved gas exchange and oxygen delivery in a porcine model of ALI, presumably in part through modification of eicosanoid production with a decrease in PVR and an increase in cardiac index.

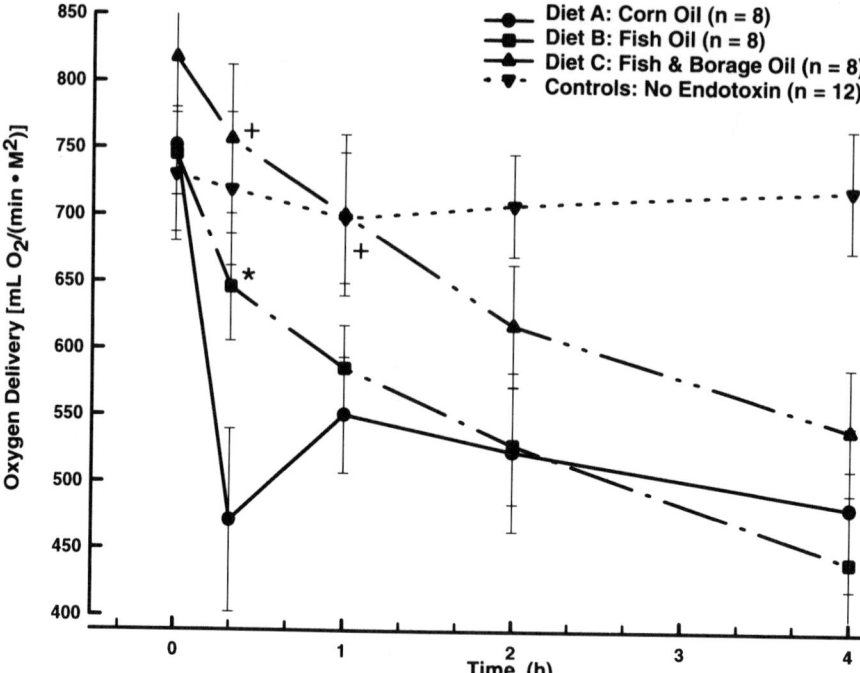

Fig. 12.5. Oxygen delivery was measured before and after endotoxin infusion in pigs fed enteral diets for 8 d containing either corn oil (Diet A), fish oil (Diet B), or a combination of fish and borage oil (Diet C). Pooled control pigs were infused with normal saline. $+P < 0.05$, Diet C compared with diet A; $*P < 0.05$, Diet B compared with Diet A.

Study II. Effects of Eicosapentaenoic and γ-Linolenic Acid on Lung Permeability, Arterial Blood Pressure, and Alveolar Macrophage Eicosanoid Synthesis in Endotoxic Rats

Endotoxin-induced ALI is characterized by an increase in pulmonary capillary permeability, pulmonary edema and hypoxemia (34,60). The AMφ is an inflammatory cell that resides in great number in the alveolar spaces of the lung and is thought to play a central role in the pathogenesis of ALI. AMφ release proinflammatory eicosanoids derived from the lipoxygenase and cyclooxygenase pathways of AA metabolism during endotoxemia. Levels of the 4-series LTs are elevated in bronchoalveolar lavage (BAL) fluid of patients with the ARDS (61). LTB_4 is a potent chemoattractant signal for neutrophils and is capable of stimulating neutrophils to adhere to pulmonary microvascular endothelial cells (62) and secrete oxygen free radicals and proteolytic enzymes that mediate microvascular lung damage and pulmonary edema (63). The cysteinyl LTs, LTC_4, and LTD_4 have been shown to directly increase pulmonary microvascular permeability and increase PVR (64,65). The 2-series PGs, including PGE_2 and TXA_2, have been implicated as important causative agents in septic shock and ALI in humans and animals (66).

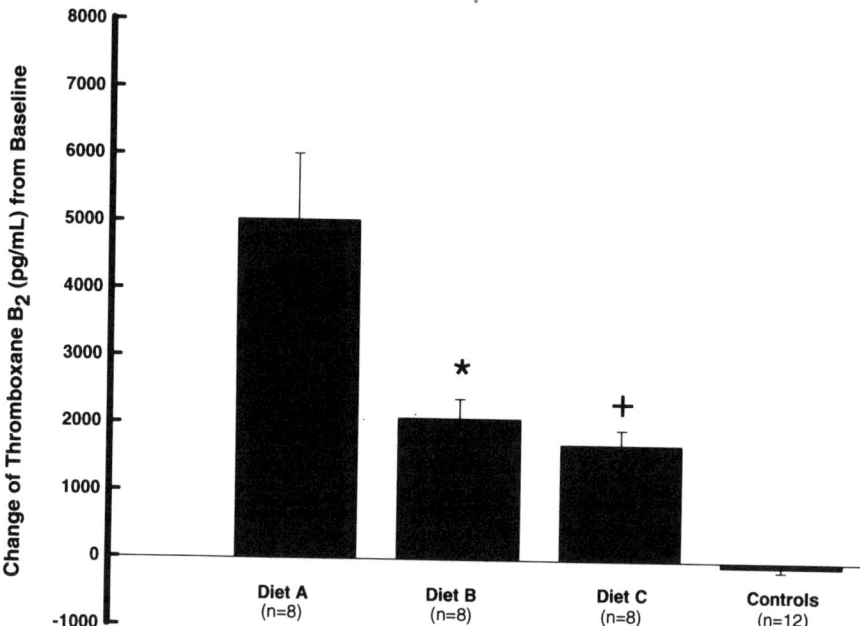

Fig. 12.6. The effects of endotoxin on plasma levels of thromboxane B2 were made at baseline and after 4 h of endotoxemia. Data are expressed as changes from baseline. +P < 0.05, Diet C compared with diet A; *P < 0.05, Diet B compared with Diet A.

Studies have shown that decreasing the AA content of tissue phospholipids can reduce the severity of inflammatory injury (27,67,68). Dietary fish oil (EPA and DHA) supplements have been used to modulate eicosanoid synthesis in a number of inflammatory states (32,69). Fish oil has been shown to reduce AA and increase EPA and DHA in tissue phospholipids (18,70). The elevated levels of EPA in tissue phospholipids can compete with AA for cyclooxygenase and 5-lipoxygenase binding sites and reduce eicosanoid formation from AA (70,71). EPA can be converted to the 3-series PG and 5-series LTs (72) which are considered less biologically active and less inflammatory than the 2-series PGs and 4-series LTs (73,74). Borage oil is a plant seed oil that contains a high level of GLA and has been shown to affect PG and

TABLE 12.2 Fatty Acid Composition of Platelet Phospholipids

Fatty Acid (%)	Diet A Corn Oil	Diet B Fish Oil	Diet C Fish & Borage Oil
18:2n-6	13.4 ± 1.0[a]	9.3 ± 1.0[b]	6.9 ± 0.5[c]
18:3n-6	0.6 ± 0.08[a]	0.6 ± 0.03[a]	0.9 ± 0.05[b]
20:3n-6	0.6 ± 0.07[a]	0.8 ± 0.09[b]	1.0 ± 0.04[b]
20:4n-6	8.5 ± 0.8[a]	5.9 ± 0.7[b]	5.6 ± 0.6[b]
20:5n-3	0.6 ± 0.2[a]	3.4 ± 1.0[b]	3.4 ± 1.0[b]
22:6n-3	3.7 ± 0.6[a]	6.5 ± 0.6[b]	9.4 ± 0.7[c]
n-6/n-3 Ratio	3.5 ± 0.3[a]	1.5 ± 0.2[b]	1.5 ± 0.1[b]

Values with different superscripts are significantly different; P < 0.05.

LT metabolism and suppress acute and chronic inflammation in animal models of injury (27,32). We recently showed in a rat model of burn and endotoxin injury that parenteral diets supplemented with borage oil modulated 2-series PG levels in plasma by reducing the ratio of TXB_2 to 6-keto-$PGF_{1\alpha}$ (29). Dietary GLA does not accumulate in tissue phospholipids because it is rapidly elongated to DGLA. DGLA incorporation into membrane phospholipids has been shown to increase PGE_1 synthesis in stimulated murine peritoneal macrophages (30) and indirectly decrease LT formation by inhibition of 5-lipoxygenase in macrophages (75). The intravenous infusion of PGE_1 in patients with ARDS has been shown to increase cardiac output and systemic oxygen delivery while reducing pulmonary artery pressure and vascular resistance (76).

Because fish and borage oil modulate different aspects of PG and LT metabolism, the potential exists to modulate by dietary intervention the production of 1-, 2-, and 3-series PGs and 4- and 5-series LTs by providing both oils in an enteral formula. Thus, fatty acids with anti-inflammatory properties, such as EPA and GLA, may modulate the production of proinflammatory eicosanoids and reduce tissue damage secondary to inflammation in endotoxin-induced ALI. Therefore, we investigated the effect of prefeeding rats for 21 d with enteral diets that provided fatty acids derived from fish oil alone and in combination with borage oil in comparison with corn oil on (1) lung microvascular protein permeability and arterial blood pressure in a model of endotoxin-induced ALI, (2) AMφ PG and LT synthesis, and (3) AMφ phospholipid fatty acid composition.

Methods

Approval to conduct this study was granted by the Animal Care and Use Committee of the University of Tennessee Graduate School of Medicine in accordance with guidelines set forth in the NIH Guide for the Care and Use of Laboratory Animals. Male Long-Evans rats (150 ± 10 g) were purchased from Charles River Laboratories (Wilmington, MA) and used for two separate experiments. Rats were randomized to receive one of the four diets. Rats were orally fed eucaloric [300 kcal/(kg·d)] and isonitrogenous diets for 21 d containing either corn oil (CO), fish oil (FO) or FO and increasing levels of borage oil. Diets were provided in sterilized feeding bottles and water was provided ad libitum. The diets provided 16.7% of calories from protein, 28.1% of calories from carbohydrate, and 55.2% of calories from lipid. The fatty acid composition of the enteral diets is shown in Table 12.3. The CO diet represents a standard high fat formula enriched with LA. The 20% FO, 20% FO/5% borage oil (FO/BOL), and 20% FO/20% borage oil (FO/BOH) diets had nearly identical levels of FO and medium-chain triglycerides. To maintain a similar n-6 to n-3 fatty acid ratio among these three diets, LA was replaced with GLA in the FO/BOL and FO/BOH diets. Due to the increased unsaturation index of the FO, FO/BOL, and FO/BOH diets, vitamins C, E and β-carotene were increased to minimize the potential of lipid peroxide formation in the diet preparations and to protect antioxidant capacity *in vivo* (77).

Experiment 1 assessed the effects of oral nutrition for 21 d with four high fat, low carbohydrate enteral diets on the development of ALI following an intravenous

TABLE 12.3 Fatty Acid Content of Enteral Diets

Fatty Acid (%)	CO	FO	FO/BOL	FO/BOH
Caproic (6:0)	ND	0.09	0.09	0.09
Caprylic (8:0)	ND	12.56	12.85	13.05
Capric (10:0)	ND	9.54	9.71	9.93
Lauric (12:0)	0.09	0.20	0.24	0.20
Myristic (14:0)	0.15	1.22	1.21	1.24
Palmitic (16:0)	11.30	6.26	6.11	5.95
Palmitoleic (16:1)	0.04	1.70	1.67	1.69
Stearic (18:0)	2.27	1.48	1.69	1.86
Oleic (18:1n-9)	24.59	28.0	27.56	25.96
Linoleic (18:2n-6)	59.35	21.67	20.31	16.68
γ-linolenic (18:3n-6)	ND	0.08	1.25	4.63
α-linolenic (18:3n-3)	1.01	3.68	3.72	3.92
Stearidonic (18:4n-3)	ND	0.70	0.69	0.71
Arachidic (20:0)	0.41	0.31	0.81	0.27
Eicosenoic (20:1n-9)	0.30	1.08	1.82	1.92
Arachidonic (20:4n-6)	ND	0.38	0.38	0.38
Eicosapentaenoic (20:5n-3)	ND	5.52	5.35	5.31
Erucic (22:1n-9)	0.04	0.57	0.72	1.12
Docosapentaenoic (22:5n-3)	ND	0.55	0.54	0.54
Docosahexaenoic (22:6n-3)	ND	2.30	2.32	2.52
Others	0.45	2.11	2.06	2.03
n-6/n-3 ratio	58.76	1.74	1.74	1.67

Abbreviations: ND, not detected. CO, corn oil; FO, 20% fish oil; FO/BOL, 20% fish and 5% borage oil; FO/BOH, 20% fish oil and 20% borage oil.

injection of 10 mg/kg *Salmonella enteritidis* endotoxin. Pulmonary microvascular protein permeability was determined by localization of ^{99m}Tc-HSA (human serum albumin) in the lungs by computerized γ-scintigraphy. Arterial blood pressure was measured from a carotid artery catheter for 2 h post-endotoxin.

Experiment 2 assessed the effect of oral nutrition for 21 d on the fatty acid composition of AMϕ phospholipids and the capacity of AMϕ to generate proinflammatory PGs and LTs *in vitro*. AMϕ were isolated by BAL. AMϕ phospholipid fatty acid composition was determined by gas chromatography (Hewlett-Packard Model #5890 Series II). AMϕ were isolated and the washed adherent cells were incubated in the presence or absence of 10 μM A23187 for 15 min. Eicosanoids were analyzed as described previously with minor modifications (70). TXB_2, PGE_2, and 6-keto-$PGF_{1\alpha}$ were analyzed by RIA (Advanced Magnetics, Cambridge, MA). LTs were separated by reverse-phase HPLC and quantified based on their molar extinction coefficients (78) using the internal standard PGB_1, with a Hewlett-Packard (Liverpool, NY) 1090M Photodiode Array scanning spectrophotometer, monitoring at 280 nm.

Results and Discussion

This study showed that prefeeding high fat enteral formulations containing dietary fatty acids derived from fish and borage oil modulated many of the pathophysiologic responses to an intravenous injection of endotoxin in rats. The results in Fig. 12.7

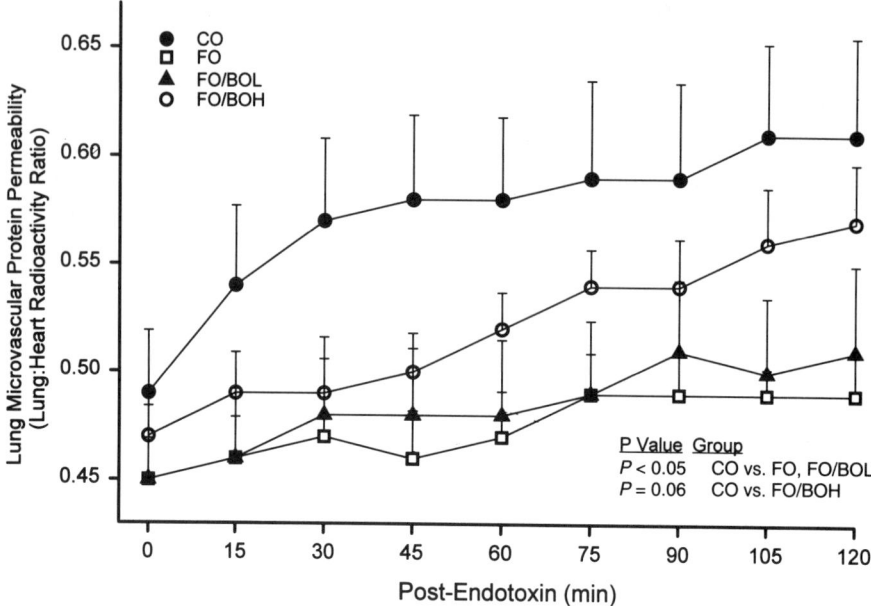

Fig. 12.7. Lung:heart radioactivity ratios following an intravenous bolus injection of *Salmonella enteritidis* endotoxin (10 mg/kg of body weight) in rats fed diets supplemented with CO (corn oil), FO (20% fish oil), FO/BOL (20% fish and 5% borage oil), or FO/BOH (20% fish and 20% borage oil) for 21 d. Values are means ± SEM for 9–11 rats. Error bars are shown in one direction for clarity.

show that the endotoxin-induced increase in pulmonary microvascular protein permeability was markedly reduced with diets containing FO, FO/BOL, and FO/BOH compared with CO. Such a reduction in permeability may have coordinated beneficial effects by decreasing transcapillary fluid flux and pulmonary edema, thereby facilitating gas exchange leading to an improvement in arterial oxygenation. The early and late hypotensive effects of endotoxin were attenuated with FO, FO/BOL, and FO/BOH compared with CO (Fig. 12.8). Although FO has been widely shown to depress vascular reactivity to agonists as well as to lower blood pressure in hypertension (79), the results of this study and that of Murray et al. (1,18) indicate that FO does not exacerbate the hypotensive effects of endotoxin but rather diminishes the fall in mean arterial blood pressure compared with CO. The results of Study I in this chapter and those previously published (1) showed sustained improvements in PVR, cardiac index, and oxygen delivery following an intravenous infusion of *E. coli* endotoxin in pigs prefed FO and BO compared with FO or CO.

Computerized γ-scintigraphy has been shown to be a sensitive, noninvasive, dynamic technique for the detection and quantitation of pulmonary microvascular leakage of protein (80). We assessed changes in protein conductance across the pulmonary microvascular endothelium by calculating the lung:heart radioactivity ratio of radiolabeled albumin before and after the intravenous administration of endotoxin. The lung:heart radioactivity ratio was constant for 2 h in rats given an intravenous

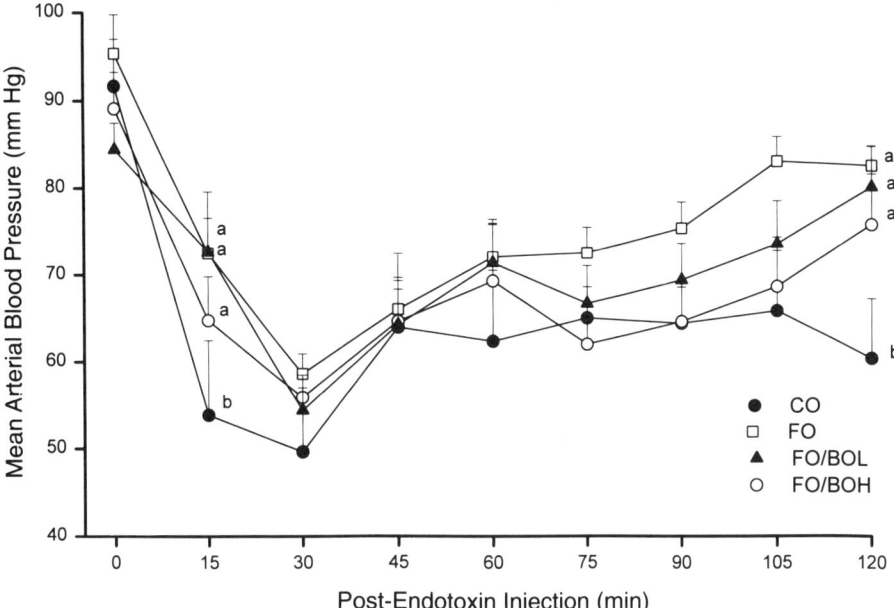

Fig. 12.8. Mean arterial blood pressure following an intravenous bolus injection of *Salmonella enteritidis* endotoxin (10 mg/kg of body weight) in rats fed diets supplemented with CO (corn oil), FO (20% fish oil), FO/BOL (20% fish and 5% borage oil), or FO/BOH (20% fish and 20% borage oil) for 21 d. Values are means ± SEM for 9-11 rats. Error bars are shown in one direction for clarity. Symbols with different letters are significantly different ($P \leq 0.05$).

injection of saline (data not shown). Previous studies have shown that an increase in the lung:heart radioactivity ratio is due to an increase in pulmonary microvascular permeability resulting from microvascular injury (80). This study shows that the greatest increase in lung microvascular permeability after endotoxin administration was with CO and that there was a significant reduction in permeability with FO and FO/BOL; this effect approached significance ($P = 0.06$) with FO/BOH.

We believe that one of the mechanisms responsible for the reduction in endotoxin-induced lung microvascular permeability with FO or FO and BO was the reduced synthesis of AA-derived proinflammatory eicosanoids as shown in Table 12.4 and Fig. 12.9. Table 12.5 shows a decrease in the level of AA that was accompanied by higher levels of EPA, docosapentaenoic (22:5n-3), and DHA in the phospholipids of AMφ with FO or FO and BO. These findings are in agreement with other studies showing that dietary FO supplementation displaces AA from tissue phospholipids (16,18,70). The incorporation of these n-3 fatty acids into tissue phospholipids is significant for many reasons. First, an increase in tissue EPA suppresses the formation of AA-derived PGs by inhibiting cyclooxygenase. Second, EPA is the precursor of the 3-series PGs which are less biologically active than the 2-series PGs. Last, EPA suppresses 4-series LT formation (derived from AA) (70). The significant increases in DGLA and the ratio of DGLA to AA in the phospholipids of AMφ with FO/BOH as

TABLE 12.4 Effect of Feeding Diets Supplemented with CO, FO, FO/BOH on Eicosanoid Release from Alveolar Macrophages Following Stimulation *in Vitro* with A23817 (ng/10^6 cells)

Eicosanoids	CO	FO	FO/BOH
LTB_5	ND	7.32 ± 0.62^a	4.69 ± 0.30^b
6-*trans*-LTB_4	8.34 ± 1.01	7.67 ± 0.82	5.95 ± 1.34
TXB_2	6.06 ± 0.16^a	4.58 ± 0.55^b	4.40 ± 0.44^b
PGE_2	1.83 ± 0.24^a	1.03 ± 0.26^b	0.95 ± 0.14^b
6-keto-$PGF_{1\alpha}$	0.15 ± 0.01	0.14 ± 0.01	0.13 ± 0.02

Abbreviations: ND, not detected; CO, corn oil; FO, 20% fish oil; FO/BOH, 20% fish and 20% borage oil; TXB_2, thromboxane B_2; LTB_5, leukotriene B_5; PGE_2, prostaglandin E_2; 6-keto-prostaglandin $F_{1\alpha}$. Values are means ± SEM; $n = 3$ pooled samples. Values in the same row with different letters are significantly different ($P \leq 0.05$).

TABLE 12.5 Effect of Feeding Diets Supplemented with CO, FO, and FO/BOH for 21 Days on Alveolar Macrophage Phospholipid Fatty Acid Composition (mole %)

Fatty Acid	CO	FO	FO/BOH
16:0	48.7 ± 1.87	52.6 ± 2.47	52.53 ± 2.13
16:1	4.11 ± 0.29	4.93 ± 0.44	5.04 ± 0.40
18:0	11.25 ± 0.54	9.48 ± 0.79	9.94 ± 0.57
18:1	7.05 ± 0.41^a	8.48 ± 0.32^b	8.19 ± 0.45^b
18:2n-6	14.49 ± 0.45^a	7.00 ± 0.51^b	5.16 ± 0.28^c
18:3n-6	0.05 ± 0.03^a	ND	0.58 ± 0.02^b
20:3n-6	0.22 ± 0.04^a	0.24 ± 0.04^a	0.62 ± 0.06^b
20:4n-6	11.99 ± 0.77^a	5.47 ± 0.24^b	8.21 ± 0.94^c
18:3n-3	0.03 ± 0.02^a	0.23 ± 0.01^b	ND
20:5n-3	ND	2.68 ± 0.23^a	1.93 ± 0.13^b
22:5n-3	0.38 ± 0.07^a	2.06 ± 0.08^b	1.82 ± 0.13^b
22:6n-3	0.96 ± 0.12^a	4.14 ± 0.13^b	3.97 ± 0.20^b
n-6/n-3 ratio	20.72 ± 1.91^a	1.48 ± 0.11^b	1.88 ± 0.09^c
DGLA/AA	0.02 ± 0.002^a	0.05 ± 0.018^b	0.07 ± 0.002^b

Abbreviations: ND, not detected; DGLA/AA, 20:3n-6/20:4n-6; CO, corn oil; FO, 20% fish oil; FO/BOH, 20% fish and 20% borage oil. Values ($n = 6$ or 7) in the same row with different letters are significantly different, $P \leq 0.05$. Values are means ± SEM.

shown in Table 12.5 suggest that DGLA was not completely converted to AA and would be available for 1-series PG synthesis. Previous studies have reported increases in DGLA in tissue phospholipids (81,82) and plasma (29) following dietary GLA supplementation. Our previous results showed that dietary supplementation with GLA modulated AA-derived 2-series PGs after burn and endotoxin injury (29).

It can be seen in Fig. 12.9 that the release of LTB_4 from AMϕ following stimulation with A23187 was significantly lower with FO and FO/BOH compared with CO. This may have been due to a combined effect of a decrease in AA, the metabolic precursor of LTB_4, in the phospholipids of AMϕ and to competitive inhibition of 5-lipoxygenase by EPA (4,83). Although there were significantly higher AA levels in the AMϕ with FO/BOH compared with FO (Table 12.5), this did not result in increases in eicosanoid synthesis. In addition, 15-OH-20:3n-6 (15-HETrE), a 15-lipoxygenase metabolite of DGLA, has been shown to attenuate LTB_4 formation by inhibiting 5-lipoxygenase (82). Importantly, DGLA cannot be converted to LT (82). LTB_4 is elevated in the BAL fluid of patients with ARDS (61,66) and has been shown to increase

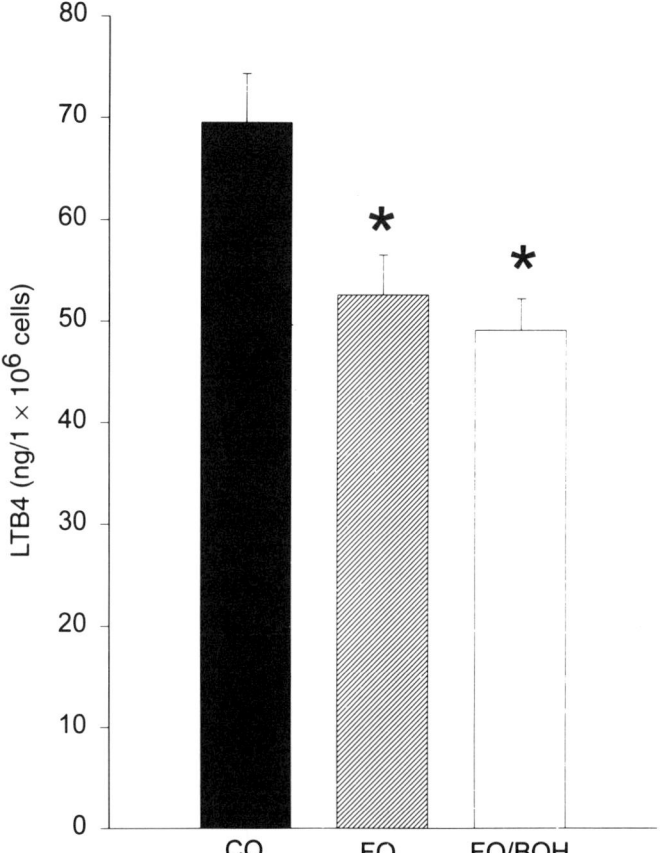

Fig. 12.9. LTB_4 levels (ng/1 × 10^6 cells) released from alveolar macrophages following stimulation *in vitro* with 10 μM A23187 for 15 min from rats fed diets supplemented with CO (corn oil), FO (20% fish oil), or FO/BOH (20% fish and 20% borage oil) for 21 d. Values are means ± SEM for 9 rats. Bars with an asterisk are significantly different than CO ($P \leq 0.05$).

pulmonary microvascular permeability in rabbits (63). LTB_4 is a potent chemoattractant of polymorphonuclear neutrophils. Neutrophil-mediated endothelial injury has been implicated in animal models of ALI (63,84). An inhibition of LTB_4 formation has been shown to significantly reduce lung microvascular permeability and edema in ALI in rats (85) and dogs (84). In addition, AMφ stimulated with A23187 produced elevated levels of LTB_5, a 5-lipoxygenase metabolite of EPA, with FO and FO/BOH. LTB_5 is much less potent as a chemoattractant for polymorphonuclear neutrophils than LTB_4 (74). Taken together, these results indicate that there was an overall decrease in the potency of the signal for neutrophil chemotaxis with FO and FO/BOH.

TXA_2 is an important mediator in the development of pulmonary hypertension in ARDS and in endotoxin-induced lung injury (66,86). Thromboxane synthase inhibitors have been shown to significantly attenuate pulmonary hypertension in a porcine model of bacteremia (87) and increase survival after endotoxin infusion in rats (88). Although TXA_2 may not have a direct effect on microvascular permeability, thromboxane receptor inhibition may indirectly inhibit neutrophil adherence, thus reducing endothelial cell damage (66). The protection against endotoxin-induced increases in lung permeability with FO or FO and BO may be due in part to reduced formation of TXA_2 *in vivo*. Table 12.4 shows that the release of this eicosanoid was reduced from AMϕ stimulated with A23187 *in vitro*.

PGE_2 is required for normal immune function and T-cell differentiation at very low concentrations ($<10^{-9}$ M). Following injury, elevated concentrations of PGE_2 ($>10^{-8}$ M) are immunosuppressive (78). In this study, PGE_2 from stimulated AMϕ was significantly lower with FO and FO/BOH than with CO (Table 12.4). Thus, modulation of PGE_2 formation by dietary FO or FO and BO may normalize immune function and T-cell differentiation.

In summary, prefeeding high fat enteral formulas enriched with FO or FO and BO compared with CO for 21 d was protective against increases in pulmonary microvascular protein permeability and hypotension in endotoxin-induced ALI in rats. Enteral nutrition with a LA-enriched diet (CO) resulted in an early and much larger increase in pulmonary microvascular permeability and more severe hypotension compared with diets containing FO or FO and BO. The addition of BO to the FO diet did not further blunt the endotoxin-induced increase in lung microvascular protein permeability and hypotension. The reduced synthesis of the proinflammatory AA-derived mediators, LTB_4, TXB_2, and PGE_2, from stimulated AMϕ was indicative of a decrease in AA and an increase in DGLA and EPA in cell membrane phospholipids. The modulation of proinflammatory eicosanoid synthesis with anti-inflammatory fatty acids, EPA and GLA, may be responsible for limiting the severity of ALI (pulmonary microvascular protein permeability) and hypotension after endotoxin administration.

Although it is not yet known if dietary intervention with high fat, low carbohydrate formulas can modulate an ongoing pulmonary inflammatory response in patients at risk of developing ARDS, the results of this study indicate that changing the fatty acid composition of tissue phospholipids by dietary intervention had beneficial effects in a rat model of endotoxin-induced ALI. It may be possible to provide a high fat, low carbohydrate formula, designed initially to reduce minute ventilation and the respiratory quotient in ventilator-dependent patients, with anti-inflammatory fatty acids (EPA and GLA) at the expense of LA to modulate eicosanoid metabolism and reduce the abnormality in pulmonary microvascular protein permeability and hemodynamic insufficiency in critically ill patients at risk of developing ARDS.

Study III. Modulation of Rat Alveolar Macrophage and Lung Tissue Phospholipid PUFA in Endotoxemic Rats After Continuous Enteral Feeding for 3 or 6 Days

Alterations in lung function have been associated with the release of lipid mediators derived from AA. Recent treatment modalities for patients with lung injury have therefore been directed toward downregulation of these lipid metabolites by pharmacologic means (81–91). However, few clinical studies have investigated the efficacy of nutrition intervention to modulate the synthesis of lipid mediators derived from immune cell phospholipid PUFA.

The capacity of select dietary PUFA to reduce the relative quantity of AA and LA present in macrophage membranes and thereby attenuate inflammatory processes driven by dienoic eicosanoids and oxygen radicals derived from the respiratory burst may prove clinically relevant for critically ill patients at risk of developing ARDS. Incorporation of dietary EPA into mononuclear cell phospholipids has been associated with decreased formation of several vasoactive eicosanoids derived from AA and reduced synthesis of TNF-α and IL-1β (13,15). Similarly, provision of GLA as a diet supplement has been associated with reduced inflammation secondary to formation of monoenoic eicosanoids derived from DGLA (26). Because the majority of commercially available enteral diets are enriched with LA, the precursor of AA, novel enteral formulations containing low levels of LA and supplemented with EPA and/or GLA have been assessed for potential application in the critical care setting. The outcome of preliminary experiments with pigs fed novel enteral preparations lends further support to the concept that pulmonary and systemic inflammation as sequelae of endotoxemia can be attenuated by short-term (<8 d) nutritional pretreatment with EPA alone (18) or EPA in combination with GLA (1,92). However, while oral nutrient pretreatment has proven advantageous in these models, whether or not provision of these formulations enterally or during septic complications would confer the same functional benefits remains unresolved. A second concern has been that such intervention therapies would be practical only if their application can impart a beneficial effect within a clinically relevant time span. In this regard, the rapidity and extent of incorporation of EPA and metabolism of GLA to DGLA within lung macrophages *in vivo* during endotoxemia has not been well characterized.

The following study was undertaken to characterize the dietary modulation of AMϕ and lung tissue phospholipid PUFA in endotoxemic rats enterally fed continuously for 3 or 6 d with enteral formulations enriched with EPA in combination with either a "low" or "high" percentage of GLA.

Methods

The following protocol was approved by the Deaconess Animal Care and Use Committee. Briefly, male (225–275 g) Sprague Dawley rats (Harlan, Altamont, NY) were randomized to dietary and endotoxin treatment groups as discussed below. After anesthetization with ether (0830 h of d –1), an 0.040" i.d. × 0.085" o.d. medical silastic catheter was inserted aseptically through a fundal gastrostomy, advanced 2.5 cm into the duodenum, and anchored to the stomach wall with a purse string suture. A 0.025" i.d. × 0.047" o.d. catheter was inserted in the left jugular vein for intravenous infusion of endotoxin or vehicle. The catheters were exteriorized at the midscapular region and attached to a flow-through dual channel swivel to permit freedom of movement as previously described (93,94). Each rat was allowed water ad libitum for the study duration.

Enteral Diets

After recovery from catheterization surgery, all rats were infused with Vital HN (Ross Products Division, Abbott Laboratories, Columbus, OH) at half the caloric requirement [125 kcal/(kg·d); lipid = 9.4% total kcal] from 1500 h of d −1 until 0900 h of d 0. Independent subsets of rats (n = 6/group) were then infused continuously by a programmable syringe pump with either Diet A, B, or C (Table 12.6) until either 0900 h of d 3 or 0900 h of d 6. Diet A represented a standard high fat enteral diet enriched with LA. Diets B and C were enriched with fish and borage oils and had reduced concentrations of LA. Although Diets B and C were nearly identical with respect to individual or total n-3 PUFA, Diet B had a relatively low level of GLA (1.25%) whereas Diet C had a higher percentage of GLA (4.63%). To maintain a similar n-6/n-3 ratio between Diets B and C, LA was replaced by GLA in Diet C. Vitamins C, E and β-carotene were increased in Diets B and C relative to Diet A to minimize the potential of lipid peroxide formation *in vivo*. All rats received an isovolemic, isonitrogenous and isocaloric [250 kcal/(kg·d)] amount of the assigned formulation. These diets provided 16.7% of calories from protein, 28.1% of calories from carbohydrate, and 55.2% of calories from lipid.

Endotoxin Infusion

Within each dietary treatment group, rats (n = 6) received an intravenous infusion of 0.4 mg/(kg·d) endotoxin (*E. coli* 026:B6) continuously by syringe pump starting at 1500 h of d −1, and ending at the time of killing (d 0, 3, or 6). This dose of endotoxin induced physical signs of endotoxicosis (conjunctival hemorrhage, lethargy, ear flattening, and piloerection) and doubling of spleen weight within 3 d, with minimal lethality.

Subsets (n = 6/group) of rats were killed on d 0 (prediet baseline), d 3 or 6 depending upon the randomization schedule. AMφ were collected by BAL as described previously (94). Following lavage, lung tissue samples (free of bronchial tissue) were excised and stored under nitrogen gas at −20°C. Frozen lung tissue was homogenized in saline immediately before lipid extraction as described below.

Quantitation of fatty acids in the phospholipid fraction of AMφ and lung tissue homogenate was determined by gas chromatography after isolation of the phospholipid band by thin layer chromatography (94).

TABLE 12.6 Polyunsaturated Fatty Acid Profiles of Enteral Diets

Fatty Acid (%)	Diet		
	CO	FO/BOL	FO/BOH(20%)
18:2n-6	59.4	20.3	16.7
18:3n-6	0	1.3	4.6
18:3n-3	1	3.7	3.9
20:5n-3	0	5.4	5.3
22:6n-3	0	2.3	2.5
n-6/n-3 Ratio	58.8	1.7	1.7

Abbreviations: CO, corn oil; FO, 20% fish oil; FO/BOL, 20% fish and 5% borage oil; FO/BOH, 20% fish oil and 20% borage oil.

Results and Discussion

The results of this study have revealed several important findings. The first was the rapidity and extent to which dietary fatty acids were incorporated or metabolized (i.e., DGLA from GLA) by AMϕ and lung tissue (Fig. 12.10 and 12.11) through continuous enteral feeding. This feeding modality optimizes the exposure of lung and liver cell membranes to dietary PUFAs that have been packaged as components of lipoproteins released either from the liver into the venous circulation or from the intestine into the lymphatic circulation. An alternative but less prominent route for distribution of dietary PUFAs would be as free fatty acids within the portal circulation (95). As reported earlier, plasma phospholipid fatty acids are also significantly affected by the dietary lipid profile as well as by the feeding pattern (29,93,96). Furthermore, remodeling of phospholipid PUFAs is facilitated by the normally extensive turnover of cell membranes *in vivo* (97). There were only a few instances in the present study in which further changes in the relative percentage of macrophage or lung tissue phospholipid PUFA occurred after the first 3 d of feeding. Given the similarities between humans and rats with regard to tissue esterification and incorporation of dietary PUFAs (98), provision of select dietary PUFAs by continuous

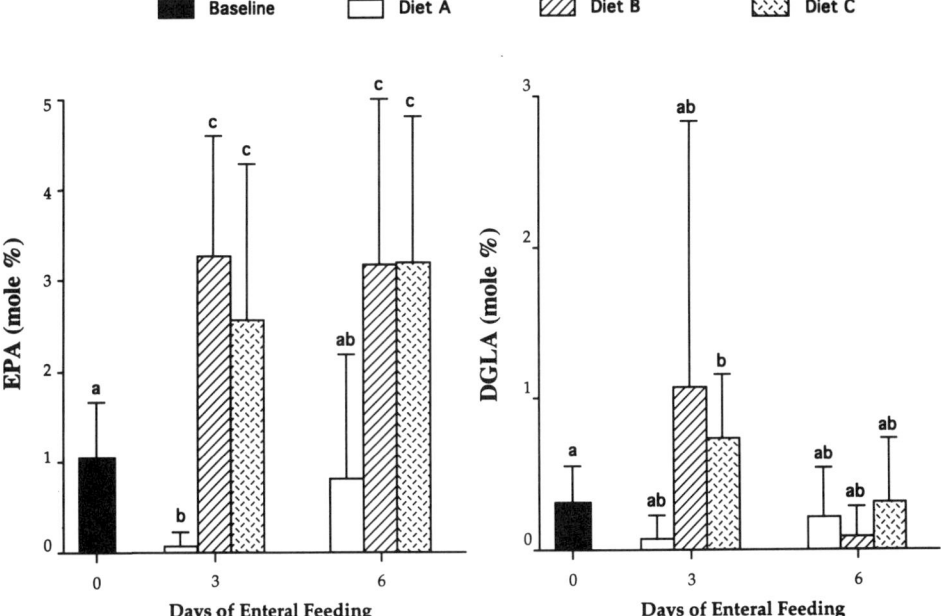

Fig. 12.10. Mean ± SD mole % of eicosapentaenoic acid (EPA; 20:5n-3) and dihomo-γ-linolenic acid (DGLA; 20:3n-6) in rat alveolar macrophage phospholipids. Endotoxemic rats were randomized to receive enteral diets enriched with either linoleic acid (LA; 18:2n-6) (Diet A), or a diet low in LA and containing EPA and one of two levels of γ-linolenic acid (GLA; 18:3n-6): Diet B = low % GLA; Diet C = high % GLA. Subsets of rats were fed enterally in a continuous manner for 3 or 6 d (n = 6/group). For a given fatty acid, values that do not share the same superscript letter are significantly different, $P < 0.05$.

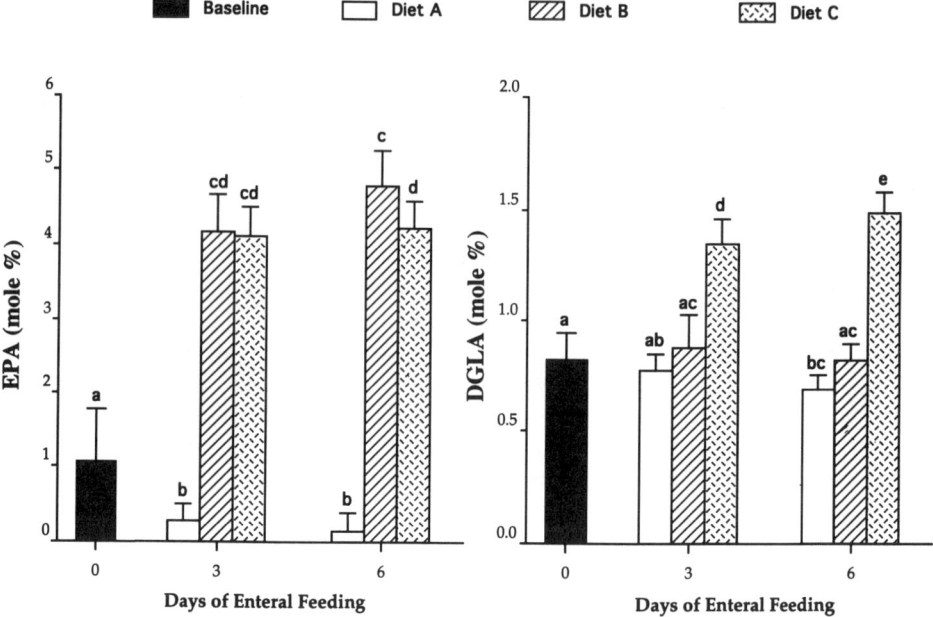

Fig. 12.11. Mean ± SD mole % of EPA and DGLA in rat lung tissue phospholipids. See legend for Fig. 12.10 for explanation of the dietary treatment groups. For a given fatty acid or ratio, values that do not share the same superscript letter are significantly different, $P < 0.05$.

enteral feeding could prove to be a practical and effective treatment modality for downregulating inflammatory processes within the lung and liver.

A second observation of potential importance was the significant displacement of endogenous LA and AA from the resident AMϕ (Fig. 12.12) and lung tissue (Fig. 12.13) phospholipids by highly unsaturated n-3 (i.e., EPA and DHA) and n-6 (i.e., DGLA) PUFA in rats given the EPA + GLA enriched diets.

A third finding was that endotoxemia did not significantly alter the dietary modification of AMϕ phospholipid PUFAs (unpublished comparisons with vehicle-infused control rats). These results suggest that application of enteral nutritional regimens for remodeling of phospholipid PUFAs may not be limited to nonstressed patients or pre-emptive situations only, but may also be employed postoperatively or during septic complications (99,100).

Interestingly, providing GLA enterally at 4.6% of the total lipid kcal (Diet C) did not foster increased formation of AA in the AMϕ (Fig. 12.12). A similar observation had been noted earlier in the peritoneal macrophage phospholipids from mice fed orally with a diet enriched with GLA (25.6% of total fatty acids) (30). Although DGLA is the immediate precursor of AA, this conversion by Δ5-desaturase appears to be tightly regulated and, under pathophysiologic conditions, may be a rate-limiting step (4,28,29). Nor was the lack of an effect of GLA on AA levels due to the incapacity of cells to further increase phospholipid AA content, given the increased relative % of AA observed in the AMϕ and lung samples (Figs. 12.12 and 12.13, respec-

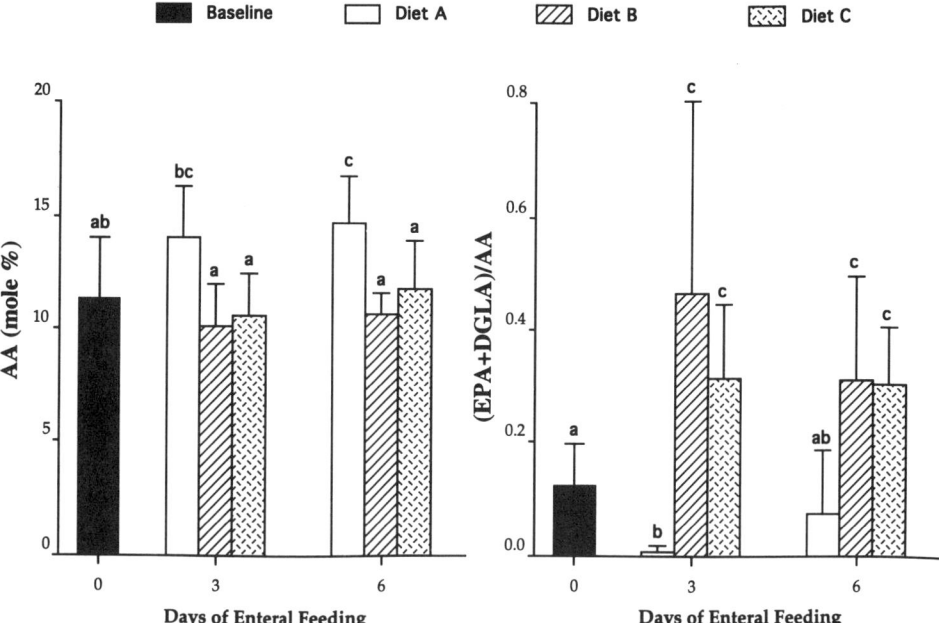

Fig. 12.12. Mean ± SD mole % of arachidonic acid (AA) and the ratio of EPA + DGLA/AA in rat alveolar macrophage phospholipids. See legend of Fig. 12.10 for explanation of the dietary treatment groups. For a given fatty acid or ratio, values that do not share the same superscript letter are significantly different, $P < 0.05$.

tively) from rats receiving the LA-enriched formulation (Diet A). The outcome observed in the present study therefore may be due in part to low Δ5-desaturase activity in macrophages during endotoxemia coupled with inhibition of this enzyme by dietary EPA (4). While the lungs from rats given Diet C tended to have higher levels of AA than those given Diet B (Fig. 12.13), this difference was relatively small compared with the difference between lungs from these groups and lungs from rats given Diet A (Fig. 12.13). The physiological significance of the difference in relative percentage of lung phospholipid AA between rats given Diet B or Diet C is not evident at this time.

As mentioned above, rats infused with Diet A had significantly higher relative percentages of AMϕ (Fig. 12.12) and lung (Fig. 12.13) phospholipid AA by d 3 than that observed in the rats at baseline (d 0). These remarkable increases are due in part to the low fat intake (lipid content of chow pellets and Vital HN = 14.5 and 9.4% of total kcal, respectively) of the rats up to Day 0 coupled with the imposition of a diet (Diet A) with a substantially higher total lipid (55% of total kcal) and LA (59%) content. In contrast, AMϕ (Fig. 12.12) from rats receiving Diets B and C (which have identical total lipid kcal but low levels of LA) for 6 d maintained relative percentage levels of AA similar to those observed in rats at baseline. Displacement of phospholipid AA to levels significantly lower than baseline was achieved only in lung tissue (Fig. 12.13) from rats given either Diet B or C for 6 d. Within these dietary groups, the mean relative percentage of lung phospholipid AA continued to decrease

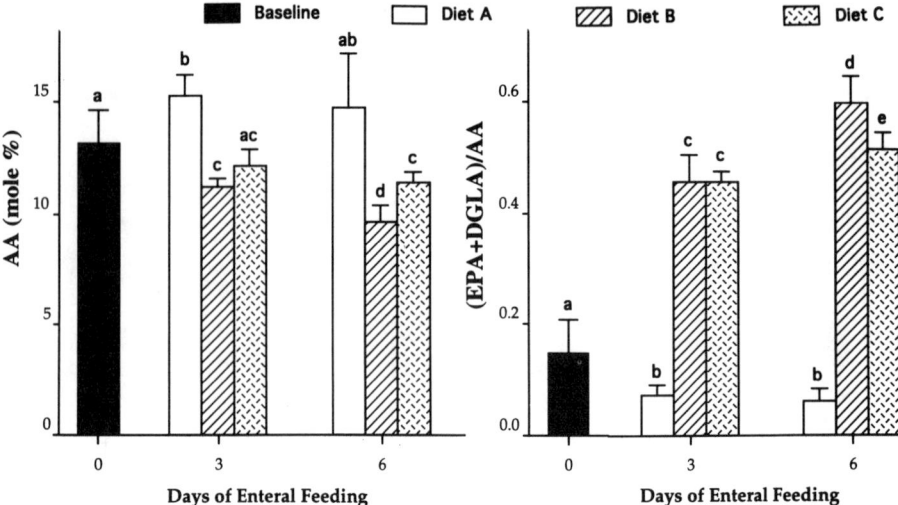

Fig. 12.13. Mean ± SD mole % of AA and the ratio of EPA + DGLA/AA in rat lung tissue phospholipids. See legent for Fig. 12.10 for explanation of the dietary treatment groups. For a given fatty acid or ratio, values that do not share the same superscript letter are significantly different, $P < 0.05$.

between d 3 and 6 in conjunction with increased incorporation of EPA ($P < 0.06$) in rats given Diet B (Fig. 12.11) or increased incorporation of DGLA ($P < 0.05$) in rats treated with Diet C (Fig. 12.11) during that interval. Also worthy of mention was the finding that any EPA (1–1.5%) present in the rat macrophages and lung tissue at baseline was effectively displaced by n-6 PUFAs within 3 d of feeding Diet A. These results emphasize the concept that the membrane phospholipids of these cells rapidly respond to changes in plasma PUFA patterns induced during continuous feeding with novel or, in this instance, conventional lipids (93).

The biologic response elicited after eicosanoid release is dependent upon the net balance of eicosanoids derived from AA, EPA, and GLA. At this time, it is not known whether concomitant alterations in eicosanoid metabolism occur in conjunction with the rapid modification of the macrophage phospholipid PUFA after short-term enteral feeding. Various ratios of n-6 and n-3 PUFAs have been utilized to predict potential formation of the respective dienoic vs. trienoic series of eicosanoids. It is important to note, however, that DGLA, the precursor of the monenoic series, is included in the n-6 family despite the fact that under pathophysiologic conditions it may not be desaturated to AA. For this reason, a more relevant ratio (i.e., EPA + DGLA/AA) was utilized to combine those PUFA, i.e., EPA and DGLA, that compete with AA for cyclooxygenase binding. Elevated values of this ratio of precursor PUFAs signify that potential formation of the trienoic and monoenoic eicosanoids relative to dienoic eicosanoids is increased. However, this ratio is useful only from the standpoint of availability of each precursor PUFA based upon relative mole percent. It cannot account for any actual differences which may exist in selective PUFA distribution among the inner and outer membrane phospholipids, or relative binding affinities or spatial proximity of the individual PUFA to membrane cyclooxygenase.

With that caveat in mind, EPA + DGLA/AA ratios calculated for the macrophage (Fig. 12.12) and lung tissue (Fig. 12.13) phospholipids in rats receiving the EPA + GLA diets (i.e., Diets B and C) were four- to ten-fold higher than those in rats infused with the LA-enriched diet (Diet A) at either d 3 or d 6.

In conclusion, this study suggests that short-term continuous enteral feeding with diets containing EPA and higher levels of GLA should potentiate AMϕ synthesis of the monoenoic and trienoic series of eicosanoids that have reduced inflammatory properties in lieu of the vasoactive dienoic eicosanoids derived from AA.

Acknowledgments

We want to acknowledge all members of the technical staffs from the institutions involved in the three studies. Study I was performed under the direction of Michael J. Murray, M.D., Ph.D. at the Department of Anesthesiology and Critical Care Service, Mayo Clinic and Mayo Foundation; Study II was performed under the direction of Michael D. Karlstad, Ph.D. at the Department of Anesthesiology, Graduate School of Medicine, University of Tennessee Medical Center; and Study III was performed under the direction of John D. Palombo, D.Sc. at the Deaconess Hospital, Harvard Medical School.

References

1. Murray, M.J., Kumar, M., Gregory, T.J., Banks, P.L., Tazelaar, H.D., and DeMichele, S.J. Diets Containing Eicosapentaenoic Acid and Gamma-linolenic Acids Attenuate Cardiopulmonary Dysfunction During Acute Lung Injury (1995) *Am. J. Physiol. 296 (Heart and Circ. Physiol. 39),* H2090–H2099.
2. Mancuso, P., Whelan, J., DeMichele, S.J., Snider, C.C., Guszcza, J.A., Claycombe, K.J., Smith, G.T., Gregory, T.J., and Karlstad, M.D. Effects of Eicosapentaenoic and Gamma-Linolenic Acid on Lung Permeability and Alveolar Macrophage Eicosanoid Synthesis in Endotoxic Rats (1996) *Crit. Care Med.* (submitted for publication).
3. Palombo, J.D., DeMichele, S.J., Lydon, E., Gregory, T.J., Banks, P.L., Forse, R.A., and Bistrian, B.R. Rapid Modulation of Lung and Liver Macrophage Phospholipid Fatty Acids in Endotoxemic Rats by Continuous Enteral Feeding with n-3 and γ-Linolenic Fatty Acids (1995) *Am. J. Clin. Nutr. 63,* 208–219.
4. Kinsella, J.E., Broughton, K.S., and Whelan, J. Dietary Unsaturated Fatty Acids: Interactions and Possible Needs in Relation to Eicosanoid Synthesis (1990) *J. Nutr. Biochem. 1,* 123–141.
5. Sibille, Y., and Reynolds, H.Y. Macrophages and Polymorphonuclear Neutrophils in Lung Defense and Injury (1990) *Am. Rev. Respir. Dis. 141,* 471–501.
6. Callery, M.P., Kamei, T., Mangino, M.J., and Flye, M.W. Organ Interactions in Sepsis: Host Defense and the Hepatic-Pulmonary Axis (1993) *Arch. Surg. 126,* 28–32.
7. Palombo, J.D., Blackburn, G.L., and Forse, R.A. Endothelial Cell Factors and Response to Injury (1991) *Surg. Gynecol. Obstet. 173,* 505–518.
8. Maridonneau-Parini, I., Tringale, S.M., and Tauber, A.I. Identification of Distinct Activation Pathways of the Human Neutrophil NADPH Oxidase (1986) *J. Immunol. 137,* 2925–2929.
9. Sakata, A., Ida, E., Tominaga, M., and Onoue, K. Arachidonic Acid Acts As an Intracellular Activator of the NADPH-oxidase in FCG Receptor-Mediated Superoxide Generation in Macrophages (1987) *J. Immunol. 138,* 4353–4359.

10. Crim, C., and Simon, R.H. Effects of Oxygen Metabolites on Rat Alveolar Type II Cell Viability and Surfactant Metabolism (1988) *Lab. Invest. 58,* 428–437.
11. Demling, R.H. Adult Respiratory Distress Syndrome: Current Concepts (1993) *New Horizons 1,* 388–401.
12. Moore, F.A., Moore, E.E., and Read, R.A. Postinjury Multiple Organ Failure: Role of Extrathoracic Injury and Sepsis in Adult Respiratory Distress Syndrome (1993) *New Horizons 1,* 538–549.
13. Billiar, T.R., Bankey, P.E., Svingen, B.A., Curran, R.D., West, M.A., Holman, R.T., Simmons, R.L, and Cerra, F.B. Fatty Acid Intake and Kupffer Cell Function: Fish Oil Alters Eicosanoid and Monokine Production to Endotoxin Stimulation (1988) *Surgery 104,* 343–349.
14. Barton, R.G., Wells, C.L., Carlson, A., Singh, R., Sullivan, J.J., and Cerra, F.B. Dietary Omega-3 Fatty Acids Decrease Mortality and Kupffer Cell Prostaglandin E_2 Production in a Rat Model of Chronic Sepsis (1991) *J. Trauma 31,* 768–773.
15. Endres, S., Ghorbani, R., Kelley, V.E., Georgilis, K., Lonnemann, G., van der Meer, J.W.M., Cannon, J.G., Rogers, T.S., Klempner, M.S., Weber, P.C., Schaefer, E.J., Wolff, S.M., and Dinarello, C.A. The Effect of Dietary Supplementation with n-3 Polyunsaturated Fatty Acids on the Synthesis of Interleukin-1 and Tumor Necrosis Factor by Mononuclear Cells (1989) *N. Engl. J. Med. 320,* 265–271.
16. Sperling, R.I., Benincaso, A.I., Knoell, C.T., Larkin, J.K., Austen, K.F., and Robinson, D.R. Dietary n-3 Polyunsaturated Fatty Acids Inhibit Phosphoinositide Formation and Chemotaxis in Neutrophils (1993) *J. Clin. Invest. 91,* 651–660.
17. Pomposelli, J.J., Flores, E.A., Blackburn, G.L., Zeisel, S.H., and Bistrian, B.R. Diets Enriched with n-3 Fatty Acids Ameliorate Lactic Acidosis by Improving Endotoxin-Induced Tissue Hypoperfusion in Guinea Pigs (1991) *Ann. Surg. 213,* 166–176.
18. Murray, M.J., Svingen, B.A., Yaksh, T.L., and Holman, R.T. Effects of Endotoxin on Pigs Prefed n-3 vs. n-6 Fatty Acid-enriched Diets (1993) *Am. J. Physiol. 265,* E920–E927.
19. Murray, M.J., Svingen, B.A., Holman, R.T., and Yaksh, T.L. Effects of a Fish Oil Diet on Pigs' Cardiopulmonary Response to Bacteremia (1991) *J. Parent. Enteral Nutr. 15,* 152–158.
20. Horrobin, D.F. The Regulation of Prostaglandin Biosynthesis by the Manipulation of Essential Fatty Acid Metabolism (1983) *Rev. Pure Appl. Pharmacol. Sci. 4,* 339–432.
21. Willis, A.L. and Smith, D.L. Dihomo-Gamma-Linolenic and Gamma-Linolenic Acids in Health and Disease (1989) in *New Protective Roles for Selected Nutrients,* Spiller, G.A., and Scala, J., eds., Alan R. Liss, New York, pp. 39–108.
22. Nassar, B.A., Huang, Y.-S., Manku, M.S., Das, U.N., Morse, N., and Horrobin, D.F. The Influence of Dietary Manipulation with n-3 and n-6 Fatty Acids on Liver and Plasma Phospholipid Fatty Acids in Rats (1986) *Lipids 21,* 652–656.
23. Das, U.N., Horrobin, D.F., Begin, M.E., Huang, Y.-S., Cunnane, S.C., Manku, M.S., and Nassar, B.A. Clinical Significance of Essential Fatty Acids (1988) *Nutrition 4,* 337–341.
24. Spielmann, D., Bracco, U., Traitler, H., Crozier, G., Holman, R., Ward, M., and Cotter, R. Alternative Lipids to Usual ω-6 PUFAS: Gamma-linolenic Acid, Alpha-Linolenic Acid, Stearidonic Acid, EPA, etc. (1988) *J. Parent. Enteral Nutr. 12 (suppl.),* 111S–123S.
25. Gunstone, F.D. Gamma Linolenic Acid—Occurrence and Physical and Chemical Properties (1992) *Prog. Lipid Res. 31,* 141–162.
26. Horrobin, D.F. Gamma Linolenic Acid: An Intermediate in Essential Fatty Acid Metabolism with Potential As an Ethical Pharmaceutical and As a Food (1990) *Rev. Contemp. Pharmacother. 1,* 1–45.

27. Tate, G., Mandell, B.F., Laposata, M., Ohliger, D., Baker, D.G., Schumacher, H.R., and Zurier, R.B. Suppression of Acute and Chronic Inflammation by Dietary γ-Linolenic Acid (1989) *J. Rheumatol. 16,* 729–733.
28. Diboune, M., Ferard, G., Ingenbleek, Y., Tulasne, P.A., Calon, B., Hasselmann, H., Sauder, P., Spielman, D., and Metais, P. Composition of Phospholipid Fatty Acids in Red Blood Cell Membranes of Patients in Intensive Care Units: Effects of Different Intakes of Soybean Oil, Medium Chain Triglycerides, and Black Currant Seed Oil (1992) *J. Parent. Enteral Nutr. 16,* 136–141.
29. Karlstad, M.D., DeMichele, S.J., Leathem, W.D., and Peterson, M.B. Effect of Intravenous Lipid Emulsions Enriched with γ-Linolenic Acid on Plasma n-6 Fatty Acids and Prostaglandin Biosynthesis after Burn and Endotoxin Injury in Rats (1993) *Crit. Care Med. 21,* 1740–1749.
30. Fan, Y.Y., and Chapkin, R.S. Mouse Peritoneal Macrophage Prostaglandin E_1 Synthesis Is Altered by Dietary γ-Linolenic Acid (1992) *J. Nutr. 122,* 1600–1606.
31. Kunkel, S.L., Ogawa, H., Conran, P.B., Ward, P.A., and Zurier, R.B. Suppression of Chronic Inflammation by Evening Primrose Oil (1981) *Prog. Lipid Res. 20,* 886–888.
32. Tate, G.A., Mandell, B.F., Karmali, R.A., Laposata, M., Baker, D.G., Schumacher, H.R., and Zurier, R.B. Suppression of Monosodium Urate Crystal-Induced Acute Inflammation by Diets Enriched with Gamma-Linolenic Acid and Eicosapentaenoic Acid (1988) *Arthritis Rheum. 31,* 1543–1551.
33. Pullman-Mooar, S., LaPosata, M., Lem, D., Holman, R.T., Leventhal, L.J., DeMarco, D.M., and Zurier, R.B. Alteration of the Cellular Fatty Acid Profile and the Production of Eicosanoids in Human Monocytes by Gamma-Linolenic Acid (1990) *Arthritis Rheum. 33,* 1526–1533.
34. Read, M.A., and Meyrick, B.O. Effects of Endotoxin on Lung Endothelium (1994) in *Endotoxin and the Lung,* Brigham, K.L., ed., Marcel Dekker, Inc., New York, pp. 83–110.
35. Kollef, M.H., and Schuster, D.P. The Acute Respiratory Distress Syndrome (1995) *N. Eng. J. Med. 332,* 27–37.
36. Dahlen, S.-E., Hedqvist, P.M., Hammarstrom, S., and Samuelsson, B. Leukotrienes Are Potent Constrictors of Human Bronchi (1980) *Nature (Lond.) 288,* 484–486.
37. Allen, E., and Gellai, M. Hemodynamic Responses to Leukotriene Receptor Stimulation in Conscious Rats (1990) *Am. J. Physiol. 258,* R1034–R1041.
38. Brigham, K.L., Woolverton, W.C., Blake, L.H., and Staub, N.C. Increased Sheep Lung Vascular Permeability Caused by Pseudomonas Bacteremia (1974) *J. Clin. Invest. 54,* 792–804.
39. Hanly, P.J., Roberts, D., Dobson, K., and Light, R.B. Effect of Indomethacin on Arterial Oxygenation in Critically Ill Patients with Severe Bacterial Pneumonia (1987) *Lancet 1,* 351–354.
40. Mozes, T., Zijlstra, F.J., Heiligers, J.P.C., Tak, C.J.A.M., Ben-Efraim, S., Bonta, I.L., and Saxena, P.R. Sequential Release of Tumour Necrosis Factor, Platelet Activating Factor and Eicosanoids During Endotoxin Shock in Anaesthetized Pigs: Protective Effects of Indomethacin (1991) *Br. J. Pharmacol. 104,* 691–699.
41. Byrne, K., Carey, P.D., Sielaff, T.D., Jenkins, J.K., Blocher, C.R., Cooper, K.R., Fowler, A.A., and Sugerman, H.J. Ibuprofen Prevents Deterioration in Static Transpulmonary Compliance and Transalveolar Protein Flux in Septic Porcine Acute Lung Injury (1991) *J. Trauma 31,* 155–164.
42. Kopolovic, R., Thrailkill, K.M., Martin, D.T., Ambrose, T., Vento, M., Carey, L.C., and Cloutier, C.T. Effects of Ibuprofen on a Porcine Model of Acute Respiratory Failure (1984) *J. Surg. Res. 36,* 300–305.

43. Carey, P.D., Leeper-Woodford, S.K., Walsh, C.J., Byrne, K., Fowler, A.A., and Sugarman, H.J. Delayed Cyclo-Oxygenase Blockade Reduces the Neutrophil Respiratory Burst and Plasma Tumor Necrosis Factor Levels in Sepsis-Induced Acute Lung Injury (1991) *J. Trauma 31*, 733–740.
44. Fink M.P., Kruithoff, K.L., Antonsson, J.B., Wang, H., and Rothschild, H.R. Delayed Treatment with an LTD_4/E_4 Antagonist Limits Pulmonary Edema in Endotoxic Pigs (1991) *Am. J. Physiol. 260*, R1007–R1013.
45. Demling, R.H., Smith, M., Gunther, R., and Gee, M.H. Pulmonary Injury and Prostaglandin Production During Endotoxemia in Conscious Sheep (1981) *Am. J. Physiol. 240*, 348–353.
46. Demling, R.H. The Role of Mediators in Human ARDS (1988) *J. Crit. Care 3*, 56–72.
47. Weiss, S.J. Tissue Destruction by Neutrophils (1989) *N. Engl. J. Med. 320*, 365–376.
48. Esbenshade, A.M., Newman, J.H., Lams, P.M., Jolles, H., and Brigham, K.L. Respiratory Failure After Endotoxin Infusion in Sheep: Lung Mechanics and Lung Fluid Balance (1982) *J. Appl. Physiol. 53*, 967–976.
49. Heflin, A.C., Jr., and Brigham, K.L. Prevention by Granulocyte Depletion of Increased Vascular Permeability of Sheep Lung Following Endotoxemia (1981) *J. Clin. Invest. 68*, 1253–1260.
50. McCaffree, D.R., Gray, B.A., Pennock, B.E., Coalson, J., Bridges, C., Taylor, F.B., and Rogers, R.M. Role of Pulmonary Edema in the Acute Pulmonary Response to Sepsis (1981) *J. Appl. Physiol. 50*, 1198–1205.
51. Winn, R., Harlan, J., Nadir, B., Harker, L., and Hildebrandt, J. Thromboxane A_2 Mediates Lung Vasoconstriction But Not Permeability After Endotoxin (1983) *J. Clin. Invest. 72*, 911–918.
52. Snapper, J.R., Hutchinson, A.A., and Ogletree, M.L. Effects of Cyclooxygenase Inhibitors on the Alterations in Lung Mechanics Caused by Endotoxemia in the Unanesthetized Sheep (1983) *J. Clin. Invest. 72*, 63–76.
53. Rinaldo, J.E., and Dauber, J.H. Effects of Methylprednisolone and of Ibuprofen, a Nonsteroidal Antiinflammatory Agent, on Bronchoalveolar Inflammation Following Endotoxemia (1985) *Circ. Shock 16*, 195.
54. Bottoms, G.D., Johnson, M., Ward, J.D., Fessler, J., Lamar, C., and Turek, J. Release of Eicosanoids from White Blood Cells, Platelets, Smooth Muscle Cells, and Endothelial Cells in Response to Endotoxin and A23187 (1986) *Circ. Shock 20*, 25–34.
55. Takahashi, R., Nassar, B.A., Huang, Y.-S., Begin, M.E., and Horrobin, D.F. Effects of Different Ratios of Dietary n-6 and n-3 Fatty Acids on Fatty Acid Composition, Prostaglandin Formation and Platelet Aggregation in the Rat (1987) *Thrombosis Res. 47*, 135–146.
56. Metz, C., and Sibbald, W.J. Anti-Inflammatory Therapy for Acute Lung Injury (1991) *Chest 100*, 1110–1119.
57. Ogletree, M.L. Overview of Physiological and Pathophysiological Effects of Thromboxane A_2 (1987) *Fed. Proc. 46*, 133–138.
58. Perlman, M.B., Johnson, A., and Malik, A.B. Ibuprofen Prevents Thrombin-Induced Lung Vascular Injury: Mechanism of Effect (1987) *Am. J. Physiol. 252, (Heart Circ. Physiol.)* H605–H614.
59. Rinaldo, J.E., and Pennock, B. Effects of Ibuprofen on Endotoxin-Induced Alveolitis: Biphasic Dose Response and Dissociation Between Inflammation and Hypoxemia (1986) *Am. J. Med. Sci 291*, 29–38.
60. Brigham, K.L., and Meyrick, B. Endotoxin and Lung Injury (1986) *Am. Rev. Respir. Dis. 133*, 913–927.

61. Stephenson, A.H., Lonigro, A.J., Hyers,T.M. Webster, R.O., and Fowler, A.A. Increased Concentrations of Leukotrienes in Bronchoalveolar Lavage Fluid of Patients with ARDS or at Risk for ARDS (1988) *Am. Rev. Respir. Dis. 138*, 714–719
62. Hoover, R.L., Karnovsky, K.F., Austen, E.J., Corey, E.J., and Lewis, R.A. Leukotriene B_4 Action on Endothelium Mediates Augmented Neutrophil/Endothelial Adhesion (1984) *Proc. Natl. Acad. Sci. U.S.A. 81*, 2191–2193.
63. Yoshimura, K., Nakagawa, S., Koyama, S., Kobayashi, T., and Homma,T. Leukotriene B_4 Induces Lung Injury in the Rabbit: Role of Neutrophils and Effect of Indomethacin (1993) *J. Appl. Physiol. 74*, 2174–2179.
64. Abela, A., and Daniel, E.E. Neural and Myogenic Effects of Leukotrienes C_4, D_4, and E_4 on Canine Bronchial Smooth Muscle (1994) *Am. J. Physiol. 266*, L414–L425.
65. Cohn, S.M., Kruithoff, K.L., Rothchild, H.R., Wang,H., Antonsson, J.B., and Fink, M.P. Beneficial Effects of LY203647, a Novel Leukotriene C_4/D_4 Antagonist, on Pulmonary Function and Mesenteric Perfusion in a Porcine Model of Endotoxic Shock and ARDS (1991) *Circ. Shock 33*, 7–16.
66. Makhlouf, M., Durando, M., Cook, J.A., and Halushka, P.V. Role of Eicosanoids in Endotoxin-Induced Lung Dysfunction (1994) in *Endotoxin and the Lungs*, Brigham, K.L., ed., Marcel Dekker, Inc., New York, pp. 153–169.
67. Burton, J.L. Dietary Fatty Acids and Inflammatory Skin Disease (1989) *Lancet 7*, 27–31.
68. Teo, T.C., Selleck, K.M., Wan, J.M.F., Pomposelli, J.J., Babayan, V.K., Blackburn, G.L., and Bistrian, B.R. Long-Term Feeding with Structured Lipid Composed of Medium-Chain and n-3 Fatty Acids Ameliorates Endotoxic Shock in Guinea Pigs (1991) *Metabolism 40*, 1152–1159.
69. Simopoulos, A.P. Omega-3 Fatty Acids in Health and Disease and in Growth and Development (1991) *Am. J. Clin. Nutr. 54*, 438–463.
70. Whelan, J., Broughton, K.S., and Kinsella, J.E. The Comparative Effects of Dietary Alpha-Linolenic Acid and Fish Oil on 4- and 5-Series Leukotriene Formation *in Vivo* (1991) *Lipids 26*, 119–126.
71. Lands, W.E.M., LeTellier, P.R., Rome, L.H., and Vanderhoek, J.Y. Inhibition of Prostaglandin Biosynthesis (1972) *Adv. Biosci. 9*, 15–27.
72. Lands, W.E.M. Biochemistry and Physiology of n-3 Fatty Acids (1992) *FASEB J. 6*, 2530–2536.
73. Fischer, S., and Weber, P.C. Prostaglandin I_3 Is Formed *in Vivo* in Man After Dietary Eicosapentaenoic Acid (1984) *Nature 307*, 165–168.
74. Lee, T.H., Mencia-Huerta, J., Shih, C., Corey, E.J., Lewis, R.A., and Austen, K.F. Characterization and Biologic Properties of 5,12-Dihydroxy Derivatives of Eicosapentaenoic Acid, Including Leukotriene B_5 and the Double Lipoxygenase Product (1984) *J. Biol. Chem. 259*, 2383–2389.
75. Chapkin, R.S., Miller, C.C., Somers, S.D., and Erickson, K.L. Ability of 15-Hydroxy-eicosatrienoic Acid (15-OH-20:3) to Modulate Macrophage Arachidonic Acid Metabolism (1988) *Biochem. Biophys. Res. Comm. 153*, 799–804.
76. Appel, P.L., and Shoemaker, W.C. Hemodynamic and Oxygen Transport Effects of Prostaglandin E_1 in Patients with Adult Respiratory Distress Syndrome (1984) *Crit. Care Med. 12*, 528–529.
77. Lenz, P.H., Watkins, T., and Bierenbaum, M. Effect of Dietary Menhaden, Canola and Partially Hydrogenated Soy Oil Supplemented with Vitamin E upon Plasma Lipids and Platelet Aggregation (1991) *Thromb. Res. 61*, 213–224.

78. Santoli, D., Phillips, P.D., Colt, T.L., and Zurier, R.B. Suppression of Interleukin 2-Dependent Human T Cell Growth *in Vitro* by Prostaglandin E and Their Precursor Fatty Acids (1990) *J. Clin. Invest. 85,* 424–432.
79. Chin, J.P.F., and Dart, A.M. How Do Fish Oils Affect Vascular Function? (1995) *Clin. Exper. Pharm. 22,* 71–81.
80. Sugerman, H.J., Strash, A.M., Hirsch, J.I., Glauser, F.L., Shirazi, K.K., Sharp, D.E., and Greenfield, L.J. Sensitivity of Scintigraphy for Detection of Pulmonary Capillary Albumin Leak in Canine Oleic Acid ARDS (1991) *J. Trauma 21,* 520–527.
81. Chapkin, R.S., and Coble, K.J. Utilization of Gammalinolenic Acid by Mouse Peritoneal Macrophages (1991) *Biochim. Biophys. Acta 1085,* 365–370.
82. Ziboh, V.A., and Fletcher, M.P. Dose-Response Effects of Dietary γ-Linolenic Acid-Enriched Oils on Human Polymorphonuclear-Neutrophil Biosynthesis of Leukotriene B_4 (1992) *Am. J. Clin. Nutr. 55,* 39–45.
83. Holman, R.T., and Mohrhauer, H. A Hypothesis Involving Competitive Inhibitions in the Metabolism of Polyunsaturated Fatty Acids (1963) *Acta Chem. Scand. 17,* 584–590.
84. Sprague, R.S., Stephenson, A.H., and Lonigro, A.J. OKY-046 Prevents Increases in LTB_4 and Pulmonary Edema in Phorbol Ester-Induced Lung Injury in Dogs (1992) *J. Appl. Physiol. 73,* 2493–2498.
85. Ball, H.A., Cook, J.A., Spicer, K.M., Wise, W.C., and Halushka, P.V. Essential Fatty Acid-Deficient Rats Are Resistant to Oleic Acid-Induced Pulmonary Injury (1989) *J. Appl. Physiol. 57,* 811–816.
86. Wisner, D., Sturm, J., Sutter, G., Ellendorf, B., and Nerlich, M. Thromboxane Receptor Blockade in an Animal Model of ARDS (1988) *Surgery 104,* 91–97.
87. Svartholm, E., Bergqvist, D., Hedner, U., Ljungberg, J., and Haglund, U. Arachidonic Acid Cascade Metabolites in Porcine *E. coli* Shock (1988) *Acta Chir. Scand. Suppl. 154,* 133–139.
88. Cook, J.A., Wise, W.C., and Halushka, P.V. Elevated Thromboxane Levels in the Rat During Endotoxic Shock: Protective Effects of Imidazole, 13-Azaprostanoic Acid, or Essential Fatty Acid Deficiency (1980) *J. Clin. Invest. 65,* 227–230
89. Christman, B.W., and Bernard, G.R. Antilipid Mediator and Antioxidant Therapy in Adult Respiratory Distress Syndrome (1993) *New Horizons 1,* 623–630.
90. Koike, K., Moore, E,E., Moore, F.A., Carl, V.S., Pitman, J.M., and Banerjee, A. Phospholipase A_2 Inhibition Decouples Lung Injury from Gut Ischemia-Reperfusion (1992) *Surgery 112,* 173–180.
91. Said, S.I., and Foda, H.D. Pharmacologic Modulation of Lung Injury (1989) *Am. Rev. Respir. Dis. 139,* 1553–1564.
92. Murray, M.J., DeMichele, S.J., Kanazi, G., Warner, D.O., Moxley, M.A., Longmore, W.J., and Gregory, T.J. The Effects of Eicosapentaenoic and γ-Linolenic Acid on Surfactant Composition and Function and Pulmonary Compliance During Porcine Endotoxemia (1993) *Am. Rev. Respir. Dis. 147,* A988 (abstract).
93. Palombo, J.D., Bistrian, B.R., Fechner, K.D., Blackburn, G.L., and Forse, R.A. Rapid Incorporation of Fish or Olive Oil Fatty Acids into Rat Hepatic Sinusoidal Cell Phospholipids after Continuous Enteral Feeding During Endotoxemia (1993) *Am. J. Clin. Nutr. 57,* 643–649.
94. Palombo, J.D., Lydon, E.E., Chen, P.L., Bistrian, B.R., and Forse, R.A. Fatty Acid Composition of Lung, Macrophage and Surfactant Phospholipids after Short-Term Enteral Feeding with n-3 Lipids (1994) *Lipids 29,* 643–649.
95. Mansbach, C.M., Dowell, R.F., and Pritchett, D. Portal Transport of Absorbed Lipids in Rats (1991) *Am. J. Physiol. 261,* G530–G538.

96. Mascioli, E.A., Smith, M.F., Trerice, M.S., Meng, H.C., and Blackburn, G.L. Effect of Total Parenteral Nutrition with Cycling on Essential Fatty Acid Deficiency (1978) *J. Parent. Enteral Nutr. 3,* 171–173.
97. Mahoney, E.M., Hamill, A.L., Scott, W.A., and Cohn, Z.A. Response of Endocytosis to Altered Fatty Acyl Composition of Macrophage Phospholipids (1977) *Proc. Natl. Acad. Sci. 74,* 4895–4899.
98. Lands, W.E.M. Biosynthesis of Prostaglandins (1991) *Annu. Rev. Nutr. 11,* 41–60.
99. Kenler, A., Swails. W., Driscoll, D., DeMichele, S.J., Babineau, T., Peterson, M., and Bistrian, B.R. Early Enteral Feeding in Postsurgical Cancer Patients: Fish Oil Structured Lipid-Based Diet versus a Standard Diet (1994) *J. Parent. Enteral. Nutr. 18,* 26S (abs.).
100. Adams, S., Yeh, Y., and Jensen, G. Changes in Plasma and Erythrocyte Fatty Acids in Patients Fed Enteral Formulas Containing Different Fats (1993) *J. Parent. Enteral. Nutr. 17,* 30–34.

Chapter 13

Effects of Feeding a Supplement of γ-Linolenic Acid Containing Oils with Fish Oil on the Fatty Acid Composition of Serum Phospholipids in Healthy Volunteers

Armand Christophe

Department of Endocrinology and Metabolic Diseases, Division of Nutrition, University of Ghent, Belgium

Introduction

The effects of the administration of γ-linolenic acid (GLA) or higher unsaturated n-3 fatty acids (n-3 HUFAs) on the fatty acid composition of serum phospholipids (PL) of humans are well documented (1,2) (HUFAs are fatty acids with a chain length of at least 20 carbon atoms and having at least 3 double bonds). The effects of supplementing the diet with n-3 and n-6 fatty acids simultaneously have been studied in animals (3,4). In humans, they are less well documented. Vegetarians (5) and patients on diets low in preformed arachidonic acid (AA; 20:4n-6) (6) have lower levels of AA in their PL than do controls, and feeding meals with preformed AA and n-3 HUFAs increases these fatty acids (7). Increasing n-6 fatty acids in a diet with n-3 fatty acids has a mitigating effect on the increase of n-3 fatty acids in PL (8). The aim of this study was to document the effects of supplementing healthy individuals with a mixture containing GLA in combination with n-3 HUFA, on the fatty acid and HUFA composition of serum PL.

Materials and Methods

Eighteen healthy volunteers (students; 20–25 y) participated in this study which was approved by the Ethical Committee of this institution. They were instructed to take 3 × 3 capsules/d of a supplement containing GLA and n-3 fatty acids for 4 wk and to make no changes to their habitual Western-type diet. The supplement was a commercial preparation (Naudicelle Forte®; Bio-Oil, Nantwich, UK) containing 500 mg/capsule of a mixture of borage oil, evening primrose oil, and salmon oil. Its fatty acid composition was determined by the same methodology as that used for serum PL. Serum was obtained in the fasting state just before and at the end of the supplementation period. Lipids were extracted and the fatty acid composition of the serum triglycerides and phospholipids was analyzed as described previously (9). The daily intake of linoleic and α-linolenic acid was estimated for all individuals from the percentage of these fatty acids in the serum triglyceride fraction according to the Lands' equation (10). From the gas chromatographic data, fatty acids were calculated as a weight percentage of total fatty acids in the PL. Individual HUFA was also calculated as a percentage of total HUFA. Changes are defined as the differences between the pre- and the posttreatment values. Significance was calculated by paired Student's t-tests (before vs. after supplementation). The first-order linear regression model was used to determine correlations and their significance.

Results

The fatty acid composition of the supplement is given in Table 13.1. Intakes of GLA and of n-3 fatty acids with the supplement were about 700 mg and 390 mg/d, respectively. Calculated intakes of linoleic and α-linolenic acids with the usual nonsupplemented diets ranged from 3–11 en% (average 5.9 en%) and from 0.2 to 1.4 en% (average 0.7 en%), respectively. The linoleic acid intake correlated positively with the α-linolenic acid intake ($r = 0.78$: $P < 0.001$), and the ratio of linoleic acid intake to α-linolenic acid intake varied from 5.3 to 19.9 (mean ± SD, 9.7 ± 3.6). Table 13.2 shows that after supplementing with the GLA/n-3 mixture. GLA ($P < 0.05$), 20:5n-3 ($P < 0.01$), 22:5n-3 ($P < 0.01$), and 22:6n-3 ($P < 0.001$), which were present in the supplement, were significantly higher. The elongation product of GLA, dihomo-γ-linolenic acid (DGLA; 20:3n-6), was also significantly increased ($P < 0.01$) but 20:4n-6, the Δ5 desaturation product of 20:3n-6, was not. The levels of 16:1n-7, its elongation product, 18:1n-7, and 22:4n-6, the elongation product of 20:4n-6, were significantly lower ($P < 0.05$). The proportion of 22:5n-6, the desaturation product of 22:4n-6, was higher, however ($P < 0.01$). Total monoenes were reduced ($P < 0.05$) and total n-3 increased ($P < 0.001$). The levels of n-6 HUFA ($P < 0.05$), n-3 HUFA ($P < 0.001$) and total HUFA ($P < 0.01$) were increased. For the fatty acids that changed significantly, correlations were calculated between these changes and those of all other

TABLE 13.1 Fatty Acid Composition of the Dietary Supplements

Fatty Acid[a]	(wt %)	Fatty Acid	(wt %)
14:0	1.5[†]	18:4n-3	0.9
15:0	0.1	20:0	0.2
16:0	11.3	20:1	2.9
16:1n-7	2.1	20:3n-3	0.2
16:1n-5	0.2	20:5n-3	3.9
17:0	0.2	22:0	0.1
18Br	0.3	22:1	1.6
18:0	3.5	22:5n-3	0.4
18:1n-9	15.4	22:6n-3	2.7
18:2n-6	33.9	24:1	1.2
18:3n-6	15.6		
18:3n-3	0.3	others	2.6

[†]Average of two analyses.
[a]Fatty acid notation: number of carbon atoms: number of double bonds followed by extra information; n-x = biological series; Br = branched chain.

TABLE 13.2 Fatty Acid Composition (mean ± SD) of Serum Phospholipids Before and After Supplementation with a Mixture of Plant and Marine Oils, Rich in γ-Linolenic and n-3 Fatty Acids (composition in Table 13.1)

Fatty Acid[a]	Before (%) Mean ± SD	After (%) Mean ± SD	P
14:0	0.35 ± 0.09	0.34 ± 0.1	
15:0	0.18 ± 0.05	0.19 ± 0.06	
16Br	0.78 ± 0.14	0.81 ± 0.16	
16:0	29.05 ± 1.98	2.73 ± 1.99	
16:t	0.12 ± 0.06	0.11 ± 0.06	
16:1n-9	0.11 ± 0.05	0.09 ± 0.06	
16:1n-7	0.61 ± 0.2	0.52 ± 0.15	*
16:1n-5	0.09 ± 0.08	0.05 ± 0.08	
17:0	0.36 ± 0.05	0.35 ± 0.07	
18Br	0.64 ± 0.17	0.63 ± 0.17	
18:0	11.88 ± 1.25	1.02 ± 1.38	
18:1t	0.47 ± 0.22	0.44 ± 0.27	
18:1n-9	8.04 ± 0.77	7.61 ± 0.91	
18:1n-7	1.22 ± 0.22	1.12 ± 0.17	*
18:1n-5	0.05 ± 0.09	0.09 ± 0.16	
18:2tt	0.05 ± 0.06	0.03 ± 0.06	
18:2ct	0.03 ± 0.06	0 ± 0	
18:2n-6	21.34 ± 3.23	0.29 ± 3.13	
18:3n-6	0.07 ± 0.07	0.13 ± 0.08	*
18:3n-3	0.22 ± 0.15	0.26 ± 0.2	
20:0	0.41 ± 0.2	0.32 ± 0.21	
20:1n-9	0.12 ± 0.04	0.12 ± 0.09	
20:2n-6	0.04 ± 0.05	0.05 ± 0.05	
20:3n-9	0.34 ± 0.09	0.34 ± 0.1	
20:3n-6	2.72 ± 0.54	3.41 ± 1.17	**
20:4n-6	9.42 ± 1.57	9.37 ± 1.71	
20:0	1.37 ± 0.26	1.38 ± 0.28	
20:5n-3	0.79 ± 0.42	1.22 ± 0.61	**
22:4n-6	0.28 ± 0.07	0.23 ± 0.08	*
24:0	0.13 ± 0.13	0.10 ± 0.11	
24:1	1.07 ± 0.32	1.04 ± 0.28	
22:5n-6	1.67 ± 0.47	2.06 ± 0.40	**
22:5n-3	0.79 ± 0.27	0.93 ± 0.19	**
22:6n-3	3.41 ± 0.83	4.15 ± 0.81	***
Total SAT	43.73 ± 1.36	43.96 ± 1.23	
Unpaired	0.54 ± 0.07	0.54 ± 0.12	
Branched	1.42 ± 0.29	1.43 ± 0.31	
Total *trans*	0.67 ± 0.25	0.61 ± 0.3	
Total monoene	11.44 ± 1.04	10.69 ± 0.94	*
Total n-6	35.54 ± 2.1	35.03 ± 2.26	
Total n-3	5.21 ± 1.26	6.56 ± 1.17	***
n-6 HUFA	14.13 ± 1.89	15.11 ± 2.24	*
n-3 HUFA	5.14 ± 1.25	6.29 ± 1.16	***
Total HUFA	19.61 ± 2.76	21.74 ± 2.73	**

*$P < 0.05$; **$P < 0.01$; ***$P < 0.001$.
[a]Fatty acid notation: number of carbon atoms: number of double bonds followed by extra information; n-x = biological series: Br = branched chain.

fatty acids, and calculated en% intake of linoleic acid, α-linolenic acid and their ratio. The changes in 16:1n-7 correlated positively with that of 18:1n-9 ($r = 0.77, P < 0.001$). The changes in 20:3n-6 correlated negatively with 18:2n-6 ($r = -0.69, P < 0.0025$), and changes in 22:5n-6 correlated positively with 22:6n-3 ($r = 0.71; P < 0.001$). Other correlations between changes in fatty acids in the PL fraction had significance >0.01. Changes in fatty acids did not correlate strongly ($r < 0.5$) with either en% linoleic acid, α-linoleic acid or their ratio in the diet.

Regression analyses were done between the changes in GLA and all HUFA present in the supplement and their pretreatment values in the PL. In each case, correlations were negative but $P < 0.01$ was reached for 22:5n-3 only ($r = -0.72, P < 0.001$). When expressed as a percentage of total HUFA, the potential eicosanoid precursors 20:3n-6 and 20:5n-3 were significantly higher, whereas 20:4n-6 was significantly lower after the administration of the supplement (Table 13.3).

Discussion

We opted to evaluate the effect of the supplement in individuals who were on their usual as opposed to a standardized diet. It was anticipated that by doing so, variability in pretreatment values would be higher. High variability in pretreatment values allows us to determine if the effect induced by feeding the supplement depends on pretreatment values.

The effects of GLA/n-3 feeding obtained in this study are comparable to those described for rats (3,4). An increase of the n-3 HUFA in PL, as seen in this study after feeding the GLA/n-3 HUFA supplement, has also been demonstrated after supplemention with n-3 HUFA without GLA (2,11). Under the latter circumstances, mainly linoleic acid was reduced in compensation and there also was a small reduction of AA (2,11). In this study, AA, expressed as percentage of total fatty acids in the PL fraction, did not change significantly. Supplementation with GLA without n-3 fatty acids

TABLE 13.3 Individual Higher Unsaturated Fatty Acids[†] As a Percentage of Total Higher Unsaturated Fatty Acids

Fatty Acid[a]	Before Mean ± SD	After Mean ± SD	P
20:3n-6	13.92 ± 2.51	15.63 ± 4.89	*
20:3n-9	1.79 ± 0.53	1.59 ± 0.46	
20:4n-6	48.14 ± 5.39	43.01 ± 4.65	***
20:5n-3	3.99 ± 1.74	5.63 ± 2.82	**
22:4n-6	1.41 ± 0.29	1.06 ± 0.34	***
22:5n-6	8.53 ± 2.33	9.51 ± 1.71	*
22:5n-3	3.99 ± 1.77	4.29 ± 0.81	
22:6n-3	17.27 ± 2.98	19.1 ± 2.71	*

[†]Fatty acids with a chain length of 20–22 carbon atoms and with at least three double bonds.
*$P < 0.05$; **$P < 0.01$; ***$P < 0.001$.
[a]Fatty acid notation: number of carbon atoms: number of double bonds followed by extra information; n-x = biological series.

has been shown to result in an increase of DGLA usually accompanied by a relatively smaller increase in AA (1). It can even result in an increase of n-3 HUFAs (11). These increases were associated with a decrease in 18:1 (13). After feeding the supplement, DGLA was higher, but AA was not. This is consistent with the finding that n-3 fatty acids inhibit the conversion of DGLA to AA (14). If the main aim of a dietary intervention is to obtain maximal DGLA/AA ratios, as may be beneficial in certain diseases (Christophe et al. unpublished results), feeding GLA in combination with n-3 fatty acids seems indicated. The main determinants of the fatty acid composition of serum and tissue PL are the selectivities of the enzymes involved in their synthesis as well as the relative abundance of the different fatty acids (10). As a consequence, positive correlations are expected for changes in fatty acids which are formed from dietary precursors by the same enzymes whereas negative correlations would reflect competition for incorporation. Thus, the positive correlation between the reduction in 16:1n-7 and 18:1n-9 is an indication of reduced $\Delta 9$ desaturase activity, and the negative correlation between 20:3n-6 and 18:2n-6 indicates replacement of the latter by increased amounts of the former. The fatty acids 22:5n-6 and 22:6n-3 are formed by the same metabolic pathway. The positive correlation between the changes in these two fatty acids could mean that this peroxisomal pathway is enhanced.

Changes in a given fatty acid were found to vary considerably among the different individuals (results not shown). One obvious explanation could be differences in the composition of the background diet (14). This prompted us to calculate regressions for changes in fatty acids and biomarkers for intake and/or availability. The fraction of 18:2n-6 and 18:3n-3 in the triglyceride fraction was taken to be an estimate of the intake of these fatty acids (10). For the other fatty acids, pretreatment values in the PL were taken as a measure of their availability. The negative correlations found between changes in GLA and all HUFAs and their pretreatment values suggests, as one would anticipate, that the effect of supplementation with these fatty acids is less pronounced when they are available in larger amounts before supplementation. Intakes of linoleic and α-linolenic acid or their ratio in the diet seem to be of lesser importance because they do not correlate strongly with the changes in fatty acids found. This is in contrast with the findings in rats where the effects of n-3 feeding depend on the 18:2n-6 content of the diet (15).

On the basis of their percentage in the PL, changes in amounts of fatty acids are relatively small (e.g., 0.74% for 22:6n-3 and 0.69% for 20:3n-6, Table 13.2). The 20-22 carbon fatty acids exert many of their biological effects by being incorporated into positions in phospholipids from which eicosanoid precursors are mobilized (see references in 16) and by the types of eicosanoids they form. Although not precursors of eicosanoids themselves, the 22-carbon polyunsaturated fatty acids strongly interfere with prostaglandin synthesis (16), and many interactions between HUFAs have been demonstrated (10,16–20).

Levels and types of the different eicosanoids formed are affected by the ratio of their precursors in PL (4). Therefore, it may be more revealing to express individual HUFA as a percentage of total HUFAs. The considerable difference in HUFA composition pre- and post-supplementation suggests that GLA/n-3 supplementation could have important eicosanoid-mediated physiological effects (4,19).

Acknowledgments

Mr. A. Nollet and Mr. M. Ranschaert participated as students in this study. The supplements were obtained free of charge from NV Decola (Aast. Belgium).

References

1. Manku. M.S., Morse-Fisher, N., and Horrobin, D.F. Changes in Human Plasma Essential Fatty Acid Levels as a Result of Administration of Linoleic Acid and Gamma-Linolenic Acid (1988) *Eur. J. Clin. Nutr. 42,* 55–60.
2. Blonk, M.C., Bilo, H.J.G., Nauta, J.J.P., Popp-Snijder, C., Mulder, C., and Donker, A.J.M. Dose-Response Effects of Fish-Oil Supplementation in Healthy Volunteers (1990) *Am. J. Clin. Nutr. 52,* 120–127.
3. Nassar, B.A., Huang, Y.-S., and Horrobin, D.F. Response of Tissue Phospholipid Fatty Acid Composition to Dietary (n-6) and Replacement with Marine (n-3) and Saturated Fatty Acids in the Rat (1986) *Nutr. Res. 6,* 1397–1409.
4. Takahashi, R., Nassar, B.A., Huang, Y.-S., Begin, M.E., and Horrobin, D.F. Effect of Different Ratios of Dietary n-6 and n-3 Fatty Acids on Fatty Acid Composition. Prostaglandin Formation and Platelet Aggregation in the Rat (1987) *Thromb. Res. 47,* 135–146.
5. Phinney, S.D., Odin, R., Johnson, S.B., and Holman, R.T. Reduced Arachidonate in Serum Phospholipids and Cholesteryl Esters Associated with Vegetarian Diets in Humans (1990) *Am. J. Clin. Nutr. 51,* 385–392.
6. Galli, C., Agostini, C., Mosconi. C., Rivi, E., Salari, P.C., and Giovannini, M. Reduced Plasma C-20 and C-22 Polyunsaturated Fatty Acids in Children with Phenylketonuria During Dietary Intervention (1991) *J. Pediatr. 119,* 562–567.
7. Sinclair, A.J., Johnson, L., O' Dea, K., and Holman, R.T. Diets Rich in Lean Beef Increase Arachidonic Acid and Long Chain Omega 3 Polyunsaturated Fatty Acid Levels in Plasma Phospholipids (1994) *Lipids 29,* 337–343.
8. Gronn, M., Gorbitz, C., Christensen, E., Levorsen, A., Ose, L., Hagve, T.A., and Christeophersen, B.O. Dietary n-6 Fatty Acids Inhibit the Incorporation of Dietary n-3 Fatty Acids in Thrombocyte and Serum Phospholipids in Humans (1991) *Scand. J. Clin. Lab. Invest. 51,* 255–263.
9. Christophe, A., Robberecht, E., De Baets, F., and Franckx, H. Increase of Long Chain Omega-3 Fatty Acids in the Major Serum Lipid Classes of Patients with Cystic Fibrosis (1992) *Ann. Nutr. Metab. 36,* 304–312.
10. Lands, W.E.M., Libelt, B., Morris, A., Kramer N.C., Prewitt, T.E., Bowen, P., Schmeisser, D., Davidson, M.H., and Burns, J.H. Maintenance of Lower Proportions of (n-6) Eicosanoid Precursors in Phospholipids of Human Plasma in Response to Added (n-3) Fatty Acids (1992) *Biochim. Biophys. Acta 1180,* 147–162.
11. Horrobin, D.F. Gamma Linoleic Acid: An Intermediate in Essential Fatty Acid Metabolism with Potential as an Ethical Food (1990) *Rev. Contemp. Pharmacother. 1,* 1–45.
12. Willis, A.L., Comai, K., Kuhn, D.C., and Paulsrud, J. Dihomo-Gammalinolenate Suppresses Platelet Aggregation When Administered *in Vitro* and *in Vivo* (1974) *Prostaglandins 8,* 509–519.
13. Holub, B.J., Bakker, D.J,. and Skeaff, C.M. Alterations in Molecular Species of Cholesterol Esters Formed via Plasma Lecithin-Cholesterol Acyltransferase in Human Subjects Consuming Fish Oil (1987) *Atherosclerosis 66,* 11–18.

14. Oxholm, P., Rasmussen, N., Manthorpe, R., and Horrobin, D. (1990) in *Omega-6 Essential Fatty Acids,* Horrobin, D.F., ed., Wiley-Liss, New York, pp. 255–260.
15. Rubin, D., and Laposata, M. Cellular Interactions Between n-6 and n-3 Fatty Acids: A Mass Analysis of Fatty Acid Elongation/Desaturation, Distribution among Complex Lipids and Conversion to Eicosanoids (1992) *J. Lipid Res. 33,* 1431–1440.
16. Garg, M.L., Thomson, A.B.R., and Clandinin, M.T. Interactions of Saturated n-6 and n-3 Polyunsaturated Fatty Acids to Modulate Arachidonic Acid Metabolism (1990) *J. Lipid Res. 31,* 271–277.
17. Nilsson, A., Hjelte, L., and Strandvik, B. Incorporation of Dietary Arachidonic Acid and Eicosapentaenoic Acid in Tissue Lipids During Absorption of a Fish Oil Emulsion (1992) *J. Lipid Res. 33,* 1295–1305.
18. Horrobin, D.F. A New Concept of Life-style Related Cardiovascular Disease: The Importance of Interactions Between Cholesterol, Essential Fatty Acids, Prostaglandin E_1 and Thromboxane A_2 (1980) *Med. Hypotheses 6,* 785–795.
19. Kirtland, S.J. Prostaglandin E_1: A Review (1988) *Prostaglandins, Leukotrienes, Essen. Fatty Acids 32,* 165–174.
20. Corey, E.J., Shih, C., and Cashman, J.R. Docosahexaenoic Acid Is a Strong Inhibitor of Prostaglandin but Not Leucotriene Biosynthesis (1983) *Proc. Natl. Acad. Sci. U.S.A. 80,* 3581–3584.

Chapter 14

Comparative Evaluation of the Hypocholesterolemic Effect of Octadecatrienoic Acids

Michihiro Sugano[a] and Ikuo Ikeda[b]

[a]Laboratory of Food Science and
[b]Laboratory of Nutrition Chemistry, Kyushu University School of Agriculture, Fukuoka 812-81, Japan

Introduction

There are two major octadecatrienoic acids in nature, α-linolenic (ALA, 18:3n-3) and γ-linolenic (GLA, 18:3n-6) acids. Although polyunsaturated fatty acids (PUFA) of the n-3 and n-6 families have distinctly different nutritional and physiological functions, it is indeed interesting that GLA manifests effects comparable to those of ALA within some metabolic parameters such as interference with the production of 2-series prostaglandins (PG) (1,2). In addition, there are at least two other, rarer types of octadecatrienoic acids as characterized by the positional and geometrical isomers of GLA, pinolenic acid ($5c,9c,12c$-18:3) (3) and columbinic acid ($5t,9c,12c$-18:3) (4). The alteration of the position and geometry of the double bond in GLA possibly modifies the metabolic fate and consequently, the nutritional and physiological functions.

It is not clear whether GLA itself is the active principle of the hypocholesterolemic effect, but a wide range of information supports the possible participation of its metabolite(s) and further, eicosanoids (2). Linoleic acid (LA, 18:2n-6), the parent molecule of n-6 PUFA, is a well-known hypocholesterolemic fatty acid. LA is converted to GLA by Δ6 desaturase. GLA is readily elongated to dihomo-γ-linolenic acid (DGLA, 20:3n-6), which is then desaturated to arachidonic acid (AA, 20:4n-6) by Δ5-desaturase. The desaturation systems, in particular the activity of the rate-limiting Δ6 desaturase, are reported to proceed inefficiently in humans and are disturbed by various nutritional, physiological and pathological factors (2,5). Some evidence suggests that GLA, DGLA, and AA take part in the hypocholesterolemic potential of LA. This is in contrast to the observations that components that depress Δ6-desaturase reduce plasma cholesterol (6,7). In addition to AA, DGLA is also the precursor of prostaglandin E_1 (PGE_1). Some PG are known to influence cholesterol metabolism (2,8). At present, however, information regarding the mechanism of action of PUFA is still not fully known.

In contrast, α-linolenic acid is hypotriglyceridemic rather than hypocholesterolemic in humans (9,10), although it has demonstrated significant cholesterol-lowering activity in experimental animals (11,12). Information concerning the effect of other octadecatrienoic acids on plasma cholesterol levels is quite limited, but these acids may have interesting effects not only on the cholesterol metabolism but also on the metabolism of LA (3,4).

This review deals with the effects on plasma cholesterol concentration of these octadecatrienoic acids with emphasis on the mechanism of action of GLA.

Effects of γ-Linolenic Acid on Plasma Cholesterol Levels

Animal Studies

Takayasu and Yoshikawa (13) were probably the first investigators to demonstrate the hypocholesterolemic effect of GLA. They observed a significant lowering of plasma and liver cholesterol concentrations by methyl-GLA in rats fed high-cholesterol diets, but this was not the case in rats fed cholesterol-free diets. The effect of GLA was then examined using a triglyceride form. Huang et al. (14) fed hydrogenated coconut oil, safflower oil or evening primrose oil (EPO) to rats. When cholesterol was added to the diets, the plasma cholesterol level was lowest and liver cholesterol was highest with EPO, whereas, in cholesterol-free diets, no effect on plasma cholesterol was observed, but liver cholesterol was lowered by EPO. They speculated that in cholesterol-fed rats, EPO stimulated the transfer of plasma cholesterol into the liver, either via LDL-receptors or via one of the alternative routes. In rats fed cholesterol-free diets, EPO might reduce endogenous cholesterol synthesis in the liver. In another trial (15), the reduction of plasma cholesterol 2 d after feeding PUFA in rats (previously made hypercholesterolemic by dietary cholesterol) was greater in those given GLA than in those given LA.

The effect was studied in spontaneously hypertensive rats (SHR) (16), but no difference in serum cholesterol level was found among rats fed diets containing sunflower oil, linseed oil and EPO. However, HDL-cholesterol was highest and triglyceride was lowest in EPO-fed rats. Similar results were obtained in rabbits fed EPO at a level of less than 1% of calorie intake (17). These observations are of importance for reducing the risk of atherosclerosis.

In studies with rats fed a cholesterol-containing diet, serum cholesterol level was lower with EPO than with safflower oil or soybean oil (18), or olive oil and safflower oil (Fig. 14.1) (19). In addition, the ratio of HDL-cholesterol to total cholesterol was highest and that of VLDL-cholesterol to total cholesterol was lowest in EPO-fed rats, indicating the antiatherogenic nature of GLA.

Although GLA appeared to exert a significant effect on cholesterol metabolism, two problems remain to be resolved concerning the use of EPO as a source of GLA. First, EPO contains a relatively large amount of plant sterols (approximately 15 mg/g vs. 3 mg/g in safflower oil), which are also hypocholesterolemic. This possibility was ignored because EPO, in which the plant sterol content was reduced to the level of safflower oil, produced a greater hypocholesterolemic effect compared with safflower oil (19), and liver cholesterol also tended to be lower. Thus, the effect of EPO was attributed exclusively to the occurrence of GLA. When ethyl GLA (94% purity) was added to the cholesterol-enriched diet, plasma cholesterol decreased in

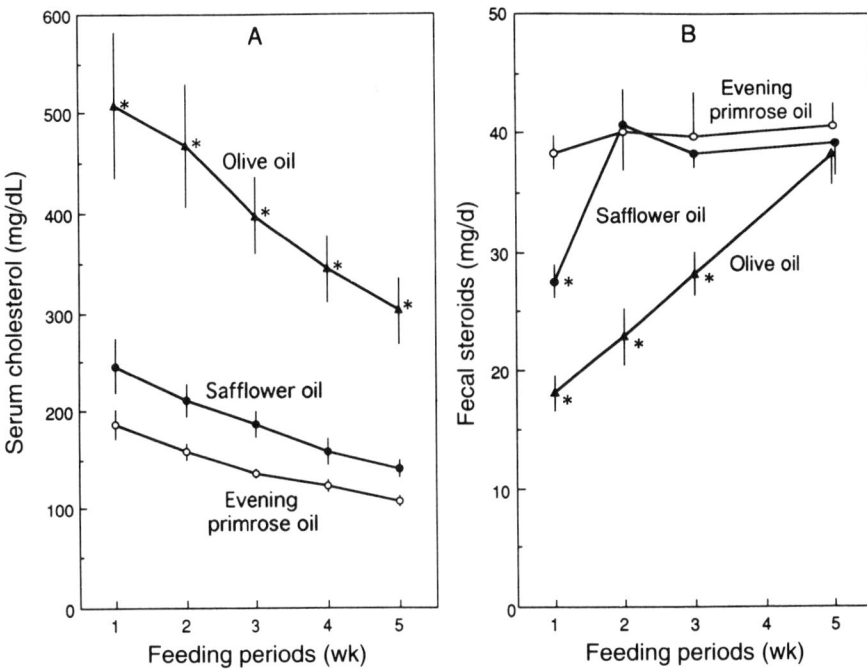

Fig. 14.1. Effects of dietary polyunsaturated oils on concentrations of serum cholesterol (A) and fecal excretion of neutral steroids (B) of rats. Dietary fat level was 10%. Values are mean of 6 rats. *Significantly different from the evening primrose oil and safflower oil groups (A) or from the evening primrose oil group (B) at $P < 0.05$ (19).

a dose-dependent manner at relatively low levels, whereas HDL-cholesterol increased (Fig. 14.2). Second, because EPO contains more than 70% LA as well as 9% GLA, the combined effect of these two PUFA should not be ruled out. This possibility can also be virtually ignored if the effect was compared between EPO and safflower oil. EPO contains GLA at the expense of LA in safflower oil. In this respect, the hypocholesterolemic effect of other GLA sources, borage oil and black currant oil, should be compared with EPO (2).

Another interesting question is whether GLA is able to exert its preferable effect even when the dietary LA level is low. To solve this question, the effect of GLA was examined in rats fed mold oil prepared from *Mortierella rammanniana* var. *angulispora* which contains about 30% palmitic acid, 45% oleic acid, 10% LA and 6% GLA (20). The hypocholesterolemic activity of mold oil was comparable to that of safflower oil containing 75% LA and was greater than palm olein containing a comparable amount of polyunsaturated fatty acid, 16% LA. These effects were not observed with LA. With the addition of more than 1% ethyl GLA to the diet, the effect on plasma total and HDL-cholesterol became significant compared with ethyl LA. These observations indicate the preferable hypocholesterolemic effect of EPO, although the absorption efficiency may differ between ethyl esters and triglyceride (21).

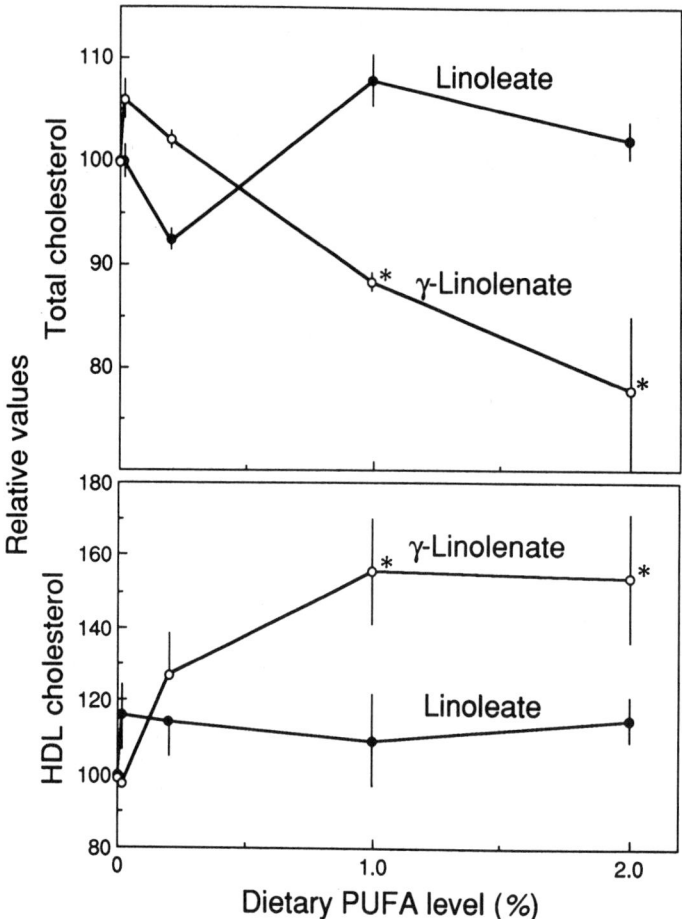

Fig. 14.2. Dose-dependent effects of dietary ethyl-linoleate and ethyl-γ-linolenate on concentrations of serum total and HDL-cholesterol. Values are means ± SE of 6 rats. Total cholesterol levels in rats fed palm oil alone (the control groups) were 140 ± 4 and 143 ± 13 mg/dL for experiments with GLA and LA, respectively. The corresponding values for HDL-cholesterol were 18.1 ± 0.8 and 21.2 ± 2.1 mg/dL. *Significantly different from the ethyl-linoleate group at $P < 0.05$ (18).

In an experiment with a cholesterol-free diet (22), the hypocholesterolemic activity of EPO was not observed in rats. However, the concentration of liver cholesterol was significantly lower in rats fed EPO or EPO + palm oil (1:1) than in those fed palm oil. The comparable effect of EPO with safflower oil in a cholesterol-free diet was also shown in an experiment in which rats of different ages (3 wk and 8 mo old) were fed EPO, safflower oil or a mixture of safflower oil and linseed oil (10% α-linolenic acid and 68% LA) (23).

When the effect of mold oil (10% LA and 6% GLA) was compared with that of palm olein (16% LA) in rats fed cholesterol-free diets containing casein or soybean protein as a source of dietary protein, mold oil prevented the elevation of plasma cholesterol due to casein in relation to soybean protein (24). The concentration of liver cholesterol in rats fed a casein-mold oil diet was lower than in those fed a casein-palm olein diet. From these observations, it is evident that GLA is effective in lowering liver cholesterol even when it does not show a hypocholesterolemic effect under a cholesterol-free regimen.

The effects of GLA as a form of triglyceride or phospholipid prepared from mold oil were compared in rats fed a high-cholesterol diet (25). Both types of mold lipids were equally effective in lowering the plasma cholesterol level when compared with soybean phospholipid which is also known to have a hypocholesterolemic effect (26). Interestingly, the concentration of liver cholesterol tended to be lower in the triglyceride form than in the phospholipid form and in soybean phospholipid. This observation deserves further study.

There are, however, a few reports that failed to show any significant hypocholesterolemic potential of EPO. When hydrogenated coconut oil, safflower oil, linseed oil or EPO were fed with or without cholesterol to guinea pigs, the hypocholesterolemic effect of EPO was comparable with other PUFA (27). When the cholesterol-lowering effect of mold oil was compared with palm oil in hamsters receiving cholesterol-free diets, plasma and liver cholesterol levels did not differ between the two oils (28). No beneficial effect of EPO compared with safflower oil was observed on the plasma cholesterol level of rabbits fed a high-cholesterol diet (29). Like humans, these animals demonstrate low activity of the fatty acid desaturation system, making them a better model for this line of research. However, the results were not supportive. The reason for these unexpected observations is not clear at present, but because the cholesterol-lowering effect of EPO was compared with other vegetable oils in these studies, these observations do not mean that GLA is not hypocholesterolemic. The existence of a large proportion of LA in EPO may conceal the effect of GLA. On the other hand, in study with rats fed GLA-rich oil extracted from fungi for 4 wk diets containing 2.88 or 7.68 g GLA/kg increased plasma total cholesterol level significantly (30). The reason for this unique result is not apparent.

Human Studies

Studies in humans are relatively limited. Horrobin and Manku (31) evaluated the effect of GLA on the plasma cholesterol level in humans. They gave EPO capsules (2–6 g/d) to hypercholesterolemic and normocholesterolemic subjects. EPO was more effective in patients having higher serum cholesterol concentrations (Table 14.1). The effect of EPO was dose-dependent and was estimated to be 170 times more effective than LA when calculated according to the Hegsted's equation (32). The cholesterol-lowering action was attributed to a fall in LDL-cholesterol, while HDL-cholesterol remained unchanged. The authors suggested that the hypocholesterolemic effect of LA becomes evident after it is converted to GLA and/or further metabolites. When hyperlipidemic men were given EPO (3 g/d including 2.2 g of LA and 0.24 g of GLA) for 4 mo, a marked reduction of total and LDL-cholesterol and triglyceride was observed (33). In contrast, HDL-cholesterol increased.

TABLE 14.1 The Effect of γ-Linolenic Acid in the Form of Evening Primrose Oil on Total Plasma Cholesterol Levels of Humans

All Starting Values (mmol/L)	n	Beginning (mean ± SD)	End	Fall (mmol/L)	Fall (mg/dl)	P
Above 8.0	7	10.90 ± 2.43	7.64 ± 1.71	3.26	125.4	0.0001
Above 7.0	15	9.15 ± 2.46	6.92 ± 1.57	2.23	85.8	0.0001
Above 6.0	31	7.79 ± 2.21	5.98 ± 1.54	1.81	69.6	0.0001
Above 5.0	50	6.94 ± 2.07	5.58 ± 1.37	1.36	52.3	0.0001
Below 5.0	34	4.32 ± 0.56	4.27 ± 0.69	0.05	1.9	NS

Mean ± SD of 12 patients receiving 6 or 8 capsules (0.5 g/capsule) per day for not more than 12 wk (31). NS, not significant.

The effectiveness of GLA is also shown in other diseases. Chaintreuil et al. (34) studied patients with type 1 diabetes by supplementing either 0.5 g or 2 g GLA/d for 6 wk and showed that 2 g GLA was effective in lowering plasma cholesterol and triglyceride levels. Although they used GLA itself instead of EPO, the magnitude of the effect was generally comparable to that reported by Horrobin and Manku (31).

In contrast to these studies, two groups of investigators failed to show any preferable effect of GLA. In one study, elderly people were given 2 g of sunflower oil (61% LA) or 1 g of sunflower oil plus 1 g of modified EPO (41% GLA and 41% LA) for 2 mo in a cross-over study (35). The authors of this study reported no changes in plasma total and HDL-cholesterol and apoA-I, A-II and B with EPO administration, although no data were shown. Viikari and Lehtonen (36) were also unable to show the hypocholesterolemic effect of GLA. They gave EPO to 20 hyperlipidemic patients for 3 mo at a dose of 2.4, 4.8 and 7.2 mL/d during the 1st, 2nd, 3rd mo, respectively. Serum total and HDL-cholesterol did not change during the treatment.

Dillon (37) gave 10 g of black currant oil containing 15% GLA to 30 elderly people for 3 mo. The control group received a mixture of linseed oil and corn oil, in which the content of LA was adjusted to that of the currant oil. There was a significant decrease in VLDL-cholesterol, but not total cholesterol in serum after feeding the currant oil. When borage oil was given to healthy males for 6 wk no significant changes of total and HDL-cholesterol and triglyceride concentration were observed (38). Borage oil contains 21.8% GLA and 35.5% LA and daily GLA intake was 5.23 g on average.

Limited data from human studies indicate the effectiveness of GLA in lowering plasma cholesterol at least in those who are hypercholesterolemic as in the case of animal studies with cholesterol-enriched diets. Although some experiments failed to show the greater hypocholesterolemic effect of GLA compared with LA, the results may indicate that the plasma cholesterol levels reached a bottom level in these subjects.

Cholesterol Metabolism and γ-Linolenic Acid

Because only a few studies are concerned with the effect of GLA and its metabolites on the dynamics of cholesterol metabolism, the mechanism of the hypocholesterolemic effect of GLA is rarely revealed.

Huang et al. (14) suggested that the decrease in liver cholesterol by EPO in rats fed a cholesterol-free diet can be attributed to a reduction in 3-hydroxy-3-methylglutaryl Coezyme A (HMG-CoA) reductase activity, the rate-limiting enzyme of cholesterol biosynthesis. However, there is no evidence supporting this assumption. When young (3 wk) and adult (8 mo) rats were fed a cholesterol-free diet containing either EPO, safflower oil or a mixture of safflower oil and linseed oil for 4 wk, the activity of liver microsomal HMG-CoA reductase was comparable between young and adult rats (Fig. 14.3) (23). However, the magnitude of the age-related decline of reductase activity was small in rats fed EPO. In contrast, Dib and Carreau (39) demonstrated an increase in HMG-CoA reductase activity in pregnant rats fed EPO compared with those fed sunflower oil.

Cholesterol 7α-hydroxylase, the rate-limiting enzyme of bile acid biosynthesis, was not influenced by EPO compared with safflower oil in young and adult rats fed a cholesterol-free diet (Fig. 14.3) (23). In rats fed a cholesterol-enriched diet, fecal excretion of neutral steroids was increased by EPO compared with safflower oil during the 1st wk of feeding (Fig. 14.1) (19). Although this increase disappeared at the

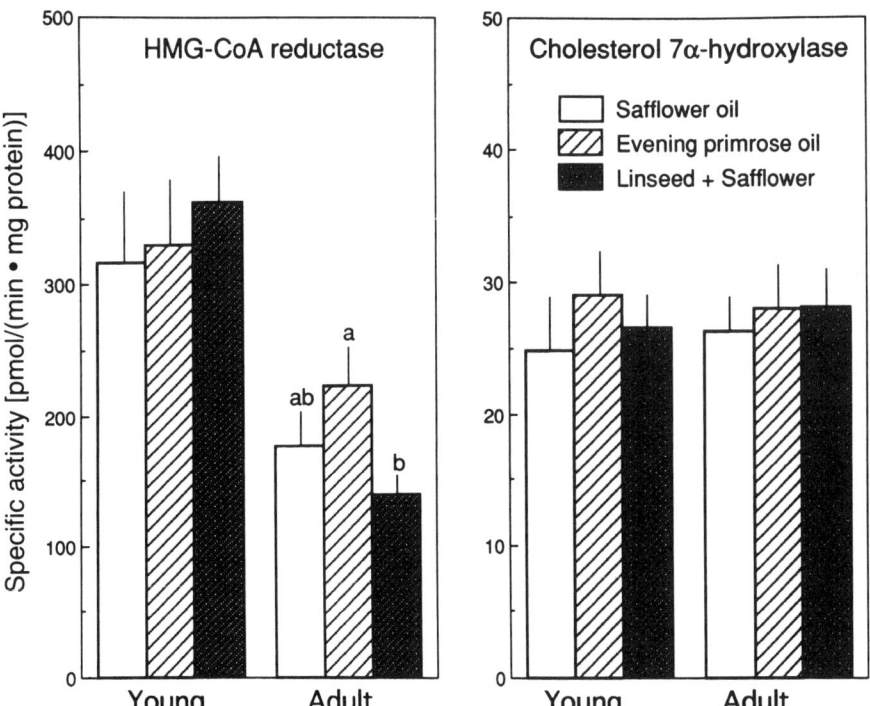

Fig. 14.3. Effects of dietary fats on the activities of HMG-CoA reductase and cholesterol 7α-hydroxylase of rat liver microsomes. Rats were fed diets containing 10% fat for 4 wk. Values are mean ± SE of 8 rats.
[a,b]Values not sharing a common letter are significantly different at $P < 0.05$ (23).

2nd wk and thereafter, the difference in steroid excretion during the first week reflected the decrease in the serum cholesterol level. The excretion of acidic steroids was not influenced by the type of dietary fat as expected from the response of cholesterol 7α-hydroxylase. In contrast, when mold oil was used as a source of GLA, no increase in fecal excretion of neutral steroids was observed, whereas the excretion of acidic steroids was rather high in rats fed safflower oil (20). Even under the dietary manipulation by which fecal steroid excretion is modified, GLA appears to exert its effect. Thus, mold oil stimulated the excretion of neutral steroids in rats fed soybean protein, but not in rats fed casein, whereas the excretion of acidic steroids remained unchanged (24).

There is a possibility that altered lipoprotein metabolism is responsible for the plasma cholesterol-lowering effect of GLA, but no information is available regarding this issue as in the case of LA (40). Because vegetable oils increase the LDL-receptor level in comparison with animal fats (41), the hypocholesterolemic effect of GLA may be directly attributable to a redistribution of plasma cholesterol to body tissues through an increase in tissue receptors, rather than a change in endogenous cholesterol synthesis or catabolism. This appears reasonable because, in a study with baboons, saturated fat sustained a significant reduction of hepatic LDL-receptor mRNA compared with unsaturated fats (42).

More information is necessary to establish the effect of GLA on hepatic LDL-receptor activity. However, when one considers greater hypocholesterolemic activity of GLA compared with LA, GLA may have a greater potential than its parent molecule in stimulating receptor activity.

Possible Effects of Metabolites of γ-Linolenic Acid

Effects of DGLE and AA

The administration of GLA increases DGLA significantly and AA to a lesser extent in tissue phospholipids (2). Horrobin (1,5) suggested the importance of the desaturation system in the cholesterol-lowering activity of LA. His suggestion is based on the following observations: (i) animals susceptible to atherosclerosis, such as rabbits and guinea pigs, convert LA to AA very slowly, (ii) low tissue level of DGLA and AA is epidemiologically shown to be an independent risk factor for the development of ischemic heart disease, (iii) LA, when administered to hypercholesterolemic patients, is not readily converted to DGLA and AA compared with normal subjects, and (iv) various factors inhibiting the Δ6-desaturation system may also be risk factors for ischemic heart disease.

DGLA (1 g/d) was administered for 4 wk to hyper- and normocholesterolemic patients with atherosclerosis (43). Hypercholesterolemic patients treated with DGLA showed significantly decreased serum cholesterol levels, and this fall was due to the reduction of cholesterol in LDL and VLDL. Because the elongation of GLA to DGLA proceeds readily, whereas Δ5-desaturation of DGLA to AA is restricted in humans, DGLA may be another possible effective metabolite of GLA. However, knowledge of the mechanism of the cholesterol-lowering activity of this fatty acid is again limited. In this connection, AA also appears to lower the plasma cholesterol concentration more efficiently than its parent molecule in humans (44) and in rats (45).

Effects as Prostaglandins

The interrelated effects of PUFA and PG on cholesterol metabolism are well known. Because DGLA and AA are the precursors of PG, an increase of these fatty acids in tissue phospholipids may seemingly influence PG production. The increased production of 1-series PG via DGLA is readily anticipated after administration of GLA. The most important PG of the 1-series is PGE_1 which has a wide range of desirable effects (1,2). Several studies have shown the increase of PGE_1 by dietary GLA and DGLA (46,47), but others failed to observe any change (17,19,33,45).

In addition, GLA and DGLA influence the formation of 2-series PG. The aortic production of PGI_2 increased in rats fed EPO or more directly GLA, compared with fats containing LA or α-linolenic acid (17,19,23,24,28). In contrast, dietary GLA appeared to reduce the production of PGE_2 and TXA_2 (2), although this result is controversial (33,48–50).

The results of these studies at least indicate that changes in PG profiles may influence cholesterol metabolism in several tissues. Dionyssiou-Asteriou et al. (8) administered a huge amount (1 mg/kg for 5 d) of PGE_1 intraperitoneally to rats and found significant decreases in cholesterol, triglyceride and phospholipid in serum and HDL.

Horrobin suggested that PGE_1 inhibits cholesterol biosynthesis (2,51). In fact, Krone et al. (52) showed that the prostacyclin analogue "iloprost" and PGE_1, but not $PGF_{2\alpha}$, suppress sterol synthesis from labeled acetate in freshly isolated human mononuclear leukocytes probably through an increase in cyclic AMP. Cyclic AMP inhibits HMG-CoA reductase and suppresses sterol synthesis (52,53), and also decreases binding, uptake and degradation of LDL by decreasing the number of LDL receptors in several cell lines (54,55).

Perturbation of the cholesterol ester metabolism in arterial walls by altered PG formation in atherosclerotic animals and humans is alleviated by several of the PG, including PGI_2 and PGE_1. In atherosclerotic rabbits, a decrease in artery PGI_2 and an increase in TXA_2 in platelets have been observed repeatedly (56). It is possible that GLA can improve such unfavorable circumstances in arterial vessels by increasing PGI_2 and PGE_1. PGE_1 markedly inhibited pigeon aorta cholesterol ester hydrolase and slightly inhibited the cholesterol ester synthetase activity in the aorta (57).

These studies indicate the possibility that GLA reduces the risk of atherosclerosis by increasing the formation of PGE_1. However, because GLA may occasionally increase the production of other PG, such as PGE_2 and TXA_2 simultaneously, attention should be paid to the dosage of GLA. In this respect, the combination of GLA with fish oil is recommended, because the synthesis of 2-series PG, in particular TXA_2, is inhibited by fish oil (58), and eicosapentaenoic acid interferes with the conversion of GLA to AA and the production of 2-series PG (59). Also, simultaneous administration of sesamin, a specific $\Delta 5$ desaturase inhibitor with hypocholesterolemic potential, seems effective (60). However, dietary indomethacin, the inhibitor of cyclooxygenase, did not modify the plasma cholesterol-lowering effect of EPO in rats (18).

Conclusions

Studies concerning the hypocholesterolemic effect of various octadecatrienoic acids were reviewed with an emphasis on γ-linolenic acid (GLA). α-Linolenic acid (ALA) is hypotriglyceridemic rather than hypocholesterolemic in humans, although it lowers both plasma cholesterol and triglyceride in experimental animals. The observation that GLA exerts a greater cholesterol-lowering activity than LA suggests that GLA and/or its elongated and desaturated metabolites may be the active principle of LA. GLA is readily metabolized to dihomo-γ-linolenic acid (DGLA) and then arachidonic acid (AA) to a lesser extent. However, it is difficult as yet to explain the mechanism by which these fatty acids lower the plasma cholesterol level. DGLA and AA are the precursors of 1- and 2-series prostaglandins (PG), respectively, and limited observations indicate that PG may also influence cholesterol metabolism and decrease the risk of ischemic heart disease. However, we should take into consideration that the formation of various PG, which exert diverse effects in many tissues and organs, is also altered by the intake of various PUFA. In any case, because Δ6-desaturation from LA to GLA is inefficient in humans and is inhibited by various factors such as diabetes, atherosclerosis, alcohol consumption and aging, the intake of GLA instead of LA is recommended to escape the side effects arising from the excessive intake of LA. Pinolenic acid ($5c,9c,12c$-18:3) exerts a cholesterol-lowering action similar to that of ALA or GLA without influencing the metabolism of LA to AA (Table 14.2) (3). In this context, columbinic acid ($5t,9c,12c$-18:3) would be interesting if it could exert a hypocholesterolemic effect, because it may not be converted to eicosanoids due to the presence of *trans* double bond in its molecule. Further study of the mechanism of the hypocholesterolemic effect of various octadecatrienoic acids, in particular GLA, will expand their application.

TABLE 14.2 Effects of Different Dietary Fats on Plasma and Liver Lipid Levels of Rats

Dietary Group	Cholesterol	
	Serum (mg/dL)	Liver (mg/g)
Cholesterol-enriched diets		
Safflower oil	155 ± 11[a]	86.0 ± 3.3
Flaxseed oil	116 ± 10[b]	85.0 ± 4.6
Pine-seed oil	132 ± 10[a,b]	79.4 ± 6.5
Cholesterol-free diets		
Safflower oil	73.9 ± 2.5	3.39 ± 0.37
Evening primrose oil	79.9 ± 2.8	2.82 ± 0.12
Pine-seed oil	78.6 ± 2.8	3.06 ± 0.13

Means ± SE of 6–7 rats. Rats were fed diets containing 10% fat for 30 d.
[a,b]Values not sharing a common letter are significantly different at $P < 0.05$ (3).

References

1. Horrobin, D.F. Gamma Linolenic Acid: An Intermediate in Essential Fatty Acid Metabolism with Potential as an Ethical Pharmaceutical and as a Food (1990) *Rev. Contemp. Pharmacother. 1,* 1–45.
2. Horrobin, D.F. Nutritional and Medical Importance of Gamma-linolenic Acid (1992) *Prog. Lipid Res. 31,* 163–194.
3. Sugano, M., Ikeda, I., Wakamatsu, K., and Oka, T. Influence of Korean Pine (*Pinus Koraiensis*)-Seed Oil Containing *cis*-5, *cis*-9, *cis*-12 Octadecatrienoic Acid on Polyunsaturated Fatty Acid Metabolism, Eicosanoid Production and Blood Pressure of Rats (1994) *Brit. J. Nutr. 72,* 775–783.
4. Houtsmuller, U.M.T. Columbinic Acid, a New Type of Essential Fatty Acid (1981) *Prog. Lipid Res. 20,* 889–896.
5. Horrobin, D.F., and Huang, Y.-S. The Role of Linoleic Acid and Its Metabolites in the Lowering of Plasma Cholesterol and the Prevention of Cardiovascular Disease (1987) *Int. J. Cardiol. 17,* 241–255.
6. Huang, Y.-S., Koba, K., Horrobin, D.F., and Sugano, M. Interrelationship Between Dietary Protein, Cholesterol and n-6 Polyunsaturated Fatty Acid Metabolism (1993) *Prog. Lipid Res. 32,* 123–137.
7. Sugiyama, K., Akachi, T., and Yamanaka, A. Eritadenine-induced Alteration of Hepatic Phospholipid Metabolism in Relation to Its Hypocholesterolemic Action in Rats (1995) *J. Nutr. Biochem. 6,* 80–87.
8. Dionyssiou-Asteriou, A., Triantafyllou, A., Lekakis, J., and Kalofoutis, A. Influence of Prostaglandin E_1 on High Density Lipoprotein-fraction Lipid Levels in Rats (1986) *Biochem. Med. Metab. Biol. 36,* 114–117.
9. Harris, W.S. Fish Oil and Plasma Lipid and Lipoprotein Metabolism in Humans: A Critical Review (1980) *J. Lipid Res. 30,* 785–807.
10. Schmidt, E.B., Kristensen, S.D., De Caterina, R., and Illingworth, D.R. The Effects of n-3 Fatty Acids on Plasma Lipids and Lipoproteins and Other Cardiovascular Risk Factors in Patients with Hyperlipoproteinemia (1993) *Atherosclerosis 103,* 107–121.
11. Kinsella, J.E., Lokesh, B., and Stone, R.A. Dietary n-3 Polyunsaturated Fatty Acids and Amelioration of Cardiovascular Disease: Possible Mechanisms (1990) *Am. J. Clin. Nutr. 52,* 1–28.
12. Simopoulos, A.P. Omega-3 Fatty Acids in Health and Disease and in Growth and Development (1991) *Am. J. Clin. Nutr. 54,* 438–463.
13. Takayasu, K., and Yoshikawa, I. The Influence of Exogenous Cholesterol on the Fatty Acid Composition of Liver Lipids in the Rats Given Linoleate and γ-Linolenate (1971) *Lipids 6,* 47–53.
14. Huang, Y.-S., Manku, M.S., and Horrobin, D.F. The Effect of Dictary Cholesterol on Blood and Liver Polyunsaturated Fatty Acids and on Plasma Cholesterol in Rats Fed Various Types of Fatty Acid Diet (1984) *Lipids 19,* 664–672.
15. Huang, Y.-S., McAdoo, K.R., and Horrobin, D.F. Comparison of Short-Term Feeding of Dietary Linoleic and Gamma-Linolenic Acid on Plasma and Liver Cholesterol and Fatty Acids in Hypercholesterolemic Rats (1988) *Nutr. Res. 8,* 389–399.
16. Singer, P., Hoffmann, P., Beitz, J., Forster, W., Wirth, M., and Godicke, W. Serum Triglycerides and HDL Cholesterol from SHR after Evening Primrose Oil and Other Polyunsaturated Fats (1986) *Prostagland. Leuk. Med. 22,* 173–177.

17. Frogoso, Y.D., and Skinner, E.R. The Effect of Gammalinolenic Acid on the Subfractions of Plasma High Density Lipoprotein of the Rabbit (1992) *Biochem. Pharmacol. 44,* 1085–1090.
18. Sugano, M., Ishida, T., and Ide, T. Effect of Various Polyunsaturated Fatty Acids on Blood Cholesterol and Eicosanoids in Rats (1986) *Agric. Biol. Chem. 50,* 2335–2340.
19. Sugano, M., Ide, T., Ishida, T., and Yoshida, K. Hypocholesterolemic Effect of Gamma-Linolenic Acid as Evening Primrose Oil in Rats (1986) *Ann. Nutr. Metab. 30,* 289–299.
20. Sugano, M., Ishida, T., Yoshida, K., Tanaka, K., Niwa, M., Arima, M., and Morita, A. Effect of Mold Oil Containing γ-Linolenic Acid on the Blood Cholesterol and Eicosanoid Levels in Rats (1986) *Agric. Biol. Chem. 50,* 2483–2491.
21. Nelson, G.J., and Ackman, R.G. Absorption and Transport of Fat in Mammals with Emphasis on n-3 Polyunsaturated Fatty Acids (1988) *Lipids 23,* 1005–1014.
22. Lee, J. H., Taguchi, S., Ikeda, I., and Sugano, M. The P/S Ratio of Dietary Fats and Lipid Metabolism in Rats: Gamma-Linolenic Acid as a Source of Polyunsaturated Fatty Acid (1988) *Agric. Biol. Chem. 52,* 3137–3142.
23. Choi, Y. S., and Sugano, M. Effects of Dietary Alpha- and Gamma-Linolenic Acids on Lipid Metabolism in Young and Adult Rats (1988) *Ann. Nutr. Metab. 32,* 169–176.
24. Sugano, M., Ishida, T., and Koba, K. Protein-fat Interaction on Serum Cholesterol Level, Fatty Acid Desaturation and Eicosanoid Production in Rats (1988) *J. Nutr. 118,* 548–554.
25. Imaizumi, K, Sakono, M., Nagata, J., Sugano, M., Kikutsugi, H., and Amano, K. Lipid and Eicosanoid Levels in Rats Fed γ-Linolenic Acid as Triglyceride or Phospholipid of the Mold Origin (1988) *Nutr. Rep. Int. 38,* 767–772.
26. Imaizumi, K., Mawatari, K. Murata, M., Ikeda, I., and Sugano, M. The Contrasting Effect of Dietary Phosphatidylethanolamine and Phosphatidylcholine on Serum Lipoproteins and Liver Lipids in Rats (1983) *J. Nutr. 113,* 2403–2411.
27. Huang, Y.-S., and Horrobin, D.F. Effect of Dietary Cholesterol and Polyunsaturated Fats on Plasma and Liver Lipids in Guinea Pigs (1987) *Ann. Nutr. Metab. 31,* 18–28.
28. Ide, T., Sugano, M., Ishida, T., Niwa, M., Arima, M., and Morita, A. Effect of Gamma-Linolenic Acid on Fatty Acid Profiles and Eicosanoid Production of the Hamster (1987) *Nutr. Res. 7,* 1085–1092.
29. Renaud, S., McGregor, L., Morazain, R., Thevenon, C., Benoit, C. Dumont, E., and Mendy, F. Comparative Beneficial Effects on Platelet Functions and Atherosclerosis of Dietary Linoleic and γ-Linolenic Acids in the Rabbit (1982) *Atherosclerosis 45,* 43–51.
30. Takada, R., Saitoh, M., and Mori, T. Dietary γ-Linolenic Acid-enriched Oil Reduces Body Fat Content and Induces Liver Enzyme Activities Relating to Fatty Acid β-Oxidation in Rats (1994) *J. Nutr. 124,* 469–474.
31. Horrobin, D.F., and Manku, M.S. How Do Polyunsaturated Fatty Acids Lower Plasma Cholesterol Levels? (1983) *Lipids 18,* 558–562.
32. Hegsted, D.M., McGandy, R.B., Myers, M.L., and Stare, F.J. Quantitative Effects of Dietary Fat on Serum Cholesterol in Man (1965) *Am. J. Clin. Nutr. 17,* 281–295.
33. Guivernau, M., Meza, N., Barja, P., and Roman, O. Clinical and Experimental Study on the Long-term Effect of Dietary Gamma-linolenic Acid on Plasma Lipids, Platelet Aggregation, Thromboxane Formation, and Prostacyclin Production (1994) *Prostaglandins Leukotrienes Essent. Fatty Acids 51,* 311–316.
34. Chaintreuil, J., Monnier, L., Colette, C., Crastes de Paulet, P., Orsetti, A., Spielmann, D., Mendy, F., and Crastes de Paulet, A. Effects of Dietary γ-Linolenate Supplementation on

Serum Lipids and Platelet Function in Insulin-dependent Diabetic Patients (1984) *Hum. Nutr. Clin. Nutr. 38C,* 121–130.

35. Vericel, E., Lagarde, M., Mendy, F., Courpron, Ph., and Dechavanne, M. Comparative Effects of Linoleic Acid and Gamma-linolenic Acid Intake on Plasma Lipids and Platelet Phospholipids in Elderly People (1987) *Nutr. Res. 7,* 569–580.
36. Viikari, J., and Lehtonen, A. Effect of Primrose Oil on Serum Lipids and Blood Pressure in Hyperlipidemic Subjects (1986) *Int. J. Clin. Pharm. Therapy Toxicol. 24,* 668–670.
37. Dillon, J.C. Essential Fatty Acid Metabolism in the Elderly. Effect of Dietary Manipulation (1987) in *Lipids in Modern Nutrition,* Horisberg, M., and Bracco, U., eds., Raven Press, New York, pp. 93–106.
38. Barre, D.E., and Holub, B.J. The Effect of Borage Oil Consumption on Human Plasma Lipid Levels and the Phosphatidylcholine and Cholesterol Ester Composition of High Density Lipoprotein (1992) *Nutr. Res. 12,* 1181–1194.
39. Dib, A., and Carreau, J.-P. Effect of γ-Linolenic Acid Supplementation on Lipogenesis Regulation in Pregnant Zinc-Deficient Rat and Fetus (1986) *Int. J. Biochem. 18,* 1053–1056.
40. Grundy, S.M. Lipids and Cardiovascular Diseases (1993) in *Nutrition and Disease Update: Heart Disease,* Kritchevsky, D., and Carroll, K.K., eds., AOCS Press, Champaign, IL, pp. 211–279.
41. Ibrahim, J.B.T., and McNamara, D.J. Cholesterol Homeostasis in Guinea Pigs Fed Saturated and Polyunsaturated Fat Diets (1988) *Biochim. Biophys. Acta 963,* 109–118.
42. Fox, J.C., McGill, H.C., Jr., Carey, K.D., and Getz, G.S. In Vivo Regulation of Hepatic LDL Receptor mRNA in the Baboon: Differential Effects of Saturated and Unsaturated Fat (1987) *J. Biol. Chem. 262,* 7014–7020.
43. Kingsbury, K.J., Morgan, D.M., Aylott, C., and Emmerson, R. Effects of Ethyl Arachidonate, Cod-Liver Oil, and Corn Oil on the Plasma-Cholesterol Level (1961) *Lancet i,* 739–741.
44. Szczeklik, A., Gryglewski, R.J., Sladek, K., Kostka-Trabka, E., and Zumuda, A. Dihomo-γ-Linolenic Acid in Patients with Atherosclerosis: Effects on Platelet Aggregation, Plasma Lipids and Low-Density Lipoprotein-Induced Inhibition of Prostacyclin Generation (1984) *Thromb. Haemostas. 51,* 186–188.
45. Peifer, J.J. Hypocholesterolemic Effects Induced in the Rat by Specific Types of Fatty Acid Unsaturation (1966) *J. Nutr. 88,* 351–358.
46. Manku, M.S., Soma, M., and Jenkins, D.K. Effects of Feeding Gamma-Linolenic Acid on Mesenteric and Urinary Prostaglandin Outflow in Guinea-Pigs (1986) *Prog. Lipid Res. 25,* 309–310.
47. Miller, C.C., and Ziboh, V.A. Gammalinolenic Acid-Enriched Diet Alters Cutaneous Eicosanoids (1988) *Biochem. Biophys. Res. Commun. 154,* 967–974.
48. Mikhailidis, D.P., Kirtland, S., Barradas, M.A., and Dandona, P. Dihomogammalinolenic Acid Inhibits Platelet Aggregation and Stimulates Platelet Prostaglandin E_1 Production in Healthy Subjects but Not in Insulin Dependent Diabetics (1986) *Prog. Lipid Res. 25,* 303–304.
49. Stone, K.J., Willis, A.L., Hart, M., Kirtland, S.J., Kernoff, P.B.A., and McNicol, G.P. The Metabolism of Dihomo-γ-Linolenic Acid in Man (1979) *Lipids 14,* 174–180.
50. Larsson-Backstrom, C., Arrhenius, E., Sagge, K., Lindmark, L., and Svensson, L. Influence of α-Linolenic and γ-Linolenic Acid Enriched and Fat Free Diets on Fatty Acid Profile and Prostaglandin Biosynthesis and on the Outcome of Rat Intraperitoneal Sepsis (1986) *Prog. Lipid Res. 25,* 197–201.

51. Horrobon, D.F. A New Concept of Lifestyle-Related Cardiovascular Disease: The Importance of Interactions Between Cholesterol, Essential Fatty Acids, Prostaglandin E_1 and Thromboxane A_2 (1980) *Med. Hypothesis 6*, 785–800.
52. Krone, W., Kaczmarczyk, P., Muller-Wieland, D., and Greten, H. Prostacyclin Analogue Iloprost and Prostaglandin E_1 Suppress Sterol Synthesis in Freshly Isolated Human Mononuclear Leukocytes (1985) *Biochim. Biophys. Acta 835*, 154–157.
53. Krone, W., Betteridge, D.J., and Galton, D.J. Mechanism of Regulation of 3-Hydroxy-3-methylglutaryl Coenzyme: A Reductase Activity by Low Density Lipoprotein in Human Lymphocytes (1979) *Eur. J. Clin. Invest. 9*, 405–410.
54. Maziere, C., Maziere, J.-C., Salmon, S., Auclair, M., Mora, L., Moreau, M., and Polonovski, J. Cyclic AMP Decreases LDL Catabolism and Cholesterol Synthesis in the Human Hepatoma Cell Line HepG2 (1988) *Biochem. Biophys. Res. Commun. 156*, 424–431.
55. Stout, R.W., and Bierman, E.L. Dibutyryl Cyclic AMP Inhibits LDL Binding in Cultured Fibroblasts and Arterial Smooth Muscle Cells (1983) *Atherosclerosis 46*, 13–20.
56. Gryglewski, R.J., Dembinska-Kiec, A., Zmuda, A., and Gryglewska, T. Prostacyclin and Thromboxane A_2 Biosynthesis Capacities of Heart, Arteries, and Platelets at Various Stages of Experimental Atherosclerosis in Rabbits (1978) *Atherosclerosis 31*, 385–394.
57. Subbiah, M.T.R., and Dicke, B.A. Effect of Prostaglandins E_1 and $F_{1\alpha}$ on the Activities of Cholesteryl Ester Synthetase and Cholesteryl Ester Hydrolases of Pigeon Aorta *in Vitro* (1977) *Atherosclerosis 27*, 107–111.
58. Tertov, V.V., Orekhov, A.N., Repin, V.S., and Smirnov, V.N. Dibutyryl Cyclic AMP Decreases Proliferative Activity and the Cholesteryl Ester Content in Cultured Cells of Atherosclerotic Human Aorta (1982) *Biochem. Biohphys. Res. Res. Commun. 109*, 1228–1233.
59. Nassar, B.A., Manku, M.S., Huang, Y.-S., Jenkins, D.K., and Horrobin, D.F. The Influence of Dietary Marine Oil (Polepa) and Evening Primrose Oil (Efamol) on Prostaglandin Production by the Rat Mesenteric Vasculature (1987) *Prostagland. Leuk. Med. 26*, 253–263.
60. Hirose, M., Inoue, T., Nishihara, K., Sugano, M., Akimoto, K., Shimizu, S., and Yamada, H. Inhibition of Cholesterol Absorption and Synthesis in Rats by Sesamin (1991) *J. Lipid Res. 32*, 629–638.

Chapter 15

γ-Linolenic Acid Attenuates Blood Pressure Responses to Environmental Stimuli: Implications for Human Essential Hypertension

David E. Mills,[a] Yung-Sheng Huang,[b] and Jean-Pierre Poisson[c]

[a]Scientific Laboratory Division, New Mexico Department of Health, Albuquerque, NM and Department of Physiology, University of New Mexico School of Medicine, Albuquerque, NM
[b]Medical Nutritional Research and Development, Ross Products Division, Abbott Laboratories, Columbus, OH
[c]Unite de Nutrition Cellulaire et Metabolique, Universite de Bourgogne, Dijon Cedex, France

Many of the medications currently used in the treatment of essential hypertension produce unacceptable side effects in a significant proportion of users, leading to reduced compliance and poor management of the disorder. As a result, there has been a growing interest in recent years in the potential use of nonpharmaceutical interventions for both the treatment and prevention of hypertension, including stress management, exercise, and dietary manipulation. Among the dietary interventions investigated, based upon the results of animal and preliminary human trials, the manipulation of dietary n-6 essential fatty acids and their metabolites appears to demonstrate promise for the attenuation of blood pressure (BP) development in individuals at risk for hypertension.

γ-Linolenic Acid and Blood Pressure in the SHR

Much of the evidence for a relationship between dietary intake of various levels and types of n-6 fatty acids and systemic blood pressure (BP) has derived from work conducted on rats. Much of that work, in turn, has derived from studies comparing the effects of different dietary fatty acids on blood pressure development in the genetically hypertensive spontaneously hypertensive rat (SHR), a commonly used animal model for human essential hypertension. Early studies in these models demonstrated that long-term feeding of diets low in n-6 fatty acids, i.e., 18:2n-6 and 20:4n-6, exacerbates BP development under normal and salt-loaded conditions (1,2). The reversal of pressor responses in these animal models upon administration/replacement of dietary 18:2n-6 suggests a protective role of the n-6 fatty acids in the regulation of BP. Perhaps the strongest evidence for a role of dietary n-6 fatty acids as a treatment modality in essential hypertension has derived from studies on SHR in which the dietary levels of various n-6 fatty acids were manipulated by the use of oil sources varying in their fatty acid composition. In general, these studies demonstrate that long-term supplementation of the diet with n-6 fatty acids (18:2n-6 or 18:3n-6) attenuates BP development (3–6).

In the SHR studies, the antihypertensive activity of dietary 18:3n-6 has been consistently shown to be more potent than that of its metabolic precursor, 18:2n-6 (see Chapter 16). This probably reflects the fact that the conversion of 18:2n-6 to 18:3n-6 by Δ6-desaturase (D6D) is the rate-limiting step in the metabolism of 18:2n-6, and is slower in the SHR than in the normotensive parent strain of the SHR, the Wistar Kyoto rat (WKY) (7–11). Thus, the provision of 18:3n-6 in the diet of the SHR by-passes this metabolic "roadblock," increasing the relative amounts of the fatty acid precursors (20:3n-6 and 20:4n-6) of eicosanoids effective in lowering blood pressure (5,12,13).

γ-Linolenic Acid and Blood Pressure in the Borderline Hypertensive Rat

Extrapolation of data derived from studies using the SHR regarding the efficacy of dietary 18:3n-6 for lowering blood pressure to the case of human essential hypertension must be viewed with great caution, because there are several significant differences between spontaneous genetic hypertension in the rat and human essential hypertension which limit the suitability of the SHR as an animal model for human hypertension (14). A fundamental species difference between rats and humans is the absence in rats of a renal prostaglandin-based mechanism for lowering blood pressure (15). A second difference concerns the natural history of genetic spontaneous hypertension in rats vs. essential hypertension in humans. Unlike human essential hypertension, hypertension in the SHR is universal throughout the strain, is present at birth, and occurs independently of environmental factors (16). Recently, Lawler et al. reported the development of a borderline genetic hypertensive rat (BHR) as an alternative to the SHR for use as an animal model for human hypertension (17–20). The BHR, which represents the F_1 generation of the backcross between the SHR and its normotensive parent strain (the WKY), has the advantage over the SHR that in the absence of additional environmental stimuli, the adult rat develops a systemic BP in the range of 150–160 mm Hg. However, when exposed to environmental stimuli, such as those demonstrated to influence the development of essential hypertension (e.g., chronic psychosocial stress, elevated salt intake, social conflict), the BHR develops a significant and irreversible exacerbation of BP which is not alleviated by the removal of the triggering stimulus, and which approaches that seen in the SHR. In contrast, BP-exacerbating stimuli in the WKY (as well as SHR) appear to be effective only for the duration of exposure to the pressor stimuli.

Because essential hypertension in humans is not present from birth, appears to result from an interplay of genetic factors with environmental stimuli (21), and is more likely to occur in individuals who are either borderline hypertensive and/or exhibit a family history of the disorder (22), an examination of the effects of dietary n-6 fatty acids on the course of BP development in the BHR might be useful to ascertain the potential role for dietary 18:3n-6 in the prevention of hypertension in genetically susceptible individuals.

Both repeated exposure to chronic psychological stress and exaggerated physiological reactivity to stress have been implicated in the development of essential hypertension in genetically susceptible individuals (23,24). Conversely, both hypertensive humans and SHR have been demonstrated to manifest exaggerated reactivity to psychological stressors. To investigate the ability of dietary fatty acid manipulation to alter physiological responses to stress, a model of chronic (4 wk) psychosocial stress involving social isolation of group-reared animals was utilized. This type of stressor has been shown to chronically and reversibly elevate systemic BP in genetically normotensive rats, initially via an adrenal-dependent elevation in sympathetic activity, later (approaching 4 wk of exposure) followed by an adrenal-independent, renal-dependent mechanism (25–27). In addition, such stress has been shown to depress the activity of liver microsomal D6D, which would interfere with the conversion of 18:2n-6 to 18:3n-6 and potentially augment BP responses (28). In a series of studies, the effects of various n-6 fatty acids on BP and heart rate responses to chronic isolation were studied (29,30). In the first of these, various purified, nonesterified n-6 fatty acids (18:2n-6, 18:3n-6, 20:4n-6) dissolved in olive oil (vehicle) were administered by constant intraperitoneal infusion by osmotic minipump at a rate of 2.4 mg/(kg·day) to genetically normotensive WKY. In rats implanted with either dummy pumps, pumps releasing vehicle only, or pumps releasing 18:2n-6, BP (Fig.

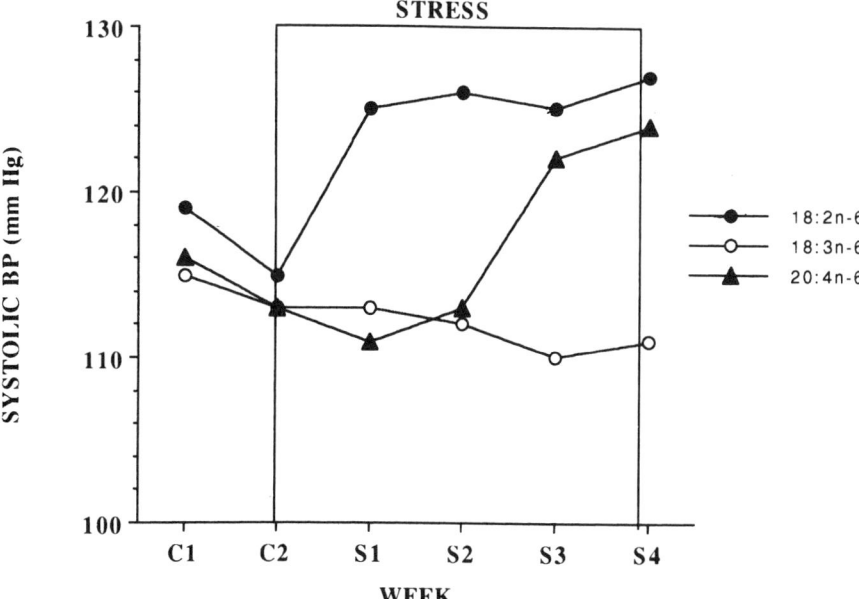

Fig. 15.1. Systolic BP responses of adult male BHR rats prior to (C1 and C2) and during 4 wk of social isolation stress (S1–S4). Rats were implanted intraperitoneally with osmotic pumps releasing vehicle (olive oil), or vehicle plus 18:2n-6, 18:3n-6, or 20:4n-6 at a dose of 2.4 mg/(kg·day) over the course of the study (n = 6/group).

15.1) and heart rate rose similarly during the 4 wk of isolation vs. the pre-isolation period. In contrast, administration of 18:3n-6 completely abolished BP and heart rate responses to isolation stress. Administration of 20:4n-6 resulted in a transient (2-wk) attenuation of BP and heart rate responses to isolation. However, by wk 3 of isolation, the protective effect of 20:4n-6 disappeared, and BP and heart rate increased similarly to animals receiving 18:2n-6. Administration of 18:3n-6 in the diet in the form of evening primrose oil (9% 18:3n-6) by pump achieved the same result as the pure 18:3n-6 (31), abolishing the BP and heart rate responses to chronic isolation. The fact that 18:3n-6 suppressed both BP and heart rate responses to stress suggests that it was acting via an alteration of central BP regulatory mechanisms. For if it had been acting solely on peripheral mechanisms, e.g., depressing peripheral vascular reactivity to catecholamines, a baroreflex increase in heart rate would have followed the initial BP attenuation. In fact, such a response was seen when an n-3 fatty acid (20:5n-3), known to act via depression of vascular reactivity, was used in the same model (32). To determine where 18:3n-6 was acting to suppress the stress response, circulating catecholamine levels and the pressor responses to intra-arterial infusions of an ED_{50} of norepinephrine and angiotensin were assessed. Whereas 18:3n-6 differentially suppressed norepinephrine responses to stress (Fig. 15.2), it had no significant effect on either circulating epinephrine levels or vascular responses to norepinephrine or angiotensin (30,31).

In the BHR, administration of 18:3n-6 intraperitoneally by osmotic pump was also effective in abolishing the chronic rise in both BP (Fig. 15.3) and heart rate asso-

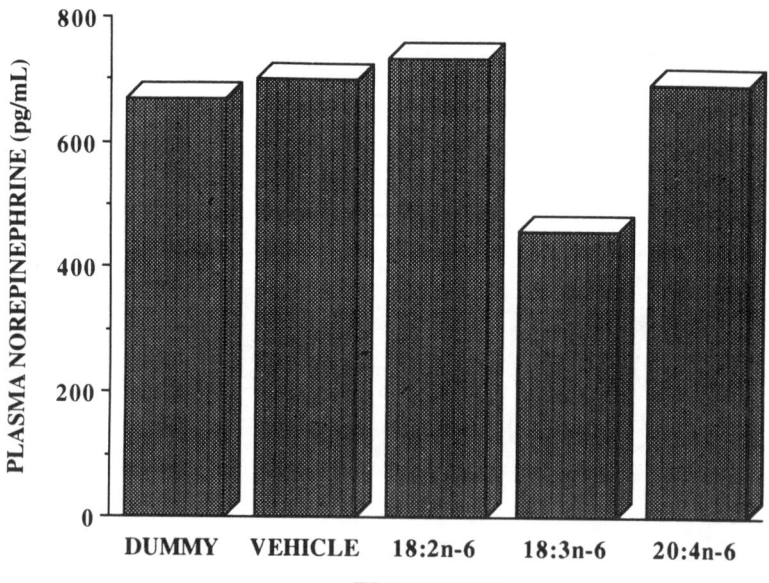

Fig. 15.2. Plasma norepinephrine levels in adult male WKY rats exposed to 2 wk of social isolation stress. Animals were treated with either either dummy pumps, or osmotic pumps releasing vehicle (olive oil), or vehicle plus 18:2n-6, 18:3n-6, or 20:4n-6 at a dose of 2.4 mg/(kg·day) over the course of the study (n = 8/group).

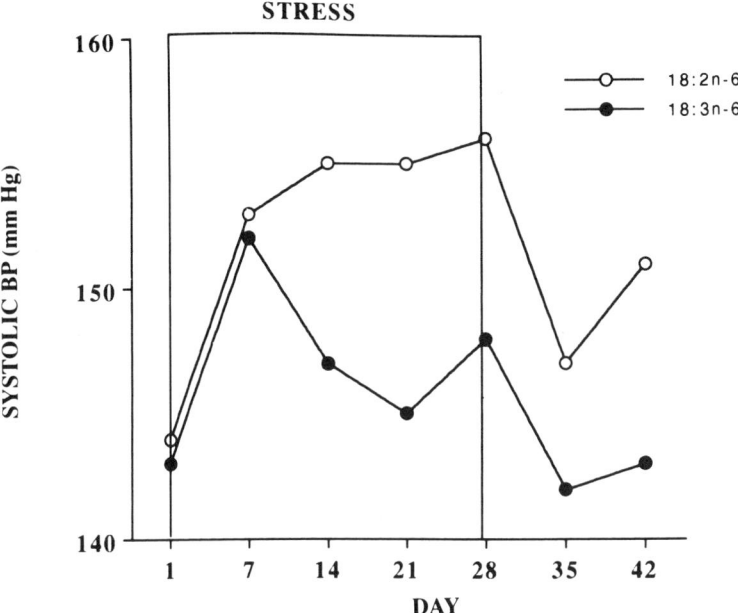

Fig. 15.3. Effects of 4 wk of isolation stress on systolic BP in adult male BHR treated with osmotic pumps releasing vehicle (olive oil) plus either 18:2n-6 or 18:3n-6 at a dose of 2.4 mg/(kg·d) over the course of the study (n = 8/group).

ciated with chronic isolation stress (4 wk) in control animals, which could not be explained by changes in vascular responsiveness to norepinephrine or angiotensin (33). In addition, after a 2-wk postisolation recovery period, BP in the control group remained elevated in comparison with prestress values, whereas BP in the 18:3n-6-treated group was similar to prestress values. This suggests that 18:3n-6 administration prevented persistent pressor effect of the stimulus in this genetically susceptible animal model. The effectiveness of dietary 18:3n-6 in preventing stress-induced hypertension in the BHR was then evaluated by examining BP responses to chronic isolation stress in BHR receiving rat chow supplemented with 10% (cal) of either sunflower oil (rich in 18:2n-6), canola oil (rich in 18:3n-3), evening primrose oil (rich in 18:3n-6), or fish oil (rich in 20:5n-3 and 22:6n-3). As expected, only those animals receiving evening primrose oil avoided an increase in BP in response to stress (Fig. 15.4).

Another pressor stimulus believed to play a role in the development of essential hypertension in humans and known to be a potent BP stimulus in rats is elevated dietary salt intake. In light of the observation that salt-loading depresses the activity of liver microsomal D6D (9), 18:3n-6 might be expected to attenuate pressor responses to salt-loading. The effects of 18:3n-6 administration both as a nonesterified fatty acid via osmotic pump and as dietary evening primrose oil on pressor responses to chronic elevation of salt intake in BHR were examined. In both experiments, salt-loading was accomplished by replacing drinking water with 1% NaCl. In the first experiment, salt loading significantly increased BP in animals implanted with dummy

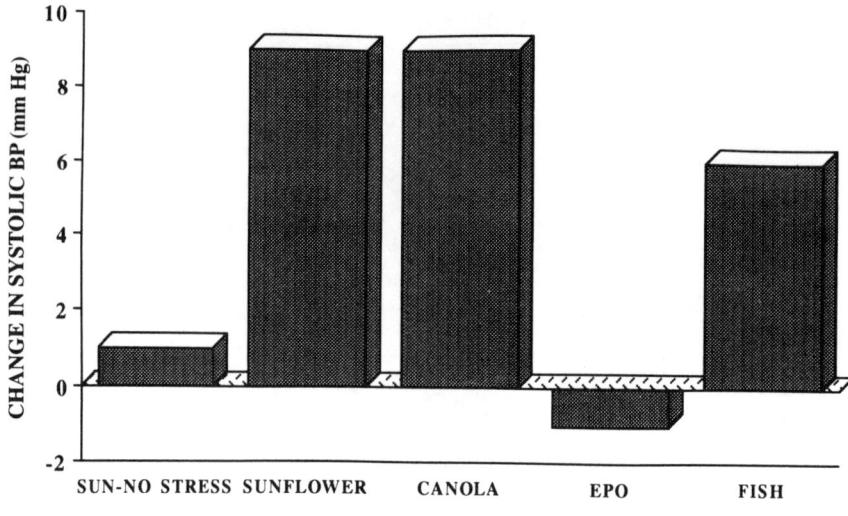

Fig. 15.4. Maximal BP response to social isolation stress in adult male BHR with ad libitum access to rat chow supplemented with 10% (cal) of either sunflower, canola, evening primrose, or fish oil during the course of the study. An additional group receiving sunflower oil served as the unstressed controls (n = 8/group).

pumps (controls) over a 12-wk period vs. both pre-salt-loading values and non-salt-loaded animals (34). Upon cessation of salt-loading, BP in these animals remained significantly elevated relative to the BP level prior to salt-loading, as well as vs. BP levels in non-salt-loaded animals, suggesting the "neurogenic triggering" effect of the stimulus, as described by Lawler (20). In contrast, the administration of 18:3n-6 by osmotic pump significantly attenuated the BP response to salt-loading (50%) and allowed BP to return to baseline levels following the removal of the salt. The protective effect of 18:3n-6 in this model was not associated with consistent changes in either food, water and electrolyte intake or water and electrolyte output.

When 18:3n-6 was administered by dietary supplementation with evening primrose oil (10% cal), BP fell significantly during a 6-wk period of salt-loading vs. pre-salt-loading values. In contrast, salt-loading significantly increased BP in rats fed diets supplemented with either olive, sunflower, or fish oil (Fig. 15.5).

To examine the potential use of dietary n-6 fatty acids in the attenuation of drug-induced hypertension, the effects of dietary supplementation (10% cal) with safflower oil (rich in 18:2n-6), evening primrose oil (rich in 18:3n-6), and fish oil (rich in 20:5n-3 and 22:6n-3) on BP and renal function were examined in animals treated with either 0.1 or 10 mg/kg cyclosporine/(kg·day) over a 5-wk period (35). Cyclosporine A is the standard immunosuppressant drug used in human organ transplantation to prevent rejection of the transplanted organ by the recipient. Although extremely effective in preventing rejection, its use is limited by its toxic side effects, which include nephrotoxicity and cardiotoxicity (hypertension). Cyclosporine A significantly and steadily increased BP over the 5-wk treatment period in animals

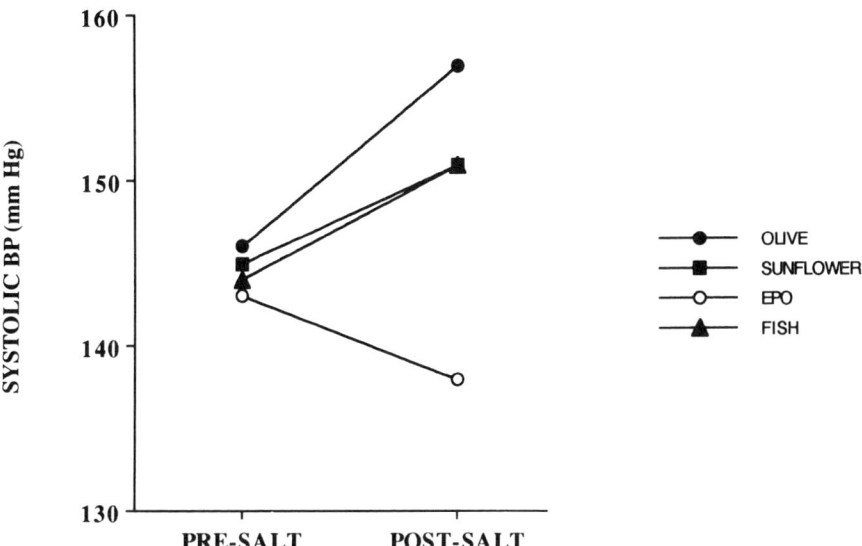

Fig. 15.5. Maximal systolic BP responses of adult male BHR to 6 wk of chronic salt-loading. Rats had ad libitum access to rat chow supplemented with 10% (cal) of either olive, sunflower, evening primrose, or fish oil during the course of the study (n = 10/group).

supplemented with safflower or fish oil. In contrast, supplementation with evening primrose oil abolished the pressor response at both drug dosages. Furthermore, dietary supplementation with evening primrose oil prevented the cyclosporine-associated 28% decline in glomerular filtration rate, which was observed in the safflower-fed animals, and which is an indicator of cyclosporine-related nephrotoxicity. In subsequent studies focusing on the renal effects of cyclosporine, 18:3n-6 was again shown to protect the kidney from the toxic effects of cyclosporine, and indicated that 18:3n-6 specifically improved the single nephron plasma flow rate and the glomerular capillary ultrafiltration coefficient, offsetting those decreases caused by cyclosporine (36). These 18:3n-6–related changes are consistent with a dilation of the afferent arteriole entering the glomerulus. Analysis of the fatty acid composition of various tissues in the cyclosporine/dietary-treated animals indicated that cyclosporine administration is associated with multiple changes in tissue fatty acid composition, most notably in the renal phospholipid fractions (37). Dietary evening primrose oil feeding during the period of cyclosporine administration was able to reverse the cyclosporine-related changes in fatty acid composition in liver, brain, and kidney. This normalization of tissue phospholipid fatty acids by 18:3n-6 may play a role in its ability to prevent cyclosporine toxicity (37).

γ-Linolenic Acid and Blood Pressure Regulation in Humans

Very little work has been completed to date examining the effects of dietary supplementation with 18:3n-6 on BP regulation in humans, and most of the studies which have been reported contain confounding variables which make interpretation problematic. Recently, Deferne et al. reported a significant reduction in systemic BP over a 6-wk period in mild hypertensives taking a dietary supplement consisting of 4 g/d of a mixture containing 18:3n-6 (58%), 20:5n-3 (9%), and 22:6n-3 (1%), as well as lithium, tocopherols and citric acid vs. a sunflower oil control (38). However, given the number of active agents contained in the supplement, it is impossible to assign the antihypertensive effect observed to 18:3n-6 itself. A second study by Venter et al., utilizing a crossover design, reported a significant fall in BP in mildly essential hypertensives after 8 wk of treatment with a combination of 18:3n-6, 20:5n-3 and 22:6n-3 contained in a mixture of evening primrose oil and fish oil vs. a control supplement consisting of a mixture of sunflower and linseed oil (39). These data are problematic because 4 of the 25 subjects in the study were dropped from the analysis as a result of their being designated as "therapeutic failures" subsequent to increases in their BP during the active treatment phase. In a third study, no effect of evening primrose oil supplementation vs. olive oil supplementation was observed in hypertriglyceridemic patients in a double-blind crossover study (40). However, it should be noted that the latter study did not target patients with essential hypertension.

In contrast to the inconclusive results in the human studies on effects of dietary 18:3n-6 on resting BP in essential hypertensives, there is a growing body of literature supporting the observations from animal studies that dietary 18:3n-6 is able to attenuate pressor stimuli. The first study in this area (41) examined the effects of 4 wk of dietary supplementation with either olive oil (control), borage oil (23% 18:3n-6), or fish oil (18% 20:5n-3 and 11% 22:6n-3) on cardiovascular reactivity to acute psychological stress (Stroop color-word conflict task) in normotensive men (10/group). Borage oil supplementation alone attenuated BP and heart rate responses to the stress by 30 and 33%, respectively. In addition, borage oil supplementation increased skin temperature during exposure to the stressor, suggesting that it increased peripheral blood flow by enhanced vasodilation. The attenuation of stress reactivity by 18:3n-6 in this study was accompanied by a significant increase in performance on the test. Borage oil supplementation similarly uniquely attenuated BP and/or heart rate reactivity vs. olive and fish oils in a variety of other stressors, including mental arithmetic, cold pressor challenge, and favorable impression task (42).

In another study, the effects of dietary 18:3n-6, in the form of borage oil, on baroreflex responses to simulated hemorrhage were studied in normotensive men (43). In this study, borage oil, but not olive oil or fish oil, enhanced both the peripheral vasoconstrictor and plasma norepinephrine responses to a reduction of cardiopulmonary blood volume which was achieved by the application of lower body negative pressure. These findings supported the concept that dietary 18:3n-6 supplementation augments the arterial baroreflex control of vascular resistance. Arterial baroreflexes have been shown to "reset" to a higher BP during the development of essential hypertension. The enhancement of this central regulatory process by 18:3n-6 may be useful as a prevention strategy by countering reflex changes in cardiovascular regulation associated with the onset of essential hypertension. As such, it could play a role in prevention strategies in individuals at risk for the disorder.

One study on humans has also investigated the effects of 18:3n-6 on peripheral vascular reactivity to pressor hormones. Broughton Pipkin et al. demonstrated in women with pregnancy-induced hypertension (characterized by exaggerated pressor responses to angiotensin) that dietary 18:3n-6, in the form of evening primrose oil, is capable of attenuating diastolic pressor responses to angiotensin II infusion, as well as reducing plasma renin concentration *vs.* untreated control patients (44). These data support those observations reported by Engler (see Chapter 16) in SHR.

Conclusions

Numerous studies in both animals and humans support the concept that 18:3n-6 is capable of modulating cardiovascular responses to a variety of endogenous and exogenous pressor stimuli. This physiological action may be useful as a primary preventive approach in individuals who are at elevated risk for the development of essential hypertension, e.g., those exhibiting hyperreactive responses to stress and/or labile BP, those having BP in the upper 10% of the normal age- and gender-adjusted population range, or having a family history of the disorder. Using diet to intervene at this stage in the development of the disorder might prove more effective than after the hypertension has established itself, because the body adapts to the elevation in BP with physical and structural changes which help perpetuate the higher pressure and which are difficult to reverse. At this point in time, however, the existing studies have not advanced to a point at which conclusions can be made regarding the potential of 18:3n-6 in this area.

References

1. Hoffman, P., and Forster, W. Influence of Dietary Linoleic Acid Content on Blood Pressure Regulation in Salt-Loaded Rats (1981) *Adv. Lipid Res. 18*, 203–227.
2. Church, J.P., Reeves, V.B., and Schoene, N.W. Effects of Essential Fatty Acid Deficiency on Blood Pressure in the Spontaneously Hypertensive Rat (1977) *Fed. Proc. 36*, 1159.
3. Singer, P., Naumann, E., and Hoffman, P. Attenuation of High Blood Pressure by Primrose Oil, Linseed Oil, and Sunflower Seed Oil in SHR (1984) *Biomed. Biochim. Acta 43*, S243–S246.
4. Soma, M., Manku, M.S., and Horrobin, D.F. The Effects of Hydrogenated Coconut Oil, Safflower Oil, and Evening Primrose Oil on Development of Hypertension and Sodium Handling in SHR (1985) *Can. J. Physiol. Pharmacol. 63*, 325–330.
5. Hoffman, P., Block, H.U., Beitz, J., Taube, C., Forster, W., Wortha, P., Singer, P., Naumann, E., and Heine, H. Comparative Study of the Blood Pressure Effects of Four Different Fats on Young, Hypertensive Rats (1986) *Lipids 21*, 733–737.
6. St. Louis, C., Lee, R., Rosenfeld, J., and Fargas-Babjak, A. Anti-Hypertensive Effect of Gamma-Linolenic Acid in SHR (1992) *Hypertension 19 (Suppl. II)*, II 111–II 115.
7. Huang, Y-S., Cantrill, R.C., DeMarco, A., Lin, X., Horrobin, D.F., and Mills, D.E. Differences in the Metabolism of 18:2n-6 and 18:3n-6 by the Liver and Kidney May Explain the Anti-Hypertensive Effect of 18:3n-6 (1994) *Biochem. Med. Metabol. Biol. 51*, 27–34.
8. Mills, D.E., and Huang, Y.-S. Metabolism of n-6 and n-3 Polyunsaturated Fatty Acids in Normotensive and Hypertensive Rats (1992) in *The Third International Congress on*

EFAs and Eicosanoids, (Sinclair, A., and Gibson, R., eds.), American Oil Chemists' Society, pp. 345–348.

9. Poisson, J.-P., Huang, Y.-S., Mills, D.E., de Antueno, R.J., Redden, P.R., Lin, X., Narce, M., and Horrobin, D.F. Effect of Salt-Loading and Spontaneous Hypertension on *in Vitro* Metabolism of [1-^{14}C] Linoleic and [2-^{14}C] Dihomo Gamma Linolenic Acids (1993) *Biochem. Med. Metabol. Biol. 49,* 57–66.

10. Narce, M., and Poisson, J.-P. In Vitro Studies of Delta-6 and Delta-5 Desaturation of Linoleic and Dihomo Gamma Linolenic Acids During the Development of Hypertension in SHR vs. WHY Rats (1984) *C R Soc. Biol. 178,* 458–466.

11. Narce, M., and Poisson, J.-P. Age-Related Depletion of Linoleic Acid Desaturation in the Liver Microsomes from Young SHR (1995) *Prost. Leuk. EFAs 53,* 59–63.

12. Engler, M.M., and Koops, R.R. Effects of Dietary Borage Oil on Plasma and Tissue Fatty Acids in SHR and Normotensive Rats (1994) *Circulation 90,* I 590.

13. Mtabaji, J.P., Manku, M.S., and Horrobin, D.F. Abnormalities in Dihomo Gamma Linolenic Acid Release in the Pathogenesis of Hypertension (1993) *Am. J. Hypertension 6,* 458–462.

14. McGiff, J.C., and Quilley, C.P. The Rat with Spontaneous Genetic Hypertension is Not a Suitable Model of Human Essential Hypertension (1981) *Circ. Res. 48,* 455–463.

15. Vane, J.R., and McGiff, J.C. Possible Contributions of Endogenous Prostaglandins to the Control of Blood Pressure (1975) *Circ. Res. 36/37 (Suppl. I),* 68–75.

16. Bruno, L., Azar, S., and Weller, D. Absence of a Pre-Hypertensive Stage in Post-Natal Kyoto Hypertensive Rats (1979) *Jpn. Heart J. 20 (Suppl. 1),* 90–92.

17. Lawler, J.E., Barker, G.F., Hubbard, J.W., and Schaub, R.G. Effects of Stress on Blood Pressure and Cardiac Pathology in Rats with Borderline Hypertension (1981) *Hypertension 3,* 496–505.

18. Lawler, J.E., and Cox, R.H. The BHR: A New Model for the Study of Environmental Factors in the Development of Hypertension (1985) *Pavlov J. Biol. Science 20,* 101–115.

19. Lawler, J.E., Cox, R.H., Sanders, B.J., and Mitchell, V.P. The BHR: A Model for Studying the Mechanisms of Environmentally Induced Hypertension (1988) *Health Psychol. 7,* 137–147.

20. Lawler, J.E., Sanders, B.J., Chen, Y.-F., Nagahame, S., and Oparil, S. Hypertension Produced by a High Sodium Diet in the BHR (1987) *Hypertension: Clin. Exper. A9,* 1713–1731.

21. Kaplan, N.M. Primary Hypertension-Natural History (1986) in *Clinical Hypertension,* (Kaplan, N.M., ed.), Williams and Wilkins, Baltimore, pp. 123–146.

22. Kooperstein, S.I., Schifrin, A., and Leahy, T.J. Level of Initial Blood Pressure and Subsequent Development of Essential Hypertension: A 10 and 15 Year Follow-Up Study (1962) *Am. J. Cardiol. 10,* 416–423.

23. Jorgensen, R.S., and Houston, B.K. Family History of Hypertension, Gender, and Cardiovascular Reactivity and Stereotypy During Stress (1981) *J. Behav. Med. 4,* 175–189.

24. Krantz, D.S., and Durel, L.A. Psychobiological Substrates of the Type A Behavior Pattern (1983) *Health Psychol. 2,* 393–411.

25. Gardiner, S.M., and Bennett, T. The Effects of Short Term Isolation on Systolic Blood Pressure and Heart Rate in Rats (1977) *Med. Biol. 55,* 325–329.

26. Gardiner, S.M., Milmer, K.E., and Bennett, T. Effect of Adrenalectomy on the Development of Isolation-Induced Hypertension in Rats (1981) *Clin. Sci. 61,* 511–519.

27. Bennett, T., and Gardiner, S.M. Maintenance of Hypertension After Long-Term Isolation in Rats: The Effect of Adrenalectomy (1981) *J. Physiol. 309,* 16P–17P.

28. Mills, D.E., Huang, Y.-S., Narce, M., and Poisson, J.-P. Psychosocial Stress, Catecholamines, and Essential Fatty Acid Metabolism in Rats (1994) *Proc. Soc. Exp. Biol. Med. 205,* 56–61.
29. Mills, D.E., and Ward, R.P. Attenuation of Psychosocial Stress-Induced Hypertension by Gamma Linolenic Acid in Rats (1984) *Proc. Soc. Exp. Biol. Med. 182,* 32–37.
30. Mills, D.E., and Ward, R.P. Effects of Essential Fatty Acid Administration on Cardiovascular Responses to Stress in the Rat (1986) *Lipids 21,* 139–142.
31. Mills, D.E., Ward, R.P., and Huang, Y.-S. Effects of n-3 and n-6 Fatty Acid Supplementation on Cardiovascular and Endocrine Responses to Stress in the Rat (1989) *Nutr. Res. 9,* 405–414.
32. Mills, D.E., and Ward, R.P. Effects of Eicosapentaenoic Acid on Stress Reactivity in Rats (1986) *Proc. Soc. Exp. Biol. Med. 182,* 127–131.
33. Mills, D.E., Summers, M.R., and Ward, R.P. Gamma Linolenic Acid Attenuates Cardiovascular Responses to Stress in Borderline Hypertensive Tats (1985) *Lipids 20,* 573–577.
34. Mills, D.E., Ward, R.P., Mah, M., and DeVette, L. Dietary n-6 and n-3 Fatty Acids and Salt-Induced Hypertension in the BHR (1989) *Lipids 24,* 17–24.
35. Mills, D.E., Ward, R.P., McCutcheon, D., Dixon, H., Ly, H., and Scholey, J. Attenuation of Cyclosporine-Induced Hypertension by Dietary Fatty Acids in the BHR (1992) *Transplantation 53,* 649–655.
36. Mills, D.E., de Antueno, R., and Scholey, J. Interaction of Dietary Fatty Acids and Cyclosporine A in the BHR: Tissue Fatty Acids (1994) *Lipids 29,* 27–32.
37. Scholey, J.W., and Mills, D.E. Dietary Fatty Acids and the Glomerular Hemodynamic Response to Cyclosporine in BHR (1995) *Kidney Int. 47,* 611–617.
38. Deferne, J.-L., and Leeds, A.R. The Antihypertensive Effect of Dietary Supplementation with a 6-Desaturated Essential Fatty Acid Concentrate as Compared with Sunflower Oil (1992) *J. Hum. Hypertension 6,* 113–119.
39. Venter, C.P., Joubert, P.H., and Booyens, J. Effects of Essential Fatty Acids on Mild to Moderate Essential Hypertension (1988) *Prost. Leuk. EFAs 33,* 49–51.
40. Boberg, M., Vessby, B., and Selinus, I. Effects of Dietary Supplementation with n-6 and n-3 Long-Chain Polyunsaturated Fatty Acids on Serum Lipoproteins and Platelet Function in Hypertriglyceridaemic Patients (1986) *Acta Med. Scand. 220,* 153–160.
41. Mills, D.E., Prkachin, K.M., Harvey, K.A., and Ward, R.P. Dietary Fatty Acid Supplementation Alters Stress Reactivity and Performance in Man (1989) *J. Hum. Hypertension 3,* 111–116.
42. Mills, D.E., and Ward, R.P. Dietary n-6 and n-3 Fatty Acids and Stress-Induced Hypertension (1990) in *Omega-6 Essential Fatty Acids: Pathophysiology and Roles in Clinical Medicine,* (Horrobin, D.F., ed.), Alan R. Liss, Inc., London, pp. 145–156.
43. Mills, D.E., Mah, M., Ward, R.P., Morris, B.L., and Floras, J.S. Alteration of Baroreflex Control of Forearm Vascular Resistance by Dietary Fatty Acids (1990) *Am. J. Physiol. 259,* R1164–R1171.
44. Broughton Pipkin, F., Morrison, R.A., and O'Brien, P.M.S. The Effect of Dietary Supplementation with Linoleic and Gamma-Linolenic Acids on the Pressor and Biochemical Response to Exogenous Angiotensin II in Human Pregnancy (1986) *Prog. Lipid Res. 25,* 425–429.

Chapter 16

γ-Linolenic Acid: A Potent Blood Pressure Lowering Nutrient

Marguerite M. Engler

University of California, San Francisco, San Francisco, CA 94143-0610

Introduction

Hypertension is a highly prevalent risk factor for cardiovascular disease. Factors such as heredity, obesity, and diet have been implicated in the development of hypertension (1). Control of hypertension decreases the risk of cardiovascular disease (2). Although pharmacologic therapy has proven effective in controlling high blood pressure, it can be associated with a range of adverse side effects. Nonpharmacologic interventions such as reducing body weight, increasing physical activity, and changing dietary intake may be more appropriate and have recently been recommended for the prevention of hypertension (1,3). An exciting area of research is the role of dietary fat intake, specifically n-6 polyunsaturated fatty acids (PUFAs), in hypertension. Early human studies demonstrated a beneficial effect of a high dietary intake of n-6 PUFA, linoleic acid, on blood pressure (4–6).

Linoleic acid is found in high concentrations in seeds (e.g., corn, safflower) and is the major fatty acid in vegetable oils. It is an essential fatty acid derived primarily from the diet because it cannot be synthesized *in vivo*. Through a series of metabolic steps, linoleic acid is converted to long-chain n-6 PUFAs which have important physiological functions as constituents of cell membranes and precursors of eicosanoids (Fig. 16.1).

Several known risk factors for cardiovascular disease including hypertension (7), diabetes (8), smoking, and stress (9) impair Δ6-desaturase enzyme activity. The resulting deficiencies of long-chain n-6 PUFAs, dihomo-γ-linolenic (DGLA, 20:3n-6) and arachidonic (AA, 20:4n-6) acids, in cell membranes and tissues may contribute to disease. Of particular interest is γ-linolenic acid (GLA, 18:3n-6) which may be used as a nutritional approach to bypass the crucial enzymatic step in the metabolism of DGLA and AA. Dietary intake of GLA provides the fatty acid directly for the metabolism.

The purpose of this review is to examine the effects of dietary GLA on blood pressure in normotensive and hypertensive states. Potential mechanisms which contribute to the blood pressure effects including pressor responsiveness, vascular reactivity, and compositional changes in tissue fatty acids are investigated.

Natural Sources of γ-Linolenic Acid

GLA is derived in large amounts from the seed oils of specific plants as well as fungi. The concentrations of GLA vary in seed oils with 21–25% in borage, 15–20% in black cur-

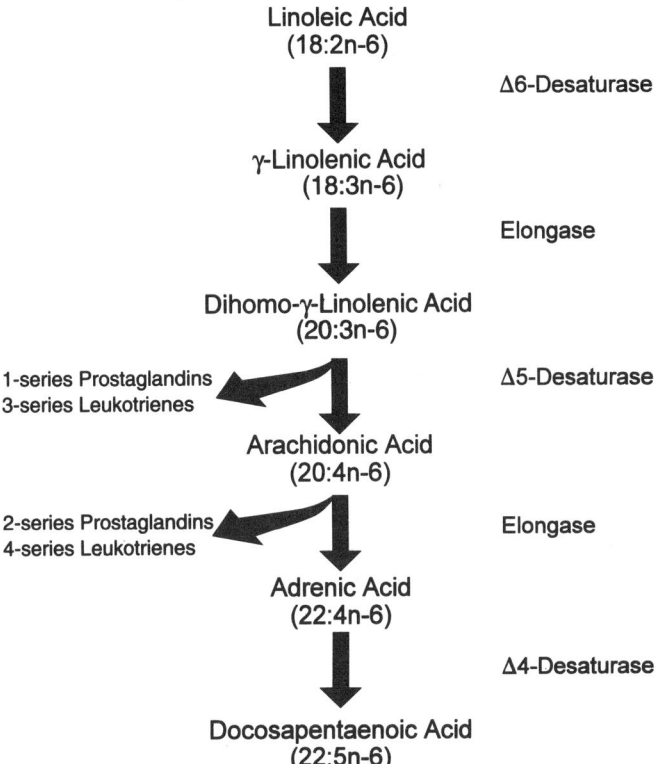

Fig. 16.1. Metabolic pathway of n-6 polyunsaturated fatty acids.

rant, 10–12% in gooseberry, 7–10% in evening primrose, and 4–5% in red currant (10). The fungal sources of GLA include *Mucor javanicus* with 23–26% and *Mortierella isabellina* with 8.3% of the fatty acid (11). GLA in seed and fungal oil sources is found distributed between the 1- and 3-positions of the triacylglycerol structure (12). For example, in evening primrose and blackcurrant oil, GLA is predominately in the 3-position, whereas it is primarily in the 2-position of borage oil and the 2- and 3-positions of *Mucor javanicus* fungal oil (12). The positional specificity may predetermine the metabolism of the faty acids in the oil.

Blood Pressure Effects of γ-Linolenic Acid in Normotensive and Hypertensive Rats

Normotension Study

Methods. Twenty male Sprague-Dawley rats (160–180 g) were fed diets enriched with 11% by weight of either sesame oil (control) or borage oil for 7 wk (13). The other dietary constituents included casein, DL-methionine, sucrose, cornstarch, cellulose, and vitamin and mineral mix. The fatty acid composition of the diets is shown in Table 16.1. Systolic blood pressure was determined weekly by the tail cuff technique.

TABLE 16.1 Major Fatty Acids in the Diet*

Fatty Acid	Sesame	Borage
Palmitic	9	9
Stearic	6	3
Oleic	35	14
Linoleic	48	40
γ-Linolenic	—	24

*Represents area % of total fatty acids.

Because changes in systemic pressor responses to vasoconstrictor hormones can influence blood pressure, the effects of angiotensin II and norepinephrine on blood pressure were assessed. Femoral arterial and venous catheters were inserted following the dietary treatments, and blood pressure responses to intravenous doses of angiotensin II (1.25–80 ng/kg) and norepinephrine (31–2000 ng/kg) were recorded.

To investigate intrinsic contractility of vascular smooth muscle as a mechanism for the blood pressure effects, vascular reactivity of thoracic aortic rings was determined. The aortic rings were suspended in a heated (37°C), water-jacketed, oxygenated tissue bath in a physiological solution of Krebs' Ringer bicarbonate buffer. Isometric tension was measured and a concentration-response relationship for potassium chloride (5–35 mM), norepinephrine (1×10^{-9}M–1×10^{-6}M) and serotonin (1×10^{-7}M–5×10^{-5}M) was obtained. The contractile response to a single dose of angiotensin II (5×10^{-7}M) was also determined.

Results. The borage oil diet produced a significant 9 mmHg reduction in blood pressure by wk 7 in the normotensive rats (Fig. 16.2). Moreover, the pressor responses to angiotensin II (40, 80 ng/kg) and norepinephrine (500, 2000 ng/kg) were significantly decreased in rats fed the borage oil-based diet. With regard to vascular reactivity, there was no difference in the contractile responses to potassium chloride or serotonin in aortic rings from the control or borage oil-fed rats. However, the contractile response of aortic rings from rats fed the borage oil diet was significantly decreased to norepinephrine (1×10^{-9}–5×10^{-8}M) and angiotensin II (5×10^{-7}M) (Figs. 16.3 and 16.4).

Summary. The study demonstrates that dietary GLA in the form of borage oil lowers blood pressure in normotensive rats. The effect is likely to be a receptor-mediated mechanism because the *in vitro* contractile responses were selective for angiotensin II and norepinephrine. This is consistent with the *in vivo* pressor responses. It is proposed that dietary GLA may alter the lipid composition of vascular smooth muscle cell membranes which affects receptor-interactions. Polyunsaturated fatty acids are known to influence the regulation of membrane-bound receptors (14).

Hypertension Study

Methods. A randomized parallel-group study was conducted in 6-wk-old spontaneously hypertensive (SHR) and age-matched normotensive Wistar-Kyoto (WKY) rats (15). Similar diets and procedures (pressor responses to norepinephrine and

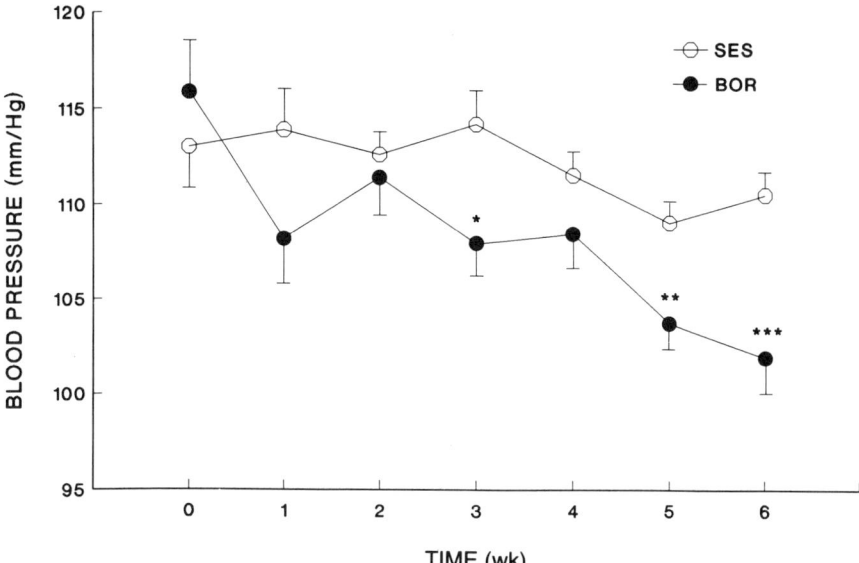

Fig. 16.2. Systolic blood pressure (mmHg) of rats fed diets enriched with sesame oil (SES, ○) or borage oil (BOR, ●). Values are expressed as means ± SEM ($n = 20$). *$P < 0.02$, **$P < 0.005$, ***$P < 0.001$. Source: M.M. Engler et al. (13). Reprinted with permission.

angiotensin II, vascular reactivity of aortic rings) were utilized as described in the normotension study. In addition, serum electrolytes, glucose, cholesterol and triglycerides were measured. To further assess whether functional alterations in vascular smooth muscle are involved in the blood pressure effects, the relaxation response to acetylcholine (10^{-5} mol/L) as well as the contractile responses to potassium chloride (10–50 mmol/L), norepinephrine (1×10^{-9}–5×10^{-6} mmol/L), and angiotensin II (5×10^{-7} mmol/L) in aortic rings from SHR and WKY rats fed the sesame and borage oil-based diets were determined.

Results. A significant 30-mmHg reduction in systolic blood pressure was found in SHR fed the borage oil-based diet for 7 wk (Fig. 16.5). Moreover, the diet produced a 10-mmHg decrease in blood pressure in WKY rats (Fig. 16.5). The pressor responses to intravenous doses of norepinephrine (62–2000 ng/kg) and angiotensin II (2.5–80 ng/kg) were not significantly different between SHR and WKY rats fed the sesame oil- or borage oil-based diets.

The contractile responses of aortic rings from borage oil-fed SHR fed the borage oil-enriched diet to potassium chloride, norepinephrine or angiotensin II were not significantly different compared with aortic rings from SHR fed the sesame oil-based diet. There was also no difference in the relaxation responses to acetylcholine in aortic rings from SHR and WKY rats on either diet. In aortic rings from WKY rats fed the borage oil-based diet, the contractile responses to potassium chloride and angiotensin II were similar to those of WKY rats fed the sesame oil-enriched diet. The borage oil diet enhanced the contractile response to norepinephrine in WKY aortic rings.

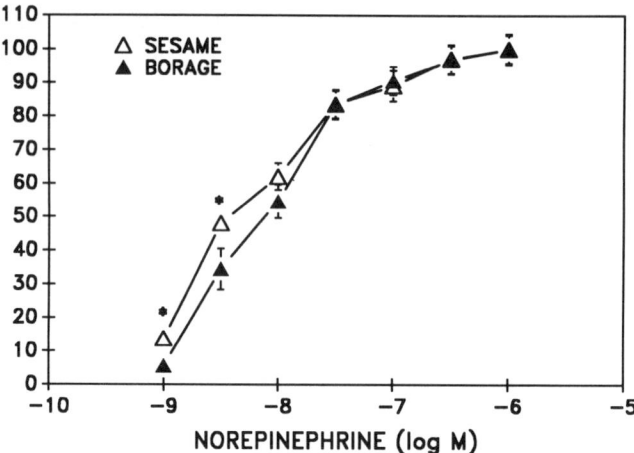

Fig. 16.3. Concentration-response curves of isolated aortic rings from rats fed diets enriched with either sesame oil or borage oil to cumulative addition of norepinephrine. Data are expressed as means ± SEM (%) of maximal response to norepinephrine (n = 7-10). *P < 0.05. *Source:* M.M. Engler et al. (13). Reproduced with permission.

There was no effect of the diet on serum levels of potassium, chloride, carbon dioxide, calcium or glucose in SHR and WKY rats (Table 16.2). In borage oil-fed WKY rats, serum sodium concentrations were lower and cholesterol concentrations were higher than in the other three groups.

Summary. Dietary GLA is a potent antihypertensive nutrient in SHR. It is also effective in lowering blood pressure in the normotensive control WKY rats, and the degree of reduction is consistent with the findings in our first study in Sprague-Dawley rats. The pressor responses to norepinephrine and angiotensin II were not dif-

TABLE 16.2 Effects of Diets on Serum Electrolytes, Glucose, Cholesterol, and Triglycerides

Parameters	SHR		WKY	
	Sesame	Borage	Sesame	Borage
Sodium (mEq/L)	141 ± 0.2	141 ± 0.3	140 ± 0.3	137 ± 0.4*
Potassium (mEq/L)	4.4 ± 0.2	4.6 ± 0.2	4.3 ± 0.1	4.2 ± 0.1
Chloride (mEq/L)	103 ± 0.5	103 ± 0.8	103 ± 0.5	101 ± 0.3
Carbon dioxide (mEq/L)	23 ± 0.6	23 ± 1	25 ± 0.5	24 ± 0.5
Calcium (mg/dL)	9.8 ± 0.1	10 ± 0.02	10 ± 0.06	10 ± 0.04
Glucose (mg/dL)	136 ± 12	168 ± 7	172 ± 9	171 ± 9
Cholesterol (mg/dL)	68 ± 4	94 ± 6	96 ± 12	137 ± 9*
Triglycerides (mg/dL)	92 ± 10	99 ± 11	144 ± 11	88 ± 20

Values expressed as means ± SEM, n = 5, *P < 0.05, vs. other groups.

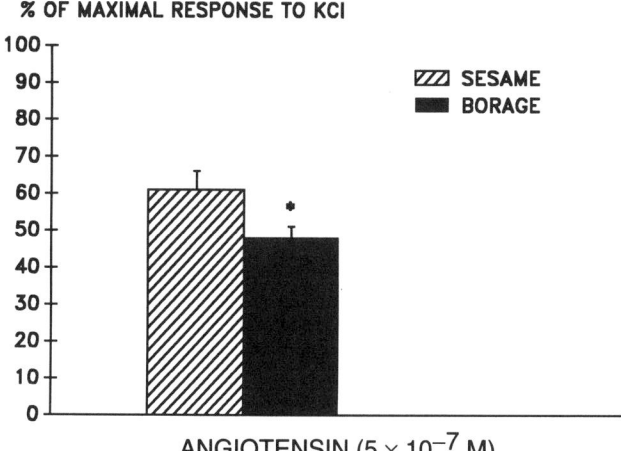

Fig. 16.4. Concentration-response of isolated aortic rings from rats fed diets enriched with either sesame oil or borage oil to addition of angiotensin II (5×10^{-7}M). Data are expressed as means ± SEM (%) of maximal response to potassium chloride (KCl) ($n = 7$–8). *$P < 0.05$. *Source:* M.M. Engler et al. (13). Reproduced with permission.

ferent in the borage oil-fed SHR and WKY rats compared with controls. Enhanced pressor responsiveness is usually indicative of a functional change in vascular smooth muscle which increases peripheral resistance and blood pressure in hypertension. Therefore, based on our results, this is not a potential mechanism for the blood pressure lowering effect of dietary GLA in SHR and WKY rats. The aortic reactivity findings rule out the possibility that dietary GLA affects the contractile elements of the excitation-contraction coupling system in vascular tissue, e.g., inhibition of intracellular calcium release or disruption of contractile protein function. Therefore, other mechanisms may be involved in the blood pressure lowering effect of dietary GLA in hypertension.

Hypertension Study: Comparison of γ-Linolenic Acid Enriched Oils

Methods. To determine the effect of seed and fungal oils with varying concentrations of GLA on blood pressure, SHR aged 6–7 wk were randomly divided into five groups and fed a fat-free basal mix diet with 11% by weight of sesame oil (SES), evening primrose oil (EPO), blackcurrant oil (BCO), borage oil (BOR), or fungal oil (FGO) for 7 wk (16). The fatty acid composition of the diet is presented in Table 16.3.

Blood pressure by the tail cuff method was measured weekly. Catheters were inserted into the femoral artery and vein, and pressor responses to norepinephrine (125, 500, 1000, 2000 ng/kg) and angiotensin II (1.25, 5, 20, 80 ng/kg) were determined. To assess whether the blood pressure responses were associated with a cellular calcium-mediated mechanism, verapamil (2.5 mg/kg), an intracellular calcium channel blocker, was injected following the maximum dose of norepinephrine

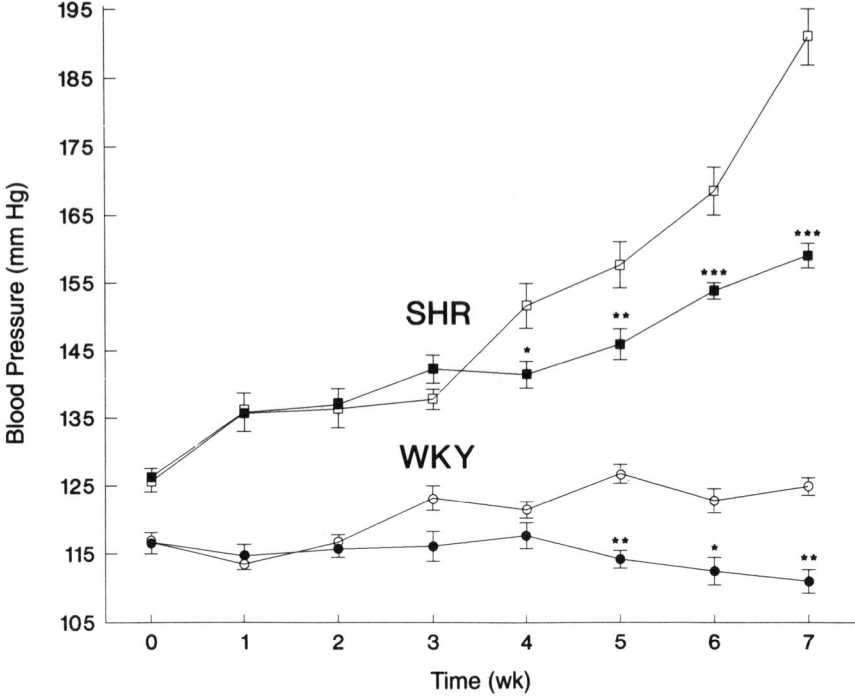

Fig. 16.5. Effect of a sesame- or borage oil-enriched diet upon the systolic blood pressure in spontaneously hypertensive (SHR) and Wistar-Kyoto (WKY) rats. Values are expressed as means ± SEM, $n = 19\text{--}24$. □, SHR fed sesame oil; ■, SHR fed borage oil; ○, WKY rats fed sesame oil; ●, WKY rats fed borage oil. $*P < 0.05$, $**P < 0.01$, $***P < 0.001$, vs. sesame oil. Source: M.M. Engler et al. (15). Reproduced with permsission.

(2000 ng/kg). Serum electrolytes, cholesterol and triglyceride levels were also measured.

Results. Dietary treatment with oils enriched with GLA for 7 wk prevented the onset of hypertension in SHR rats. The blood pressure reduction was 19 mmHg in the EPO group, 21 mmHg in the BOR group, 27 mmHg in the BCO group, and 38 mmHg in the FGO group (Fig. 16.6).

TABLE 16.3 Fatty Acids in the Diet*

Fatty Acid	Sesame	Evening Primrose	Black Currant	Borage	Fungal
Oleic	36	12	12	20	30
Linoleic	45	71	45	36	14
γ-Linolenic	—	8	17	19	26
α-Linolenic	1	—	12	—	—
Stearidonic	—	—	3	—	—

*Represents area % of total fatty acids.

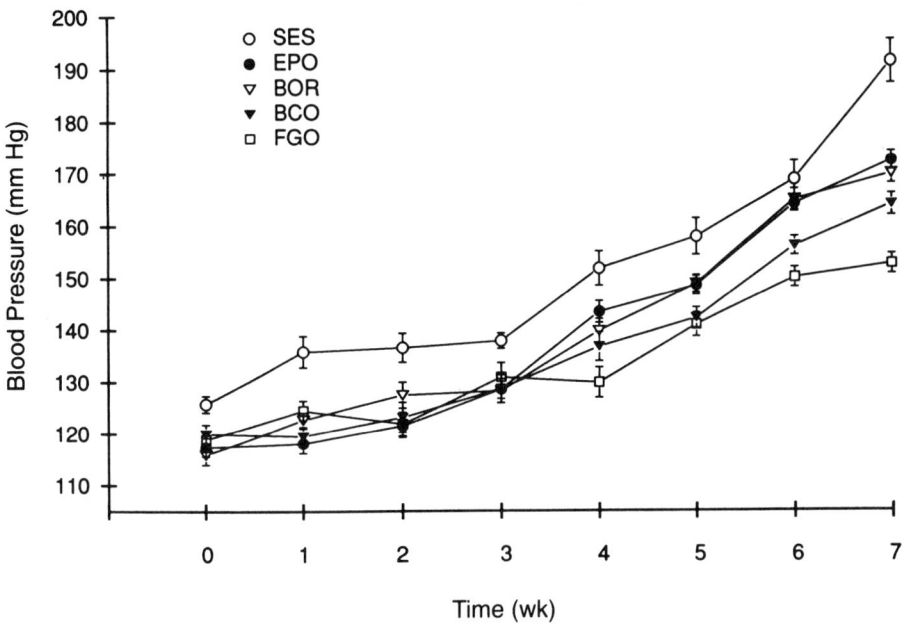

Fig. 16.6. Effect of diets enriched with SES, EPO, BCO, BOR, and FGO on systolic blood pressure in SHR. Each point represents the mean ± SEM of 16–19 rats. Significant differences at $P < 0.05$ for FGO and BCO vs. SES at wk 1, 2, 4, 5, 6, and 7; BOR vs. SES at wk 1 and 7; EPO vs. SES at weeks 1, 2, and 7. *Source:* M.M. Engler et al. (16). Reproduced with permission.

Intravenous norepinephrine and angiotensin II produced dose-dependent pressor responses in each of the dietary groups which were not significantly different from the control group. Injection of verapamil resulted in a rapid fall in blood pressure which was not significantly different among dietary groups (Table 16.4).

There was also no difference in the serum concentrations of sodium, potassium, chloride, calcium or triglycerides among dietary groups. Cholesterol levels were increased in borage oil-fed SHR compared with the SHR fed the control or fungal oil diet.

Summary. The results demonstrate that seed and fungal oils enriched with GLA effectively lower high blood pressure in SHR. Even low concentrations of GLA (8%) as found in EPO decreased blood pressure by 19 mmHg. Fungal oil with 26%

TABLE 16.4 Effect of Verapamil on Blood Pressure*

	Sesame	Evening Primrose	Black Currant	Borage	Fungal
Δ MAP (mmHg)	123 ± 4	123 ± 5	128 ± 5	136 ± 7	111 ± 8

*Values represent means ± SEM, $n = 7$–10 per group. The change (Δ) in mean arterial pressure (MAP) is the fall in blood pressure produced by verapamil following the pressor response to norepinephrine (2000 ng/kg).

GLA was the most potent of the oils with a blood pressure lowering effect of 38 mmHg.

The observed blood pressure reduction cannot be explained by depressed pressor responsiveness to vasoconstrictor hormones (i.e., norepinephrine, angiotensin II). A decrease in peripheral resistance manifested by lower pressor responses can reduce high blood pressure. To further investigate the role of peripheral resistance, the intracellular calcium channel blocker, verapamil, was used. Reportedly, calcium influx in vascular smooth muscle cells is enhanced in SHR which may increase vascular tonus or peripheral resistance (17). We hypothesized that dietary GLA through incorporation of fatty acids into the cell may alter membrane properties such as ion transport. However, because there were no differences in the blood pressure responses to verapamil among dietary groups, it is unlikely that a calcium transport mechanism is involved in the antihypertensive effect of GLA.

Effects of γ-Linolenic Acid on Tissue and Plasma Fatty Acid Composition

A series of experiments were conducted in normotensive and hypertensive rats to determine the effects of dietary GLA on tissue and plasma fatty acid profiles. n-6 PUFAs increase the fluidity of cell membranes which can influence protein functions such as receptor interactions, enzyme activities and ion transport (18). The n-6 PUFAs including DGLA and AA are also substrates for vasodilatory and antithrombotic eicosanoids (19). Therefore, dietary modification with GLA may affect important physiologic properties in the body by changing the fatty acid composition of cells, tissues, and organs.

Normotension Study

Methods. Sprague-Dawley rats (200–220 g) were fed purified diets with 11% by weight of either sesame or borage oil for 7 wk. At the end of the dietary treatments, lipids from aortic tissue and platelets were extracted and analyzed by gas chromatography (20).

TABLE 16.5 Fatty Acid Composition of Aortic Tissue[1]

Fatty Acid	Sesame	Borage
Oleic	33.9 ± 0.6	21.1 ± 0.4
Linoleic	29.0 ± 1.4	28.2 ± 1.3
γ-Linolenic	—	7.1 ± 0.3*
Dihomo-γ-Linolenic	0.2 ± 0.0	1.7 ± 0.1*
Arachidonic	2.2 ± 0.2	3.9 ± 0.3*
Adrenic	0.5 ± 0.0	1.0 ± 0.1
Docosapentaenoic	0.2 ± 0.0	0.3 ± 0.0

[1]Values given are area % of major monounsaturated and polyunsaturated fatty acids. All values represent means ± SEM, $n = 7$–8.
*Significantly different than sesame, $P < 0.05$.

TABLE 16.6 Fatty Acid Composition of Platelets[1]

Fatty Acid	Sesame	Borage
Oleic	10.3 ± 0.9	7.4 ± 0.4
Linoleic	11.1 ± 0.9	9.4 ± 0.7
γ-Linolenic	0.2 ± 0.0	1.9 ± 0.2*
Dihomo-γ-Linolenic	0.5 ± 0.0	1.1 ± 0.1*
Arachidonic	25.3 ± 0.8	28.0 ± 0.8
Adrenic	3.1 ± 0.3	2.9 ± 0.4
Docosapentaenoic	0.7 ± 0.0	1.0 ± 0.2

[1]Values given are area % of major monounsaturated and polyunsaturated fatty acids. All values represent means ± SEM, $n = 6\text{-}7$.
*Significantly different than sesame, $P < 0.05$.

Results. The fatty acid profiles of aortic tissue and platelets are presented in Tables 16.5 and 16.6. GLA from borage oil was readily incorporated into the aortic and platelet lipids after 7 wk of dietary treatment. The borage oil-enriched diet also increased the levels of DGLA and AA.

Summary. A diet rich in GLA in the form of borage oil increases the levels of n-6 PUFAs in vascular tissue and platelets. This has important implications because human studies have shown that low levels of 20-carbon n-6 PUFAs in adipose tissue, plasma, and platelets correlate strongly with high risk of cardiovascular disease (21–23). Moreover, the percentages of DGLA and AA are decreased in human coronary arteries in sudden cardiac death (24).

It is probable that the increases in DGLA and AA are due to enhanced chain elongation and desaturation of GLA because these fatty acids were not present in the diet. The borage oil diet may increase circulating plasma pools of GLA which are then metabolized in the liver to 20-carbon chain fatty acids and thus incorporated into the platelets and vascular tissue from the circulation.

Hypertension Study

Further studies examined the effect of dietary GLA on fatty acid profiles of the vasculature as well as plasma and liver in normotensive and hypertensive rats.

Methods. Spontaneously hypertensive and normotensive WKY rats (6 wk old) ($n = 28$) were fed either a sesame oil- or borage oil-enriched diet for 7 wk (25). Following the dietary treatment, total lipids were extracted from the plasma, liver, aorta, and renal artery. The fatty acid profiles were determined by gas chromatography.

Results. The composition of fatty acids in the plasma, liver, aorta, and renal artery from WKY and SHR rats are shown in Figs. 16.7–16.10. Overall, the borage oil-based diet significantly increased the levels of n-6 PUFAs, GLA, and DGLA in WKY and SHR rats. GLA levels in plasma, liver, aortic, and renal tissue were increased in SHR (4.8-, 4.6-, 2.7-, and 3.4-fold, respectively; $P < 0.001$) and WKY (5.8-, 4.2-, 4.4-, and 5.6-fold, respectively; $P < 0.001$) rats fed the borage oil-

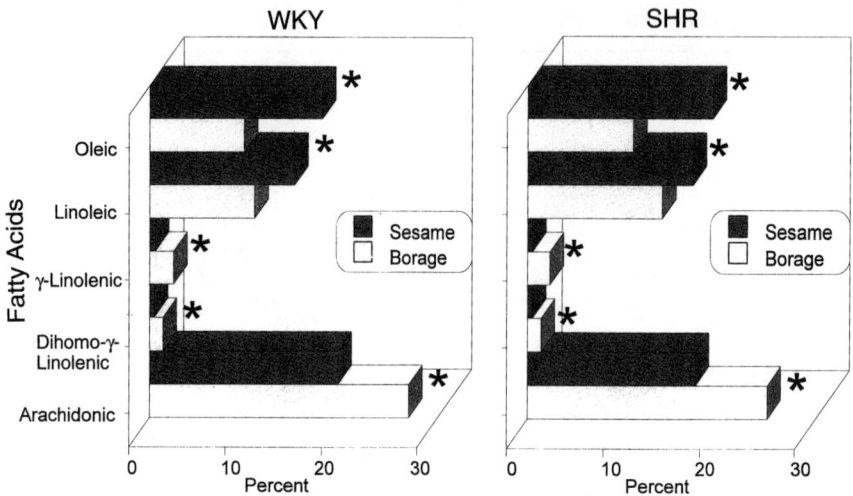

Fig. 16.7. Plasma fatty acid composition in sesame oil- and borage oil-fed WKY and SHR rats. Values given are area % of major monounsaturated and polyunsaturated fatty acids, n = 5–7. *Significantly different at $P < 0.05$. *Source:* M.M. Engler et al.

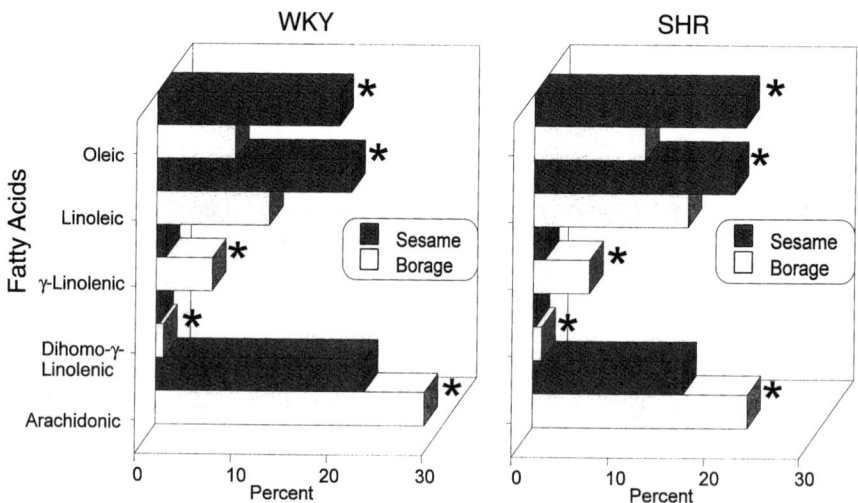

Fig. 16.8. Liver fatty acid composition in sesame oil- and borage oil-fed WKY and SHR rats. Values given are area % of major monounsaturated and polyunsaturated fatty acids. *Significantly different at $P < 0.05$. *Source:* M.M. Engler et al. (25).

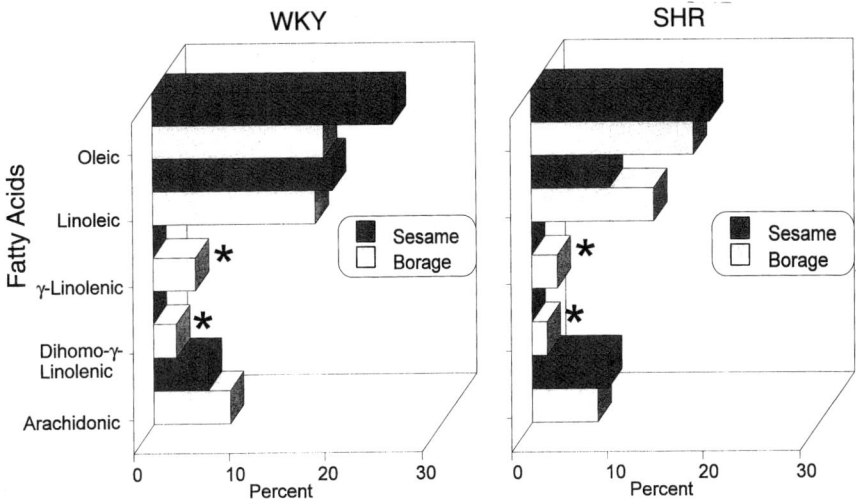

Fig. 16.9. Aortic fatty acid composition in sesame oil- and borage oil-fed WKY and SHR rats. Values given are area % of major monounsaturated and polyunsaturated fatty acids. *Significantly different at $P < 0.05$. *Source:* M.M. Engler et al. (25).

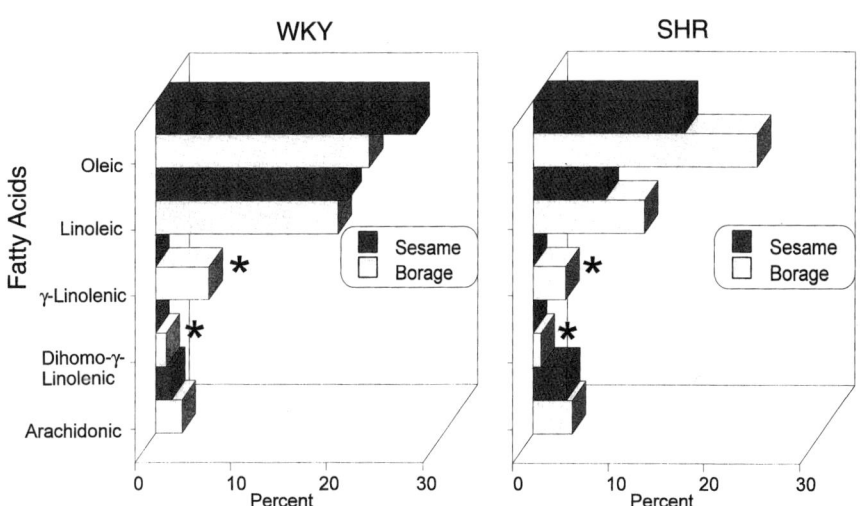

Fig. 16.10. Renal artery fatty acid composition in sesame oil- and borage oil-fed WKY and SHR rats. Values given are area % of major monounsaturated and polyunsaturated fatty acids. *Significantly different at $P < 0.05$. *Source:* M.M. Engler et al. (25).

enriched diet. The levels of DGLA were also significantly higher than controls in the same tissues with a 3-, 2.8-, 1.6-, and 0.8-fold ($P < 0.001$) increase, respectively, in SHR and a 2-, 2.8-, 2.4-, and 1.1-fold ($P < 0.01$) increase, respectively, in WKY. Moreover, AA levels were elevated in both plasma and liver of SHR (1.4- and 1.4-fold, respectively; $P < 0.05$) and WKY rats (1.3- and 1.3-fold, respectively; $P < 0.05$) fed the borage oil-based diet.

Summary. The results indicate that dietary GLA acid produces marked increases in n-6 PUFAs in the circulation, liver, and vasculature of both SHR and WKY rats. Significant reductions in blood pressure were also observed in these rats (Fig. 16.5). Eicosanoids such as vasodilatory PGE_1 and PGI_2 derived from the 20-carbon fatty acids, DGLA and AA, may contribute to the blood pressure lowering effect of GLA. One would expect that if the levels of precursor 20-carbon fatty acids are increased, especially in the vascular bed, synthesis of prostaglandins may be enhanced as well. A previous study has shown that vascular PGE_1 and PGI_2 production is increased in rats receiving DGLA (26). Evening primrose oil also increases the concentration of PGI_2 in SHR aorta (27). The role of prostaglandins in the modulation of blood pressure by GLA is further supported by a recent study in SHR. Intraperitoneal injection of GLA daily had a blood pressure lowering effect in SHR which was abolished by aspirin (28), a cyclooxygenase inhibitor which blocks prostaglandin synthesis.

Hypertension Studies: Comparison of γ-Linolenic Acid Enriched Oils

Methods. The effects of different oils enriched with GLA on plasma and tissue fatty acid profiles in hypertension were studied (29). Spontaneously hypertensive rats (6 wk old) were fed fat-free diets for 7 wk enriched with 11% by weight of SES, EPO, BCO, BOR, or FGO with respective GLA content at 0, 8, 17, 19, and 26%. The fatty acid composition of plasma, liver, aorta, and renal artery was analyzed by gas chromatography.

Results. The fatty acid profiles of plasma, liver, aorta, and renal artery lipids from SHR fed the different diets are shown in Tables 16.7–16.10. The diets enriched with GLA significantly increased the levels of GLA and DGLA in hepatic, aortic, and

TABLE 16.7 Fatty Acid Composition of Plasma[1]

Fatty Acid	Sesame	Evening Primrose	Black Currant	Borage	Fungal
Oleic	22.1 ± 1.0	9.0 ± 0.3*	10.6 ± 0.4*	12.0 ± 0.4*	22.0 ± 0.5
Linoleic	20.9 ± 1.7	24.9 ± 1.5	20.0 ± 1.8	14.5 ± 1.4	8.0 ± 0.2*
γ-Linolenic	1.2 ± 0.1	3.1 ± 0.3	5.0 ± 0.5*	5.3 ± 0.7*	7.2 ± 0.6*
Dihomo-γ-Linolenic	0.3 ± 0.0	0.5 ± 0.1	0.8 ± 0.0*	0.7 ± 0.1*	0.6 ± 0.0
Arachidonic	15.7 ± 1.6	21.7 ± 2.3	17.6 ± 0.7	21.4 ± 0.9	20.4 ± 0.8

[1]Values given are area % of major monounsaturated and polyunsaturated fatty acids. All values represent means ± SEM, $n = 5$–7.
*Significantly different than sesame, $P < 0.05$.

TABLE 16.8 Fatty Acid Composition of Liver[1]

Fatty Acid	Sesame	Evening Primrose	Black Currant	Borage	Fungal
Oleic	19.2 ± 0.7	8.9 ± 0.7*	10.4 ± 0.3*	13.5 ± 1.1*	18.1 ± 0.5*
Linoleic	17.1 ± 0.9	18.4 ± 1.0	15.2 ± 0.4	11.0 ± 1.0*	5.0 ± 0.4*
γ-Linolenic	0.5 ± 0.0	1.1 ± 0.1*	1.4 ± 0.5*	1.7 ± 0.2*	2.0 ± 0.2*
Dihomo-γ-Linolenic	0.5 ± 0.0	0.6 ± 0.0	1.2 ± 0.1*	0.9 ± 0.1*	0.9 ± 0.0*
Arachidonic	17.4 ± 0.6	23.3 ± 0.7*	22.0 ± 0.3*	22.7 ± 1.6*	25.9 ± 0.3*

[1]Values given are area % of major monounsaturated and polyunsaturated fatty acids. All values represent means ± SEM.
*Significantly different than sesame, $P < 0.05$.

renal arterial tissue. AA levels were also elevated in the liver of SHR fed the GLA-enriched diets compared with controls. With regard to the plasma, GLA was increased in SHR fed BCO-, BOR-, or FGO-enriched diets, whereas the BCO and BOR diets increased the levels of DGLA. The reductions in oleic acid in the liver and plasma reflect the composition of this fatty acid in the diet (Table 16.3).

Summary. The effects of the GLA-enriched diets were pronounced in the liver with increases in all of the n-6 PUFAs. This suggests that GLA is converted to longer-chain fatty acids in the liver. The primary effects of dietary GLA in the vasculature were increases in GLA and DGLA. The changes in fatty acid composition particularly in the arterial wall may increase cell membrane fluidity, which is important to cellular function. It has been reported that hypertensive vascular smooth muscle cell membranes contain fewer unsaturated fatty acids and have reduced fluidity (30). This may be associated with morphologic alterations such as increased media thickness which has been shown in hypertensive aortic vessels (31). It is also possible that dietary GLA affects gene expression in vascular tissue which may contribute to hypertension. For example, gene expression of a fatty acid binding protein (FABP) in hypertensive rat aorta is significantly reduced (32). The protein is believed to be involved in the uptake and metabolism of long-chain fatty acids. Therefore, dietary GLA may influence gene expression of proteins such as FABP which facilitates fatty acid utilization.

TABLE 16.9 Fatty Acid Composition of Aorta[1]

Fatty Acid	Sesame	Evening Primrose	Black Currant	Borage	Fungal
Oleic	18.7 ± 3.2	14.7 ± 3.2*	9.9 ± 2.6	17.8 ± 1.6	19.9 ± 2.6
Linoleic	8.2 ± 0.9	13.7 ± 2.1	8.3 ± 2.0	11.0 ± 0.8	4.7 ± 0.7
γ-Linolenic	—	0.8 ± 0.1*	1.3 ± 0.3*	1.9 ± 0.1*	1.9 ± 0.3*
Dihomo-γ-Linolenic	—	0.6 ± 0.0*	1.7 ± 0.5*	1.3 ± 0.1*	1.2 ± 0.2*
Arachidonic	8.0 ± 1.3	9.1 ± 1.5	10.6 ± 1.7	6.9 ± 0.7	9.0 ± 1.2

[1]Values given are area % of major monounsaturated and polyunsaturated fatty acids. All values represent means ± SEM.
*Significantly different than sesame, $P < 0.05$.

TABLE 16.10 Fatty Acid Composition of Renal Artery[1]

Fatty Acid	Sesame	Evening Primrose	Black Currant	Borage	Fungal
Oleic	15.8 ± 2.8	18.7 ± 3.9	22.4 ± 5.0	28.9 ± 1.5	32.8 ± 1.9*
Linoleic	7.5 ± 1.2	15.4 ± 3.1	14.7 ± 2.3	13.5 ± 0.9	5.5 ± 0.5
γ-Linolenic	—	1.9 ± 0.3*	2.3 ± 0.3*	3.6 ± 0.2*	3.5 ± 0.2*
Dihomo-γ-Linolenic	—	0.9 ± 0.1*	0.9 ± 0.2*	0.6 ± 0.0*	0.6 ± 0.0*
Arachidonic	3.5 ± 1.1	4.3 ± 0.9	6.7 ± 2.4	3.1 ± 0.1	3.6 ± 0.4

[1]Values given are area % of major monounsaturated and polyunsaturated fatty acids. All values represent means∆213

Conclusions

The series of studies in normotensive and hypertensive rats demonstrate the blood pressure lowering effect of oils enriched with GLA. Significant reductions in blood pressure were observed with a maximum decline of 10 mmHg in normotensive rats and 38 mmHg in spontaneously hypertensive rats. Human studies have also demonstrated an antihypertensive effect of dietary GLA (33,34).

We investigated several possible mechanisms which may explain the blood pressure lowering effect of GLA including pressor responsiveness to vasoconstrictors, intrinsic contractility of vascular smooth muscle, vascular tone dependent on intracellular calcium, and compositional changes in tissue fatty acids. Decreased pressor responsiveness to vasoconstrictors is a potential mechanism for the reduction in blood pressure in Sprague-Dawley rats. In the normotensive rat, GLA may influence blood pressure regulation through the renin-angiotensin-aldosterone axis. This is supported by our experimental results and a previous report which has shown that fatty acids inhibit receptor binding of angiotensin II and synthesis of aldosterone in rat adrenal cells (35).

In the hypertensive rat, our investigations have excluded decreased pressor responsiveness, depressed contractility of vascular smooth muscle, and calcium-mediated changes in vascular tone as possible mechanisms for the antihypertensive effect. We do, however, report significant alterations in the fatty acid composition of plasma, hepatic, and vascular tissue induced by dietary GLA. The findings were associated with the blood pressure effects and provide important information about the metabolism of GLA. Compositional changes in fatty acids can affect cell membrane fluidity and hence functional properties of the cell. It remains to be elucidated which aspect of membrane function may be affected by GLA and its metabolites. It has been suggested that GLA may affect renal Na+/K+ ATPase enzyme activity which promotes natriuresis (33). The net effect would be a reduction in blood volume which lowers blood pressure. This renal mechanism was studied in mildly hypertensive human subjects who received a concentrate of GLA (2300 mg) and smaller amounts of n-3 fatty acids daily for 6 wk (34). Blood pressure was reduced significantly, but there was no effect on urinary excretion of sodium or potassium. Therefore, the blood pressure lowering effect of GLA may not be mediated by enzymatic activity which decreases renal tubular sodium reabsorption.

Other mechanisms which may be involved include enhanced production of vasodilatory prostaglandins or modulation of the baroreceptor reflex. Prostaglandins are thought to exert a beneficial effect on blood pressure by dilating the vasculature. However, decreased production of vasodilatory prostaglandins may contribute to hypertension and has been reported in vascular smooth muscle cells of SHR (36). Our studies demonstrate that dietary GLA increases the level of precursor fatty acids in the vasculature which in turn may enhance the availability of substrate for prostaglandin synthesis.

A previous study suggests that GLA may also affect the baroreceptor reflex. Normotensive subjects were supplemented with dietary GLA for 4 wk and blood pressure was evaluated during simulated hemorrhage (37). GLA reportedly attenuated the fall in blood pressure and it was associated with an enhanced baroreceptor reflex response. Therefore, GLA may modulate blood pressure through a neurocardiovascular mechanism.

Current evidence indicates that dietary GLA is a potent blood pressure lowering nutrient which may be a useful nutritional intervention for the treatment of hypertension. Further laboratory and clinical investigations are required to define the mechanisms involved in the antihypertensive effect of GLA and to assess the long-term benefits of its use in nutritional therapy.

References

1. Joint National Committee on Detection, Evaluation, and Treatment of High Blood Pressure. The Fifth Report of the Joint National Committee on Detection, Evaluation, and Treatment of High Blood Pressure (1994) U.S. Department of Health and Human Services, Bethesda, MD: NIH publication no. 93–1088.
2. Kannel, W.B. Status of Risk Factors and Their Consideration in Antihypertensive Therapy (1987) *Am. J. Cardiol. 59,* 80A–90A.
3. WHO/ISH Guidelines Committee: Prevention of Hypertension and Associated Cardiovascular Disease: A 1991 Statement (1992) *Clin. Exp. Hypertens. A14,* 1–341.
4. Iacono, J.M., Puska, P., Dougherty, RM., Pietinen, P., Vartiainen, E., Leino, U., Mutanen, M., Moisio, S. Effect of Dietary Fat on Blood Pressure in a Rural Finnish Population (1983) *Am. J. Clin. Nutr. 38,* 860–869.
5. Rao, R.H., Rao, R.B., and Srikanba, S.G. Effect of Polyunsaturated Rich Vegetable Oils on Blood Pressure in Essential Hypertension (1981) *Clin. Exp. Hypertens. 3,* 27–38.
6. Iacono, J.M., Dougherty, R.M., and Puska, P. Dietary Fat and Blood Pressure in Humans (1990) *Klin. Wochenschr. 68 (Suppl XX),* 23–32.
7. Singer, P., Jaeger, W., Voigt, S., and Thiel, H. Defective Desaturation and Elongation of n-6 and n-3 Fatty Acids in Hypertensive Patients (1984) *Prostaglandins Leukotrienes Med. 15,* 159–165.
8. Mercuri, O., Peluffo, R.O., and Brenner, R.R. Depression of Microsomal Desaturation of Linoleic to Gamma-Linolenic Acid in the Alloxan Diabetic Rat (1966) *Biochim. Biophys. Acta 116,* 407–411.
9. Horrobin, D.F. Medical Roles of Metabolites of Precursor EFA (1995) *INFORM 6,* 428–435.
10. Traitler, H., Wille, H.J., and Studer, A. Fractionation of Blackcurrant Seed Oil (1988) *J. Am. Oil Chem. Soc. 65,* 755–760.

11. Ratledge, C. Microbial Routes to Lipids (1989) *Biochem. Soc. Trans. 17,* 1139–1141.
12. Lawson, L.D., and Hughes, B.G. Triacylglycerol Structure of Plant and Fungal Oils Containing Gamma-Linolenic Acid (1988) *Lipids 23,* 313–317.
13. Engler, M.M., Engler, M.B., and Paul, S.M. Effects of Dietary Borage Oil Rich in Gamma-Linolenic Acid on Blood Pressure and Vascular Reactivity (1992) *Nutr. Res. 12,* 519–528.
14. Spector, A.A., and Yorek, M.A. Membrane Lipid Composition and Cellular Function (1985) *J. Lipid Res. 26,* 1015–1035.
15. Engler, M.M., Engler, M.B., Erickson, S.K., and Paul, S.M. Dietary Gamma-Linolenic Acid Lowers Blood Pressure and Alters Aortic Reactivity and Cholesterol Metabolism in Hypertension (1992) *J. Hypertens. 10,* 1197–1204.
16. Engler, M.M. Comparative Study of Diets Enriched with Evening Primrose, Blackcurrant, Borage or Fungal Oils on Blood Pressure and Pressor Responses in Spontaneously Hypertensive Rats (1993) *Prostaglandins Leukotrienes Essen. Fatty Acids 49,* 809–814.
17. Bhalla, R.C., Webb, R.C., Singh, D., Ashley, T., and Broch, T. Calcium Fluxes, Calcium Binding and Adenosine Cyclic 3',5' Monophosphate-dependent Protein Kinase Activity in the Aorta of Spontaneously Hypertensive and Wistar Kyoto Rats (1978) *Mol. Pharmacol. 14,* 468–477.
18. Murphy, M.G. Dietary Fatty Acids and Membrane Protein Function (1990) *J. Nutr. Biochem. 1,* 68–79.
19. Willis, A.L., and Smith, D.L. Dihomo-Gamma-Linolenic and Gamma-Linolenic Acids in Health and Disease (1989) in *New Protective Roles for Selected Nutrients,* Spiller, G.A., and Scala, J., eds., Alan Liss, Inc., New York.
20. Engler, M.M., Karanian, J.W., and Salem, N., Jr. Influence of Dietary Polyunsaturated Fatty Acids on Aortic and Platelet Fatty Acid Composition in the Rat (1991) *Nutr. Res. 11,* 753–763.
21. Wood, D.A., Butler, S., Riemersma, R.A., Thomson, M., Oliver, M.F., Fulton, M., Birtwhistle, A., and Elton, R.A. Adipose Tissue and Platelet Fatty Acids and Coronary Heart Disease in Scottish Men (1984) *Lancet ii,* 117–121.
22. Riemersma, R.A., Wood, D.A., Butler, S., Elton, R.A., Oliver, M., Salo, M., Nikkari, T., Vartianien, E., Puska, P., Gey, F., Rubba, P., Mancini, M., and Fidanza, F. Linoleic Acid Content in Adipose Tissue and Coronary Heart Disease (1986) *Br. Med. J. 292,* 1423–1427.
23. Wood, D.A., Butler, S., Riemersma, R.A., Thomson, M., Elton, R.A., MacIntyre, C., and Oliver, M.F. Linoleic and Eicosapentaenoic Acids in Adipose Tissue and Platelets and Risk of Coronary Heart Disease (1987) *Lancet i,* 177–182.
24. Luostarinen, R., Boberg, M., and Saldeen, T. Fatty Acid Composition in Total Phospholipids of Human Coronary Arteries in Sudden Cardiac Death (1993) *Atherosclerosis 99,* 187–193.
25. Engler, M.M., and Koops, R.R. Effects of Dietary Borage Oil on Plasma and Tissue Fatty Acids in Spontaneously Hypertensive and Normotensive Rats (1994) *Circulation 90(4),* I-590 (abstract).
26. Kirtland, S.J., Buchanan, T., Cowan, I., Hooper, H., and Shawyer, C.R. Dihomo-Gamma-Linolenic Acid Increases Prostacyclin Production and Reduces Platelet Thromboxane Synthesis in the Rat (1986) *Prog. Lipid Res. 25,* 331–334.
27. Hoffman, P., Block, H.U., Beitz, J., Taube, C., Forster, W., Wortha, P., Singer, P., and Neumann, E. Comparative Study of the Blood Pressure Effects of Four Different Fats on Young, Hypertensive Rats (1986) *Lipids 21,* 733–737.

28. St. Louis, C., Lee, R., Rosenfeld, J., and Fargas-Babjak, A. Antihypertensive Effect of Gamma-Linolenic Acid in Spontaneously Hypertensive Rats (1992) *Hypertension 19 (Suppl II)*, 111–115.
29. Engler, M.M. Dietary Evening Primrose, Black Currant, Borage and Fungal Oils Influence Tissue Fatty Acid Composition in Hypertension. Second International Congress on Fatty Acids and Lipids from Cell Biology to Human Disease. The International Society for the Study of Fatty Acids and Lipids, Bethesda, MD, June, 1995.
30. Bohr, D.F., Dominiczak, A.F., and Webb, R.C. Pathophysiology of the Vasculature in Hypertension (1991) *Hypertension 18 (Suppl III)*, 69–75.
31. Engler, M.B., Engler, M.M., and Ursell, P.C. Vasorelaxant Properties of n-3 Polyunsaturated Fatty Acids in Aortas from Spontaneously Hypertensive and Normotensive Rats (1994) *J. Cardiovas. Risk 1*, 75–80.
32. Sarzani, R., Claffey, K.P., Chobanian, A.V., and Brecher, P. Hypertension Induces Tissue-specific Gene Suppression of a Fatty Acid Binding Protein in Rat Aorta (1988) *Proc. Natl. Acad. Sci. U.S.A. 85*, 7777–7781.
33. Leeds, A.R., Gray, I., and Ahmad, M. Effects of n-6 Essential Fatty Acids as Evening Primrose Oil in Mild Hypertension (1990) in *Omega-6 Essential Fatty Acids: Pathophysiology and Roles in Clinical Medicine*, Horrobin, D.F., ed., Alan Liss, Inc., New York.
34. Deferne, J.-L., and Leeds, A.R. The Antihypertensive Effect of Dietary Supplementation with a 6-Desaturated Essential Fatty Acid Concentrate as Compared with Sunflower Seed Oil (1992) *J. Hum. Hypertens. 6*, 1–7.
35. Goodfriend, T.L., Ball, D.L., Elliott, M.E., Morrison, A.R., and Evenson, M.A. Fatty Acids Are Potential Regulators of Aldosterone Secretion (1991) *Endocrinology 128*, 2511–2519.
36. Jaiswal, N., Jaiswal, R.K., Tallant, A., Diz, D.I., and Ferrario, M. Alterations in Prostaglandin Production in Spontaneously Hypertensive Rat Smooth Muscle Cells (1993) *Hypertension 21*, 900–905.
37. Mills, D.E., Mah, M., Ward, R.P., Morris, B.L., and Floras, J.S. Alteration of Baroreflex Control of Forearm Vascular Resistance by Dietary Fatty Acid (1990) *Am. J. Physiol. 259*, R1164–R1171.

Chapter 17

Impact of Dietary γ-Linolenic Acid on Macrophage-Smooth Muscle Cell Interactions: Down-Regulation of Vascular Smooth Muscle Cell DNA Synthesis

Robert S. Chapkin,[a] Yang-Yi Fan,[a] and Kenneth S. Ramos[b]

[a]Faculty of Nutrition, Molecular and Cell Biology Group, and
[b]Department of Veterinary Physiology and Pharmacology, Texas A&M University, College Station, TX 77843-2471

Effect of Dietary γ-Linolenic Acid on Macrophage Lipid Metabolism

In many animal tissues and cells, linoleic acid (18:2n-6) is converted to arachidonic acid (20:4n-6) by an alternating sequence of Δ6-desaturation, chain elongation and Δ5-desaturation, in which hydrogen atoms are selectively removed to create new double bonds and two carbon atoms are then added to lengthen the fatty acid chain (1). Reports by Chapkin et al. (2) have demonstrated that peritoneal macrophages lack Δ6-desaturase activity, the enzyme responsible for the conversion of 18:2n-6 into γ-linolenic acid (18:3n-6, GLA). This observation suggests that the availability of macrophage 20:4n-6 cannot be modulated at the level of local synthesis from 18:2n-6, its major dietary essential fatty acid antecedent. Recently, Chapkin et al. (3) have shown that peritoneal macrophages in vitro can synthesize low levels of 20:4n-6 from dihomo-γ-linolenic acid (20:3n-6), and therefore possess modest Δ5-desaturase activity. In addition, the presence of elongase activity capable of converting 18:2n-6 into 20:2n-6, 20:3n-6 into 22:3n-6, and 20:4n-6 into 22:4n-6 was noted. Although the significance of the extensive elongation (two-carbon atom chain lengthening) of polyunsaturated fatty acids (PUFAs), by macrophages in vitro remains nebulous, the pathway may serve to control the level of potential inhibitor(s) of 20:4n-6 metabolism (4). An evaluation of macrophage PUFA metabolism in vivo has also demonstrated the presence of an active long-chain PUFA elongase. In these studies, we demonstrated that the total phospholipid 20:3n-6/20:4n-6 ratio was elevated significantly ($P < 0.05$) in animals fed a GLA-rich diet (5,6). This ratio was highest in the macrophage relative to the liver, spleen, and lung. Collectively, these results clearly show that the macrophage is capable of elongating GLA into 20:3n-6 and that the Δ5-desaturase, the enzyme catalyzing the transformation of 20:3n-6 into 20:4n-6, is rate limiting. The striking elevation of macrophage phospholipid 20:3n-6 levels is of particular interest because this trienoic fatty acid can serve as a precursor for the biosynthesis of eicosanoids which possess anti-inflammatory, anti-thrombotic and potent pharmacodynamic properties (7–9).

Lipoxygenation of Dihomo-γ-Linolenic Acid

Examination of the oxidative metabolism of 20:3n-6 into lipoxygenase products has shown that peritoneal macrophages metabolize endogenous 20:3n-6 into the 15-lipoxygenase product, 15-monohydroxy-8,11,13-eicosatrienoic acid (15-OH-20:3, 15-HETrE) (3). Because there is increasing evidence to suggest that 15-lipoxygenase-derived hydroxy fatty acids regulate the synthesis of 20:4n-6 metabolites (10), experiments were conducted by Chapkin et al. (11) to determine the ability of 15-OH-20:3 to modulate macrophage 20:4n-6 metabolism in vitro. In those experiments, 15-OH-20:3 inhibited zymosan-induced leukotriene C_4 (LTC_4) and 5-hydroxy-eicosatetraenoic acid (5-HETE) synthesis. In contrast to the inhibition of macrophage 5-lipoxygenase, 15-OH-20:3 had no effect on cyclooxygenase metabolism. These observations are significant because elevated levels of 20:4n-6-derived 5-lipoxygenase products, e.g., LTC_4 and LTB_4, are associated with several pathological inflammatory, hyperproliferative processes (10). The macrophage metabolism of GLA is summarized in Fig. 17.1.

Utilization of Dietary γ-Linolenic Acid: Conversion to Prostaglandin E_1

We have previously demonstrated (6) that the feeding of borage oil (*Borago officinalis*), containing the highest level of dietary GLA of any edible oil (26% by weight), to mice resulted in the accumulation of 20:3n-6 in phosphatidylinositol (PtdIns), 1-O-alk-1'-enyl-2-acyl (PlsEtn) and 1,2-diacylglycerophosphoethanolamine (PtdEtn) and in 1-O-alkyl-2-acyl (PakCho) and 1,2-diacylglycerophosphocholine (PtdCho). However, until recently it was not known if dietary GLA could augment the macrophage production of PGE_1, a potent anti-proliferative eicosanoid in vascu-

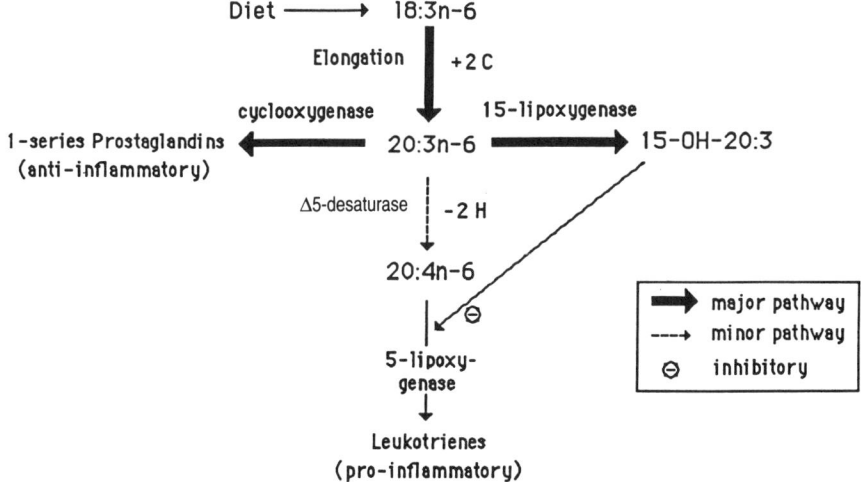

Fig. 17.1. Macrophage metabolism of γ-linolenic acid (18:3n-6).

lar smooth muscle cells (SMCs). Using combined solid phase extraction, HPLC and RIA methodologies, we determined for the first time that GLA alimentation is capable of significantly ($P < 0.05$) increasing PGE_1 synthesis in mouse peritoneal macrophages (Fig. 17.2) (12). In addition, we have recently demonstrated (13) that the activation of phospholipase A_2 in combination with the inhibition of lysophosphatidate acyltransferase (reacylation) can augment macrophage PGE_1 synthesis. Relative to phospholipase A_2 activity, the inhibition of lysophospholipid reacylation has a proportionally significant effect on enhancing macrophage PGE_1 biosynthesis. These data indicate the regulatory importance of fatty acid reacylation relative to phospholipase A_2 activity when considering macrophage prostaglandin biosynthesis.

Recently, we determined the effect of borage oil supplementation on human platelet PGE_1 and PGE_2 formation, and noted a moderate increase in platelet PGE_1 synthesis following collagen stimulation (14). A significant increase in the 20:3n-6/20:4n-6 ratio in platelet phospholipids was also observed. These data demonstrate that GLA supplementation is capable of increasing phospholipid precursor pools of PGE_1 in humans.

Biological Properties of Prostaglandin E_1

It is noteworthy that the biological properties of the monoenoic prostaglandins are markedly different from those of the dienoic 20:4n-6-derived prostaglandins (15). PGE_1 inhibits platelet aggregation via a cAMP-dependent mechanism, inhibits platelet thrombus formation in mesenteric microvessels and dilates coronary arteries, whereas PGE_2 potentiates vasoconstriction and thrombus formation (9,16). In

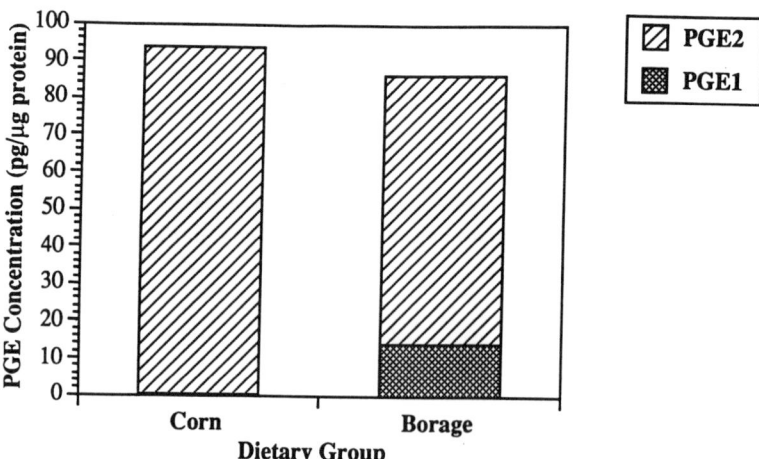

Fig. 17.2. Prostaglandin E_1 and E_2 synthesis from mouse peritoneal macrophages stimulated with zymosan. Mice ($n = 4$) were fed diets containing corn oil (CO, contains no GLA) and borage oil (BO, contains 26% w/w GLA) at 10% by weight for 2 wk.

addition, PGE_1 has been shown to inhibit vascular SMC proliferation through a cAMP-dependent mechanism, inhibit superoxide anion generation and activate the fibrinolytic system in nonhuman primates and man (9). This is significant because agents which reduce the migration and proliferation of vascular SMCs also retard the formation of atherosclerotic plaques (17). In addition, PGE_1 was far more effective than either dipyridamole or PGI_2 in inhibiting platelet deposition following angioplasty (18). The evidence reviewed above indicates that PGE_1 is synthesized in many human and animal cells, including the monocyte/macrophage (12,13), that it has a range of desirable effects at physiological concentrations which are distinct from those of other prostaglandins, and that these effects could be utilized therapeutically in battling arterial occlusive disease. One of the experimental approaches to exploit the desirable effect of PGE_1 on a variety of vascular disorders has been to infuse PGE_1 (7,8). However, because of the very short half-life of PGE_1 in the body, this method can be used only in situations in which intravascular infusions are possible. Other investigators have utilized stable analogues of PGE_1 (9,18). Unfortunately, these analogues, which are present in the circulation for hours at only slowly diminishing concentrations, have unpredictable effects (19,20). In contrast, we have recently demonstrated that dietary GLA supplementation selectively increases 20:3n-6 and the 20:3n-6/20:4n-6 ratio in human tissues and subsequently enhances PGE_1 production relative to PGE_2 (14). In the limited human studies conducted to date (21–23), GLA administration appeared to have therapeutic value with respect to coronary atherosclerosis and inflammatory disorders. However, the underlying mechanisms have not been clarified.

The Role of Macrophages and Smooth Muscle Cells in the Development of Atherosclerosis

Atherosclerosis is responsible for 50% of all the mortality in the United States, Japan and Europe (17). Atherosclerotic lesions result from an excessive inflammatory-fibroproliferative response to various forms of insults to the endothelium and smooth muscle of the arterial wall (17, 24). A large number of growth regulatory factors participate in this pathogenesis. The ability of diet to down-regulate the inflammatory-fibroproliferative response associated with atherosclerosis, or up-regulate molecular events associated with the regression of lesions, has not been adequately addressed to date.

SMCs are a major reactive cell type in atherosclerosis (17,24). The migration and proliferation of SMCs together with their capacity to produce macromolecular matrix constitute key events in the initiation and progression of atherosclerosis (24). The phenotypic spectrum of SMC has been defined based on two extreme states associated with either quiescence or unregulated proliferation. Although this concept continues to evolve, clearly important differences related to SMC phenotype have been defined. For example, in a quiescent state, SMCs respond to agents that induce vasodilation or vasoconstriction (25). In contrast, in a proliferative state, SMCs preferentially express genes for a number of growth regulatory factors and synthesize extracellular matrix. In the non-injured vessel, SMCs have a low mitotic rate, but can, in response to the appropriate stimulus, undergo migration and proliferation (25). Because proliferation of vascular SMCs is a key event in the development of atherosclerotic lesions (17), it is believed that these cells play a principal role in the fibroproliferative component of this disease. Many growth-regulatory molecules have been identified which have multiple effects with regard to SMC mitogenesis (17,26). These include platelet-derived growth factor (PDGF), basic fibroblast growth factor (bFGF), nitric oxide (NO), PGI_2, PGE_1, leukotrienes, neuropeptides, catecholamines, angiotension II, endothelia, heparin-binding epidermal growth factor-like growth factor (HB-EGF), insulin-like growth factor-1 (IGF-1), interleukin-1 (IL-1), tumor necrosis factor-α (TNF-α), and transforming growth factor-β (TGF-β). Each of these growth-regulatory molecules is capable of modulating SMC proliferation (17,25). Although an abundance of information has accumulated concerning growth mediators that stimulate vascular SMC proliferation, less is known about factors which are inhibitory to SMC growth.

Macrophages are present at all stages of atherosclerosis (17). They are considered to be the principal inflammatory mediators of cells in the atheromatous plaque environment. In regard to mitogenesis, macrophages can secrete IL-1, NO, TNF-α, TGF-β and a mitogenic factor similar to PDGF, macrophage-derived growth factor (MDGF), thus playing a role in the vascular response of SMC proliferation (17,25). Macrophages also secrete eicosanoids which have been demonstrated to regulate arterial SMC phenotype and proliferative capacity. Specifically, PGE_1 (derived from 20:3n-6) and prostacyclin (PGI_2, derived from 20:4n-6) inhibit asynchronous, cycling (growing) SMC proliferation (26). When PGE_1 or PGI_2 are added to asynchronous cycling SMC (i.e., PGE_1 is added to cells in G_1, S, G_2, and in M), this causes a pronounced elevation in cellular cyclic 3′,5′-adenosine monophosphate (cAMP) levels which results in growth arrest (28,29). Therefore, PGE_1 and PGI_2 may be potent antiproliferative therapeutic agents capable of ameliorating atheromatous plaque formation. It is noteworthy that although PGE_1, PGE_2, and PGI_2 all possess inhibitory properties with respect to SMC DNA synthesis, PGE_1 has the greatest biopotency (27,28). Interestingly, we have demonstrated that dietary GLA is capable of enhancing mouse peritoneal macrophage production of PGE_1 and PGI_2 (12) and may therefore be capable of reducing or down-regulating vascular SMC proliferation.

Development of a Macrophage-Smooth Muscle Cell Co-Culture Model to Elucidate the Mechanisms by Which Dietary γ-Linolenic Acid Modulates Macrophage Atherogenic Potential

Because the regulation of cytokine/growth factor network by eicosanoids may represent an important aspect of arterial response to injury and the progression of intimal hyperplasia (17), we examined the ability of resident peritoneal macrophages isolated from GLA-fed mice to influence mouse thoracic aortic SMC proliferation (30). Naive SMCs were isolated from thoracic aortas of chow-fed pathogen free C57BL/6 mice as previously described (31). Unstimulated macrophages (0.8 × 10^6) were placed in upper cell culture chambers separated by semi-permeable membranes (30 kDa cut-off). Cycling SMC (1×10^4) in the lower chamber, were co-cultured for 16 h and cell proliferation measured by pulse labeling with ^{3}H-thymidine. The results demonstrate (Fig. 17.3) that macrophages harvested from borage oil-fed (containing 26% w/w GLA) mice significantly suppressed ($P < 0.01$) SMC proliferation relative to corn oil (containing linoleic acid, 18:2n-6) or fish oil (containing n-3 polyunsaturated fatty acids) dietary treatments. The elevated macrophage PGE_1 synthesis in borage oil-fed mice may be responsible for the observed biological effect, because inhibition of SMC DNA synthesis was abrogated by macrophage preincubation with indomethacin (cyclooxygenase inhibitor) but not L655,238 (5-lipoxygenase inhibitor) prior to co-culture (32). Additional experiments are required to validate this hypothesis. The ability of borage oil-derived macrophages to inhibit asynchronously, cycling SMCs is noteworthy, because monocyte/macrophage-derived mitogenic factors play a role in the up-regulation of SMC proliferation and hence the promotion of atheromatous plaque formation (17,26).

Conclusions

Based on our SMC-macrophage experiments (Fig. 17.3), we have hypothesized that dietary GLA can favorably modulate the atherogenic process. Although it is unclear at this time whether macrophage-derived cyclooxygenase products are entirely responsible for the growth inhibitory effects of GLA, they are likely contributors to

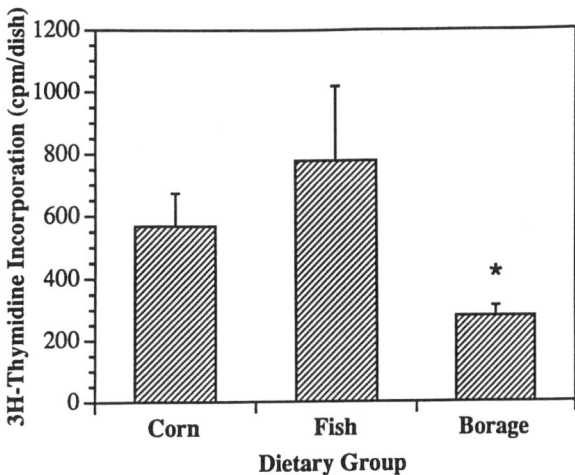

Fig. 17.3. Effect of dietary borage oil on mouse peritoneal macrophage-mediated suppression of mouse vascular SMC proliferation. SMCs were pulse labeled with ^{3}H-thymidine and processed as previously described (31). Results represent means ± SD for $n = 3$ incubations. (*) borage oil treatment significantly ($P < 0.01$) less DNA synthesis than corn oil and fish oil.

the response because only GLA-containing diets are effective, and exogenous PGE_1 mimics the diet-induced antiproliferative effects. However, the possibility exists that GLA may down-regulate the release of growth stimulatory molecules and/or up-regulate the release of other growth inhibitory molecules. Future experiments will address this question by determining the mechanism(s) by which dietary GLA modulates selected markers and mediators of SMC proliferation. These studies are essential if new approaches for the treatment and prevention of a disease responsible for enormous morbidity and mortality are to be developed.

Acknowledgments

We gratefully acknowledge the generous donations of corn oil and borage oil by Sid Tracy, Traco Labs, Seymour, IL. Vacuum-deodorized fish oil was kindly provided by the NIH Fish Oil Test Material Program, Southeast Fisheries Center, Charleston, SC. This work was supported in part by grants from Scotia Pharmaceuticals, Ltd., the Texas A&M Interdisciplinary Research Enhancement Program and NIH DK41693. Y.-Y. Fan is a recipient of the 1994 Nabisco Foods Group Predoctoral Fellowship sponsored by the American Institute of Nutrition.

References

1. Willis, A.L., and Smith D.L. (1989) in *New Protective Roles for Selective Nutrients*, Alan R. Liss, Inc., pp. 39–108,
2. Chapkin, R.S., Somers, S.D., and Erickson, K.L. Inability of Murine Peritoneal Macrophages to Convert Linoleic Acid into Arachidonic Acid (1988) *J. Immunol. 140*, 2350–2355.
3. Chapkin, R.S., Somers, S.D., Schumacher, L., and Erickson, K.L. Fatty Acid Composition of Macrophage Phospholipids in Mice Fed Fish or Borage Oil (1988) *Lipids 23*, 380–383.
4. Rosenthal, M.D. Fatty Acid Metabolism in Isolated Mammalian Cells (1987) *Prog. Lipid Res. 26*, 87–124.
5. Chapkin, R.S., Somers, S.D., and Erickson, K.L. Dietary Manipulation of Macrophage Phospholipid Classes: Selective Increase of Dihomogammalinolenic Acid (1988) *Lipids 23*, 766–770.
6. Chapkin, R.S., and Carmichael, S.L. Effect of Dietary Blackcurrant Seed Oil on Mouse Macrophage Subclasses of Choline and Ethanolamine Glycerophospholipids (1990) *J. Nutr. 120*, 825–830.
7. Sinzinger, H., Fitscha, P., Wagner, O., Kaliman, J., and Rogatti, W. Prostaglandin E_1 Decreases Activation of Arterial Smooth Muscle Cells (1986). *Lancet ii*, 156–157.
8. Sinzinger, H., O'Grady, J., Fitscha, P., Rauscha, F., and Kaliman, J. Comparable Effect of Prostaglandin E_1 in Decreasing *in Vivo* Platelet Deposition on Human Lesion Sites after Intravenous and Intraarterial Application (1988) *Thromb. Res. 50*, 749–755.
9. Simmet, T.H., and Peskar, B.A. Prostaglandin E_1 and Arterial Occlusive Disease: Pharmacological Approach (1988) *Eur. J. Clin. Invest. 18*, 549–554.
10. Feuerstein, G., and Hallenbeck, J.M. Leukotrienes in Health and Disease (1987) *FASEB J. 1*, 186–192.
11. Chapkin, R.S., Miller, C.C., Somers, S.D., and Erickson, K.I. Ability of 15-Hydroxyeicosatrienoic Acid (15-OH-20:3) to Modulate Macrophage Arachidonic Acid Metabolism (1988) *Biochem. Biophys. Res. Commun. 153*, 799–804.

12. Fan, Y.-Y., and Chapkin, R.S. Mouse Peritoneal Macrophage Prostaglandin E_1 Synthesis Is Altered by Dietary Gamma-Linolenic Acid (1992) *J. Nutr. 122*, 1600–1606.
13. Fan, Y.-Y., and Chapkin, R.S. Phospholipid Sources of Metabolically Elongated Gammalinolenic Acid: Conversion to Prostaglandin E_1 in Stimulated Mouse Macrophages (1993) *J. Nutr. Biochem. 4*, 602–607.
14. Barre, D.E., Holub, B.J., and Chapkin, R.S. The Effect of Borage Oil Supplementation on Platelet Aggregation, Thromboxane B_2, Prostaglandin E_1 and E_2 Formation (1993) *Nutr. Res. 13*, 739–751.
15. Horrobin, D.F. Gammalinolenic Acid (1990) *Rev. Contemp. Pharmacother. 1*, 1–45.
16. Kirtland, S.J. Prostaglandin E_1: A Review (1988) *Prostaglandins Leukotrienes Essen. Fatty Acids 32*, 165–174.
17. Ross, R. The Pathogenesis of Atherosclerosis: A Perspective for the 1990's (1993) *Nature 362*, 801–809.
18. See, J., Shell, W., Mathews, O., Canizales, C., Vargas, M., Giddings, J., and Cerrone, J. Prostaglandin E_1 Infusion after Angioplasty in Humans Inhibits Abrupt Occlusion and Early Restenosis (1987) *Adv. Prost. Throm. Leuk. Res. 17*, 266–270.
19. Ziboh, V.A., and Chapkin, R.S. Biologic Significance of Polyunsaturated Fatty Acids in the Skin (1987) *Arch. Dermatol. 123*, 1686a–1690a.
20. Moran, M., Mozes, M.F., Maddurx, M.S., Veremis, S., Bartkins, C., Ketel, B., Pollak, R., Wallenmark, C., and Jonasson, O. Prevention of Acute Graft Rejection by the Prostaglandin E_1 Analogue Misoprostol in Renal-Transplant Recipients Treated with Cyclosporine and Prednisone (1990) *N. Engl. J. Med. 322*, 1183–1188.
21. Kernoff, P.B.A., Willis, A.L., Stone, K.J., Davies, J.A., and McNicol, G.P. Antithrombotic Potential of Dihomo-Gamma-Linolenic Acid in Man (1977) *Br. Med. J. 3*, 1441–1444.
22. Pullman-Mooar, S., Laposata, M., Lem, D., Holman, R.T., Leventhal, L., DeMarco, D., and Zurier, R.B. Alteration of the Cellular Fatty Acid Profile and the Production of Eicosanoids in Human Monocytes by Gamma-Linolenic Acid (1990) *Arthritis Rheum. 33*, 1526–1533.
23. Sim, A.K., and McCraw, A.P. The Activity of γ-Linolenate and Dihomo-γ-Linolenate Methyl Esters *in Vitro* and *in Vivo* on Blood Platelet Function in Non-Human Primates and in Man (1977) *Thromb. Res. 10*, 385–397.
24. Badimon, J.J., Fuster, V., Chesebro, J.H., and Badimon, L. Coronary Atherosclerosis, a Multifactorial Disease (1993) Circulation 87 (suppl. II), II 3–II 16.
25. Pomerantz, K.B., and Hajjar, D.P. Eicosanoids in Regulation of Arterial Smooth Muscle Cell Phenotype, Proliferative Capacity, and Cholesterol Metabolism (1989) *Arteriosclerosis 9*, 413–429.
26. Zhang, H., Downs, E.C., Lindsey, J.A., Davis, W.B., Whisler, R.L., and Cornwell, D.G. Interactions Between Monocyte/Macrophage and Vascular Smooth Muscle Cell: Stimulation of Mitogenesis by a Soluble Factor and of Prostanoid Synthesis by Cell-Cell Contact (1993) *Arterioscler. Thromb. 13*, 220–230.
27. Owen, N.E. Effect of Prostaglandin E_1 on DNA Synthesis in Vascular Smooth Muscle Cells (1986) *Am. J. Physiol. 250*, C584–C588.
28. Nilsson, J., and Olsson, A.G. Prostaglandin E_1 Inhibits DNA Synthesis in Arterial Smooth Muscle Cells Stimulated with Platelet-Derived Growth Factor (1984) *Atherosclerosis 53*, 77–82.

29. Loesberg, C., Vanwijk, R., Zandberger, J., van Aken, W.G., van Mourik, J.A., and de Groot, P.G. Cell Cycle-Dependent Inhibition of Human Vascular Smooth Muscle Cell Proliferation by Prostaglandin E_1 (1985) *Exp. Cell Res. 160,* 117–125.
30. Fan, Y.-Y., Chapkin, R.S., and Ramos, K.S. A Macrophage-Smooth Muscle Cell Co-Culture Model: Applications in the Study of Atherogenesis. *In Vitro Cell. Dev. Biol., 31,* 492–493 (1995).
31. Ramos, K.S., and Cox, L.R. Primary Cultures of Rat Aortic Endothelial and Smooth Muscle Cells: An *in Vitro* Model to Study Xenobiotic-Induced Vascular Cytotoxicity (1987) *In Vitro Cell. Develop. Biol. 23,* 288–296.
32. Fan, Y.-Y., Ramos, K.S., and Chapkin, R.S. Dietary Gamma-Linolenic Acid Modulates Macrophage-Vascular Smooth Muscle Cell Interactions: Evidence for a Macrophage-Derived Soluble Factor Which Downregulates DNA Synthesis in Smooth Muscle Cells. *Arteriosclerosis, Thromb. Vasc. Biol. 15,* 1397–1403.

Chapter 18

Effects of γ-Linolenic Acid on Brain Fatty Acid Composition and Behavior in Mice

Patricia E. Wainwright[a] and Yung-Sheng Huang[b]

[a]Department of Health Studies and Gerontology, University of Waterloo, Waterloo, Ontario, N2L 3G1
[b]Ross Products Division, Abbott Laboratories, Columbus, OH 43215

Introduction

Polyunsaturated fatty acids (PUFA) of the n-6 and n-3 families are considered essential nutrients for humans and other animals. These essential fatty acids (EFA) are found in the body as unesterified free fatty acids or as components of cholesterol esters, triacyclglycerols, or esterified to the complex lipids of biological membranes. Following provision of the 18-C precursors, i.e., linoleic acid (LA, 18:2n-6) and α-linolenic acid (ALA, 18:3n-3) in the diet, animals have the biosynthetic capacity to convert these to longer-chain compounds through a series of desaturation and elongation reactions (reviewed in 1).

The n-3 and n-6 fatty acids compete with one another in this metabolic pathway, and there may also be competition for acylation into membrane phospholipids. The enzyme systems appear to have a higher affinity for the n-3 fatty acids, such that, given equal amounts, these will be preferentially metabolized over the n-6 fatty acids. Thus, together with the absolute amount of fatty acids available, the dietary n-6/n-3 ratio is an important factor in influencing tissue fatty acid composition (2). There are various ways in which such changes in fatty acid composition might be expected to have functional effects. The first is through effects on the structural properties of cell membranes. Depending on their chain length and the number and position of the double bonds, they alter the physical properties of the membrane, such as fluidity, flexibility and permeability, thereby influencing a variety of membrane functions. These include effects on ion channels and transport, endo- and exocytosis, and the activities of membrane bound proteins (3,4). Alternatively, the 20-carbon fatty acids also participate in the ongoing regulation of physiological activity by serving as precursors of the eicosanoids. The pathological symptoms associated with a deficiency of n-6 fatty acids include: growth retardation, scaly dermatitis, increased loss of water through the skin, and reproductive failure (5). A deficiency of n-3 fatty acids has been associated with changes in the electroretinogram in rodents, rhesus monkeys and human infants, and altered visual acuity thresholds in monkeys and human infants (6,7). EFA deficiency (n-6 and n-3), as well as n-3 deficiency alone, has also been associated with differences in performance on learning tasks in rodents (reviewed in 8). Under certain conditions desaturase activities may be impaired, thereby leading to metabolic deficiency, and in such cases, provision of the longer chain metabolites, either through the diet or as therapeutic supplements, may be necessary for optimal function.

γ-Linolenic acid (GLA, 18:3n-6) is the product of the Δ6 desaturation of LA (9). It is also available from particularly enriched plant sources, such as the seed oils of borage (*Borago officianalis*), evening primrose (*Oenothera biennis*), and black currant (*Ribes nigrum*). It is converted, through the process of chain elongation, to dihomo-γ-linolenic acid (DGLA, 20:3n-6), which is, in turn, desaturated by Δ5-desaturase to form arachidonic acid (AA). DGLA is also the precursor of the 1-series prostaglandins. Dietary supply of GLA may be of particular importance in conditions in which there is a decline in tissue levels of long-chain n-6 fatty acids, DGLA and AA, due to increased use of DGLA or reduction in the activity of Δ6-desaturase (10,11). The use of GLA to remedy a decrease in AA may be preferable to the use of AA itself, because it allows metabolic control of AA levels and subsequent eicosanoid production. In this chapter, we discuss some of our recent work on EFA and brain development. Using the mouse as an animal model, we have studied two dietary conditions which may compromise long-chain n-6 fatty acid status in the developing offspring, namely, dietary fish-oil supplementation and chronic ethanol consumption. Specifically, we have addressed the hypothesis that dietary supplementation with GLA will increase levels of 20-C and 22-C n-6 fatty acids in brain membrane phospholipids, and that these changes in fatty acid composition will have functional consequences in terms of behavioral outcomes.

γ-Linolenic Acid and Brain Fatty Acid Composition

The long-chain PUFA (LCP) predominate in brain phospholipids, particularly arachidonic acid (AA, 20:4n-6), adrenic acid (22:4n-6), and docosahexaenoic acid (DHA, 22:6n-3) (12). The membranes of the retinal rod outer segments and the synaptosomal fraction of the brain are characterized by their high DHA content. These LCP accumulate rapidly in the brain during intrauterine and early postnatal development, and dietary deficiencies during this period are reflected in changes in brain fatty acid composition (13,14). EFA deficiency results in increased tissue levels of 20:3n-9, whereas dietary n-3 deficiency or an increase in the n-6/n-3 ratio results in decreased tissue levels of 22:6n-3, with a corresponding increase in 22:5n-6 (15).

There is controversy currently about the appropriate level of supplementation of infant formulas with long-chain fatty acid (discussed in 16). Human breast milk contains small amounts of AA and DHA in addition to LA and ALA, whereas most commercial formulas provide only the 18-C compounds. The question is whether the biosynthetic capacities of the infant are able to satisfy the needs of the developing brain for long-chain n-3 fatty acids. This is of particular concern in the case of preterm infants who have very high energy needs. Supplementation of preterm formula with a marine oil concentrate that was high in eicosapentaenoic acid (EPA, 20:5n-3), while improving DHA status, was accompanied by decreases in tissue AA levels, and also a decrease in growth (17). Thus the challenge is to determine not only the absolute and relative amounts of n-6 and n-3 fatty acids required, but also the actual chain length necessary for optimal developmental outcome.

We have addressed these questions by manipulating the diet of pregnant and lactating mice, and assessing the development of 12-d-old pups. Using a dose-response design, we have shown that when the dietary n-6:n-3 ratio is decreased by supplementation with increasing amounts of fish oil concentrate containing EPA and DHA, there is an increase in DHA levels both in the brain (18) and other tissues such as the liver (19), which is accompanied by a decrease in AA (20:4n-6). These changes may be due to the inhibition of Δ6-desaturase by high levels of long-chain n-3 fatty acids. This study provided preliminary evidence suggesting that alterations in brain n-6 fatty acid composition after feeding long-chain n-3 fatty acids could be offset by the partial replacement of LA by GLA. This intervention led to increased AA levels both in the dams' milk and in the pup brain, presumably through by-passing the Δ6-desaturase. We therefore conducted the following study to explore the relationship between providing the n-6 and n-3 fatty acids either as the 18-carbon precursors, LA or ALA, or as their longer-chain metabolites, GLA and EPA (20). We hypothesized that, compared with LA and ALA, GLA and EPA would increase tissue levels of AA and DHA, respectively. However, there would also be reciprocal effects, such that GLA decreased DHA, and EPA decreased AA.

Experiment 1

Methods. In this study pregnant and lactating B6D2F$_1$ mice were maintained on a liquid diet containing sufficient minerals and vitamins and 20% (kcal) fat-free casein, 60% carbohydrate, and 20% fat. Different fat supplements were prepared from mixing variable amounts of olive oil and n-3 and n-6 fatty acid concentrates such that the n-3/n-6 ratio remained at 0.25 (n-6:n-3 ratio = 4.0), but differed in the source of the n-3 and n-6 FA. They were: (a) 18:3n-3/18:2n-6 (ALA/LA); (b) 18:3n-3/18:3n-6 (ALA/GLA); (c) 20:5n-3/18:2n-6 (EPA/LA); and (d) 20:5n-3/18:3n-6 (EPA/GLA). Twelve days after birth the animals were killed, and brains and livers were collected from the dam and one male and one female pup from each litter. Total tissue lipids were extracted with chloroform-methanol and different lipid fractions separated by thin-layer chromatography. After methylation, the fatty acid composition of the phosphatidylcholine and phosphatidylethanolamine fractions was analyzed by gas-liquid chromatography.

Results and Discussion. The results supported the hypotheses. As shown in Fig. 18.1A, in dam livers, when dietary ALA was replaced by EPA as the source of n-3 fatty acids, levels of 22:6n-3 increased and 20:4n-6 decreased; conversely, when dietary LA was replaced by GLA, 22:6n-3 decreased and 20:4n-6 increased. Similar effects of GLA but not EPA on 20:4n-6 were seen in pup liver. The effects of GLA on the brain, shown in Fig. 18.1B, were qualitatively similar but quantitatively smaller than those in liver. It is interesting to note that changes in brain fatty acid composition were seen in both the dam and pups, suggesting that it is not only the developing brain that is sensitive to dietary influences. These findings suggest that the untoward effects of diets containing long-chain n-3 fatty acids on AA status may be avoided by provision of long-chain n-6 fatty acids in the form of GLA. The possible functional effects of such alterations in brain fatty acid composition will be addressed in the following section.

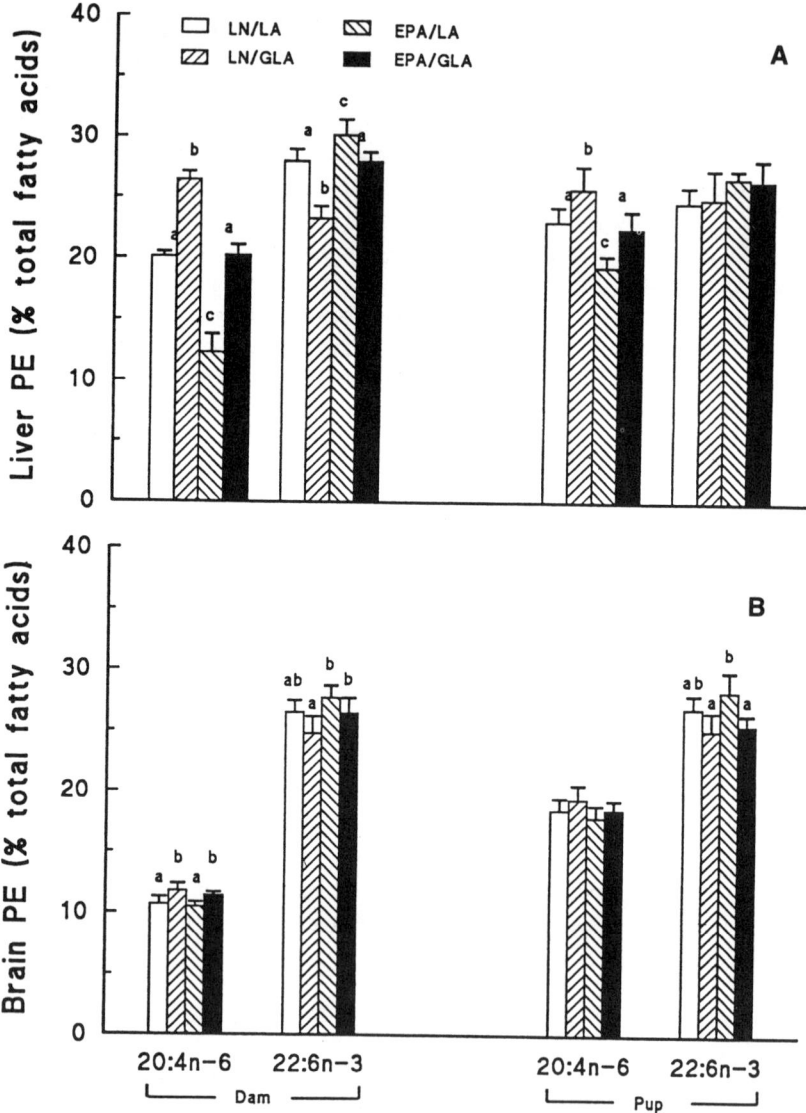

Fig. 18.1. Effect of maternal diet on fatty acid composition (wt %) of liver (A) and brain (B) phosphatidyletyhanolamine in dams and their 12-d-old suckling pups. Diets were supplemented with oil mixtures having the same n-3/n-6 ratio (0.25), but differing in source of n-3 and n-6 fatty acids (18:2n-6, LA, vs. 18:3n-6, GLA, and 18:3n-3, LN, vs. fish oil, 20:5n-3 (EPA) and 22:6n-3 (DHA). Bars with different letters are significantly different, $P < 0.05$.

γ-Linolenic Acid Supplementation and PGE$_1$ Production

The term "eicosanoids" refers collectively to a group of oxygenated 20-carbon compounds which are very active biologically and which include the prostaglandins, thromboxanes, leukotrienes, and a variety of hydroxy and hydroperoxy fatty acids (reviewed in reference 21). They are derived from either DGLA, AA or EPA, and are referred to as series 1, 2, and 3, respectively; the major precursor is AA. The fatty acids are released from the membrane phospholipids through the action of cellular phospholipases and converted to eicosanoids through the cyclooxygense, lipoxygenase, and epoxygenase pathways. Prostaglandins result from the activity of the cyclooxygenase enzymes, whereas the lipoxygenases act as catalysts in the formation of the hydroperoxy fatty acids. There is abundant evidence that dietary-induced changes in tissue fatty acid composition are associated with changes in eicosanoid production (reviewed in reference 2). Moreover, it appears that prostaglandins of the different series have different functional effects, with those derived from EPA, for example, in many cases opposing those from AA (22). Thus dietary fatty acid supply may well have important effects on overall function by altering the relative balance of these compounds. Such effects have been demonstrated by manipulating the n-6 and n-3 fatty acid content of the diet, using evening primrose or borage oil (both containing LA and GLA), and marine oil, respectively. Thus it has been shown in rat mesenteric vasculature that at high concentrations, n-3 fatty acids inhibit the conversion of both DGLA and AA to eicosanoids, but that low concentrations may increase formation of desirable 1- and 2-series eicosanoids (23). Feeding mice borage oil selectively increased the levels of DGLA in macrophage phospholipids (24), and this was converted to PGE$_1$ on stimulation (25). Similar to these findings in other organs, alterations in brain fatty acid composition associated with dietary manipulations are also accompanied by changes in eicosanoid production (26). Thus, studies on the behavioral effects of GLA (discussed below) have been based on the premise that they are mediated by the eicosanoids, specifically by increases in levels of PGE$_1$ resulting from increases in the precursor, DGLA.

Brain Fatty Acid Composition and Eicosanoid Metabolism

Neurochemical Effects of Eicosanoids

The available evidence supports a role for eicosanoids as second messengers and modulators of synaptic transmission in the brain (reviewed in references 27–31). The primary prostaglandins, PGD$_2$, PGE$_2$, PGF$_{2\alpha}$, are produced in the brain by both neuronal and glial cells, whereas TXA$_2$ and PGI$_2$ are produced from AA by cerebral microvessels and the choroid plexus. The activity of the synthetic enzymes varies by cellular location and developmental stage. PGE$_2$ and PGF$_{2\alpha}$ are potent vasoconstrictors and produce vasospasm, whereas PGI$_2$ has opposing effects: normal brain circulatory function would therefore presuppose an optimal balance among these various compounds. In rat brain, the highest basal levels of prostaglandins are found in the olfactory bulb, pineal gland and hypothalamus, and PGD_2 is quantitatively the most important cyclooxygenase product. Leukotrienes are present in small amounts, although recent work suggests caution, based on methodological concerns, in the interpretation of findings related to lipoxygenase activity in the brain (32). 12-HETE is especially high in rat pineal gland and cerebral cortex and hippocampal slices, and it has been suggested that it may be involved in the processes underlying long-term potentiation (33,34).

A high proportion of the prostaglandins in the brain are associated with synaptic terminals, and stimulation of neural pathways results in greatly increased prostaglandin synthesis and release (discussed in reference 30). The primary prostaglandins play a direct role in neural activity by modulating the release of neurohormones and neurotransmitters. They rarely act alone, but function to modulate ongoing cellular processes, particularly stimulus-secretion–coupled events. They operate through cell surface receptors which interact with and stimulate G proteins. In this way, they act as bioregulators of second messsengers, such as cAMP, inositol triphosphate and diacylglycerol. This in turn affects Ca^{++} mobilization, specific protein binding, and the activity of protein kinases. For example, it is thought that PGE inhibits neurotransmitter release in noradrenergic neurons by restricting Ca^{++} availability on the arrival of a nerve impulse. The effect of PGE_1 on calcium appears to be biphasic, with reduced release at high concentrations and enhanced release at lower concentrations. Thus different mechanisms may be operative at the two concentrations of PGE_1, thereby making dose-response relationships an important consideration.

Behavioral Effects of Eicosanoids

Prostaglandins have been shown to be involved in the regulation of body temperature, sleep-wake cycles, food and fluid intake, and autonomic reactivity (reviewed in Ref. 30,35–37). PGD_2 increases sleep time and decreases body temperature (38), whereas PGE_2 decreases sleep time and increases body temperature (39), with the preoptic area of the anterior hypothalamus being identified as the site of action. The hyperthermic response is not triggered by heat or cold exposure, but represents the febrile state induced through the production of the cytokines and mediated by the release of prostanoids (36). Induction of seizures by ECT or convulsant drugs increases the formation of PGD_2, PGE_2, and $PGF_{2\alpha}$, particularly in the cortex and hippocampus. The use of cyclooxygenase inhibitors has shown that this rise in eicosanoid production is secondary to the convulsive state. Their role is thought to be protective, in that administration of PGD_2 and PGE_2 reduces the intensity of drug-induced convulsions in rats. Because of their associated peripheral effects, the best practice in behavioral studies is to administer the prostaglandins intracerebroventricularly (ICV). ICV administration of PGE_2 and PGD_2 in the rat resulted in sedation and inhibition of locomotor and exploratory activity, with $PGF_{2\alpha}$ being less effective in producing this response (40). These compounds also increased the sleeping times induced by barbiturates, chloral hydrate, and ethanol; these effects were measured behaviorally in terms of the loss of the righting reflex (41). The behavioral sedation observed after administration of PGE would appear paradoxical in light of the work discussed above which described increased wakefulness and suggests different sensitivities and possibly different sites of action. While the prostaglandins are activators of pain at peripheral sites, they show antinociceptive properties when they are injected centrally (42). Sensory changes of this type may contribute to the effects reported on conditioned avoidance behavior (43).

Recently, there has been some interesting work done on the effects of dietary administration of PUFA on stress reactivity, which may be related to the autonomic effects of the prostaglandins. A study in spontaneously hypertensive rats demonstrated an attenuation in blood pressure following increased PUFA consumption (44). Similarly, dietary administration of EPA and GLA attenuated the pressor and tachycardiac responses to chronic psychosocial stress in rats (45–47). A further study in humans demonstrated that administration of borage oil (GLA), but not fish oil (EPA), attenuated blood pressure and heart-rate responses to stress, increased skin temperature, and improved task performance on a Stroop color-word conflict test (48).

Putative Role of PGE_1 in Alcoholism and Affective Disorder

It is thought that some of the pharmacological effects of ethanol may be related to its effects on EFA and prostaglandins (49,50). There is evidence that ethanol increases the ratio of LA to AA in various membrane fractions (reviewed in ref. 51,52). While this implies that ethanol inhibits the activity of the desaturase enzymes, an alternative explanation is that ethanol increases the utilization of the end products, DGLA and AA. This is supported by evidence that chronic administration of ethanol increases urinary PG output and amplifies indices of EFA deficiency (53). Moreover, over a range relevant to human intoxication, alcohol enhances formation of PGE_1 from DGLA in human platelets, with no effects on the PGE_2 series from AA (54). Treatment with PGE_1 potentiates some of the acute behavioral effects of ethanol and also reduces the severity of withdrawal symptoms in alcohol-addicted animals (55); similar effects are seen with evening primrose oil (EPO) and GLA (56). Furthermore, administration of PG synthetase inhibitors, such as aspirin and indomethacin, antagonizes the hypothermic (57), depressant (58) and behavioral activating (59) effects of ethanol in mice, indicating that these effects are mediated through PG production. Based on these observations, it has been suggested that PGE_1 plays an important role in alcoholism and also possibly in affective disorders (60). The hypothesis is that alcoholic intoxication, and also mania, are associated with excessive PGE_1 production, whereas depression is related to decreases in PGE_1: the putative mechanism underlying these effects is the dose-related modulation of the release and reuptake of intracellular calcium and subsequent effects on neurotransmission. Lithium reduces mania by inhibiting the mobilization of DGLA from membranes, whereas tricyclic antidepressants counteract the effects of low levels of PGE_1 on calcium release. While ethanol initially increases PGE_1 production, chronic ethanol use will result in a deficiency of DGLA and hence reduced PGE_1 by preventing the replenishment of DGLA stores through inhibition of Δ6-desaturase. It has therefore been proposed that both the physiological and behavioral sequelae of chronic alcoholism will be ameliorated by dietary supplementation of GLA (61).

γ-Linolenic Acid and Fetal Alcohol Syndrome

Chronic alcoholism is of particular concern in women of child-bearing age because of the threat it poses not only to the health of the mother, but also to that of the unborn child. Prenatal ethanol exposure in humans has been associated with a characteristic constellation of fetal effects, termed Fetal Alcohol Syndrome, which includes specific physical anomalies, pre- and postnatal growth retardation, and central nervous system dysfunction (62). Dietary deficiencies of EFA during development have also been associated with various adverse outcomes, including severe growth retardation (16), and behavioral anomalies (8). This suggests the possibility that some of the deleterious effects of ethanol consumption during pregnancy, particularly those on growth and activity, might be mediated through EFA deficiency, specifically that of DGLA and possibly AA. If so, the administration of GLA may improve EFA status and thereby improve developmental outcomes. In the following section we describe two studies from our laboratory which have addressed this hypothesis. In the first study with mice, GLA was administered by subcutaneous injection, concomitantly with ethanol, during gestation only, and treatment outcome was assessed in 12-d-old pups (63). In the second study (in press 1996, see ref. (64), the ethanol was administered during gestation only, with the GLA provided as a dietary supplement throughout the study, i.e., during gestation and lactation and throughout the life of the offspring. The treatment outcome was measured in adult animals. In addition, the design of this study allowed us to address behavioral effects of GLA independently of those of ethanol.

Experiment 1

Methods. Pregnant $B6D2F_1$ mice were fed liquid diets containing 25% ethanol-derived calories from d 7 through 17 of gestation. GLA (20, 120, and 200 mg/kg) was administered by subcutaneous injection to animals receiving ethanol, using safflower oil as the vehicle. The controls were given ethanol and vehicle only. To control for reductions in food intake in the ethanol-fed groups, all groups were pair-fed to this ethanol control, including a second control group which received sucrose substituted isocalorically for ethanol. Additional control groups included a group with ad libitum access to laboratory chow and two further ethanol groups, one treated with AA and the other with saturated fat (coconut oil). Behavioral development of the pups was measured 12 d after birth, using a standardized scale, and open-field behavior was measured at weaning.

Results and Discussion. Body and brain weight were lower in ethanol-treated pups, and ethanol also produced significant behavioral retardation on the order of 1.7 d. Open-field scores suggested that ethanol-treated males were more active than sucrose controls. Contrary to the hypothesis, in no instance was a GLA-treated group significantly different than the ethanol control. A disturbing finding was that reproductive outcome, as measured by animals that produced live pups, was worse in both the ethanol/GLA- and ethanol/AA-treated groups. Whether this reflects an effect of GLA or AA administration is not clear because, in this study, there was no administration of GLA independent of ethanol. Results obtained from the subcutaneous administration of free fatty acids may not pertain to dietary administration. Moreover, in this study, the ethanol and GLA were administered during gestation only, thereby addressing long-term effects of treatment during the well-defined *in utero* sensitive period only. In contrast, in a more recent study in rats (65), the treatment regimen of ethanol and evening primrose oil (100 mg/kg EPO, consisting of approximately 10% GLA, provided as a dietary supplement), was administered 3 wk prior to mating and throughout the study. EPO increased locomotor activity, particularly in the light cycle, and decreased the latency to find the platform in the Morris-maze, thereby offsetting the depressant effects of ongoing ethanol consumption. The design of this study, in which the animals were fed ethanol throughout, does not allow one to separate the effects of prenatal from acute ethanol exposure. This is an important point because, given that prenatal ethanol exposure is associated with hyperactivity, it is possible that GLA might in fact exacerbate rather than relieve the condition. However, some caution may be in order with respect to these findings as there was not an oil control which would allow definitive attribution of the findings to the GLA content of EPO. In addition, the statistical analysis was based on individual pups, rather than on the treatment unit, which was the litter: this has the potential to spuriously inflate the power of the study to detect treatment effects (66). Nevertheless, the observation that chronic dietary supplementation with EPO may be associated with increased activity is intriguing. Interestingly, in a related study (67), EPO attenuated the effect of ethanol on brain membrane phospholipids, suggesting an association between such changes and the effects seen on behavior.

As mentioned above, the design of this study also allows us to investigate effects of GLA independently of those of ethanol. Based on the reports of the influence of the prostaglandins on the circadian rhythm of body temperature (68,69), and sleep-wake cycles (discussed above), it is conceivable that changes in membrane fatty acid composition might also lead to changes in circadian activity. This is therefore an area in which studies of the behavioral effects of the dietary fatty acids may prove informative. Sleep disturbance is a characteristic symptom of severe affective disorders (70), and this is relieved by use of the tricyclic antidepressants (71). A recent report suggests that unsaturated free fatty acids may be involved in the regulation of antidepressant binding sites in rat brain (72). Thus the question arises whether long-term dietary GLA administration affects circadian rhythms and also whether it may act alone as an antidepressant. We therefore designed a study to address these questions (64). In addition to behavior, this study included measures of brain fatty acid composition.

Experiment 2

Specific questions addressed by this study were:

1. Will the long-term supplementation of the maternal diet with GLA counteract the effects of prenatal ethanol exposure on growth and development?

2. What are the effects of prenatal ethanol exposure and chronic dietary supplementation of GLA on adult brain fatty acid composition?
3. What are the effects of prenatal ethanol exposure and long-term dietary GLA supplementation on: (a) open-field activity and (b) circadian activity as measured in a running wheel?
4. Does long-term dietary supplementation of GLA have effects similar to that of the tricyclic antidepressant, desmethyimipramine (DMI), in decreasing the time spent immobile in a forced swimming test (Porsolt test)?

Methods. B6D2F$_1$ mice and their offspring were used in a 2 × 2 factorial design, with the addition of a fifth untreated laboratory chow control group. The factors were dietary oil composition, 18:2n-6, linoleic acid, (LA) vs. 18:3n-6, γ-linolenic acid (GLA) and ethanol (25% ethanol derived calories, EDC) vs. maltose dextrin (substituted isocalorically for ethanol). Ethanol was fed in a liquid diet, with 20% of the dietary calories provided by the experimental oils, from d 5 through 17 of gestation, and caloric equivalence was controlled during the ethanol treatment. Tail blood samples were obtained on d 15 of gestation and analyzed for blood alcohol concentration using the ultraviolet NAD/NADH determination method. For the remainder of the study, the animals were fed chow supplemented with the oils (4 g oil/100 g Purina chow, 5001). Dietary supplementation of GLA commenced 3 wk prior to mating and continued throughout the study. Thus, the design of this study addresses the effects of long-term dietary supplementation with GLA on the effects of ethanol administered during gestation only. The control oil (LA) contained n-6 fatty acids (LA, linoleic acid, 18:2n-6) from safflower oil and n-3 fatty acids (α-linolenic acid, ALA, 18:3n-3) from ALA 60; the experimental oil (GLA) contained long-chain n-6 fatty acids (GLA, γ-linolenic acid, 18-3n-6) from GLA 70 in addition to LA and ALA; ALA 60 and GLA 70 are free fatty acid concentrates (Callanish Laboratories) containing 60% LA and 70% GLA, respectively. GLA constituted 34.5% of the fatty acids in the experimental oil and 16% in the supplemented chow. The outcomes that were measured included effects on reproduction and physical development of the pups, as well as brain fatty acid composition and behavior of the adult male pups. Eye-opening in the pups was assessed 12 d after birth. One male from each litter was assigned randomly to either the open-field/wheel-running condition (starting at 7 wk of age) or to the forced swimming test. Because the Porsolt test had not been validated previously on this mouse population, a standard dose-response curve was run on a separate group of animals, using five intraperitoneally administered DMI dosage conditions, 0, 3.75, 7.5, 15, and 30 mg/kg. After testing animals in the open field, activity in the running wheels was measured by recording cumulative automated activity counts twice daily for four consecutive days, at the beginning of the 12-h light and dark cycles. Brain tisssue was obtained from these animals following behavioral testing and analyzed for fatty acid composition, as described above. The primary use of the forced swimming test is to screen for clinically effective antidepressants, which reduce the amount of time the animals spend immobile during the test, i.e., not swimming or attempting to escape (74). In this study the question asked was whether GLA, alone or in combination with the tricyclic antidepressant, DMI, might yield a similar outcome. Animals in the treatment groups were tested twice, first with saline, then 1 wk later with 7.5mg/kg DMI.

Results and Discussion

Growth and Development. Ethanol reduced the number of viable litters and decreased adult weight. While the effect of GLA on reproductive outcome was not significant, it did reduce birth weight. Adult brain weight was reduced by the joint administration of GLA and ethanol. Thus, while there is little evidence that GLA offset the effects of ethanol, the combined effects of GLA and ethanol might be viewed with some concern, particularly in light of our previous findings. Admittedly, the levels of GLA administered in the liquid diets during gestation were extremely high (7% of dietary calories), but they nevertheless suggest caution in recommending the administration of GLA to offset the effects of ethanol.

Brain Fatty Acid Composition. The selected fatty acid composition (wt %) in brain phosphatidylethanolamine is shown in Fig. 18.2. Ethanol decreased 20- and 22-carbon fatty acids, and increased levels of 16:0; in a previous study in our laboratory, similar changes were seen 12 d after birth (75). Despite their statistical significance, the magnitude of these findings was small, and their functional significance remains to be determined. GLA increased levels of dihomo-γ-linolenic acid (DGLA, 20:3n-6), particularly in PE (56%), but had no effects on AA. However, effects of dietary n-6 were seen in increases in 22:4n-6 with both GLA and safflower oil relative to chow, particularly in PE. Conversely, GLA and safflower oil decreased DHA in PE. The GLA effect predominated in the group receiving ethanol, and levels of 22:5n-6 were also higher in this group. This replicates the commonly observed finding of an inverse reciprocity between levels of 22:6n-3 and 22:5n-6 in the brain (13). Thus, in this study, the combination of GLA and ethanol resulted in a group which might be described as slightly deficient in DHA (23% of brain phosphatidylethanolamine FA vs. 28% in laboratory chow control). This again may be cause for concern, given the possible functional role of DHA in brain and retina (6).

Activity. The effects on circadian wheel-running activity, as shown in Fig. 18.3, proved interesting. While no differences were seen in the open field, wheel-running was increased by GLA in the most active phase, the dark cycle. Conversely, activity seemed to be slightly decreased by GLA in the light cycle, but this should be interpreted with caution, due to the variability in the data. Given that DGLA is a precursor of PGE_1, this suggests that these changes in the animals fed GLA might be associated with increases in PGE_1 levels. Because no behavioral sedation was observed in the open field, these differences in circadian activity are consistent with the effects of prostaglandins on sleep-wake cycles (discussed above).

Antidepressant Activity. The response of the standard animals to DMI on the Porsolt test confirmed the reliability of the test in this population of mice. However,

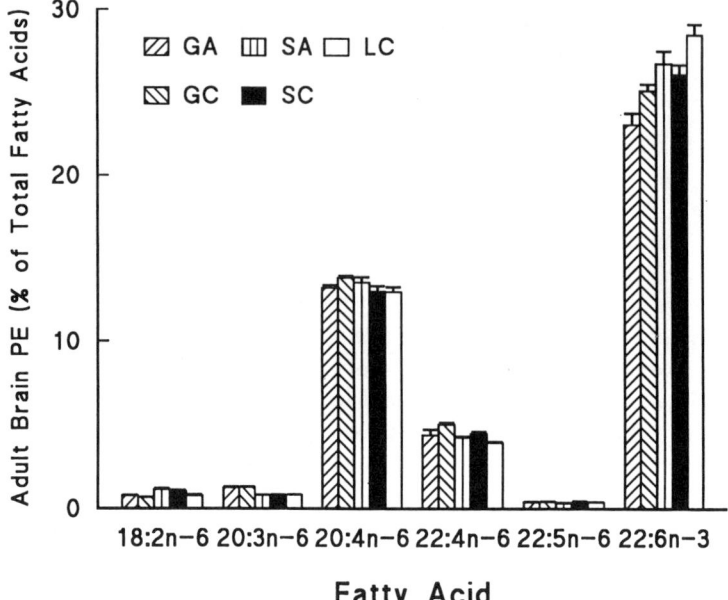

Fig. 18.2. Selected fatty acid composition of brain phosphatidylethanolamine of adult B6D2F$_2$ male mice treated with ethanol during gestation and fed diets supplemented with γ-linolenic acid. The chow group represents a reference group fed standard laboratory chow. GLA decreased 18:2n-6, and increased 20:3n-6 and 22:4n-6; it decreased 22:6n-3, particularly in combination with ETOH. ETOH decreased 18:2n-6, 22:4n-6, and 22:5n-6 ($P < 0.05$). *Source:* Ref. 64.

as shown in Figure 18.4, there were no effects of GLA or prenatal ethanol on this test, either alone, or in combination with DMI.

Summary

This chapter provides an overview of our work on the effects of dietary administration of GLA on brain fatty acid composition and behavior in mice, particularly in relation to prenatal exposure to ethanol. There was little evidence that GLA ameliorated the effects of ethanol on growth and development. On the contrary, the results suggest that the combined effects of GLA with prenatal ethanol treatment on reproductive performance may well be deleterious. This may, however, be related to the high levels of GLA used in the second study. Feeding of GLA in the diet was reflected in an increase in long-chain n-6 fatty acids in brain membrane phospholipids. No effects were seen on open-field activity, but there was an increase in circadian wheel-running activity, suggestive of modulation of sleep-wake cycles. There

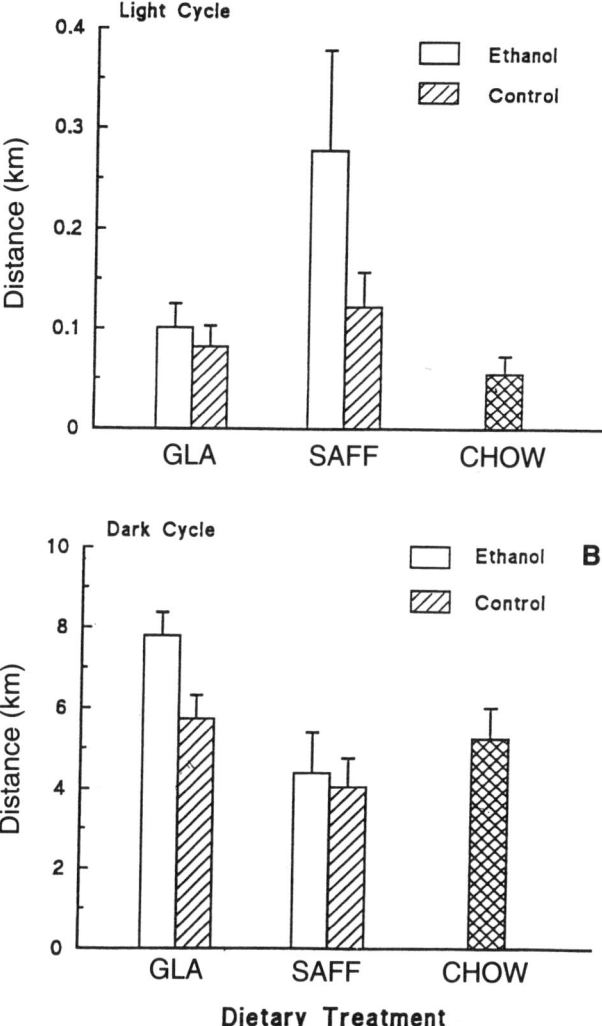

Fig. 18.3. Circadian running wheel activity of adult B6D2F$_2$ male mice treated with ethanol during gestation and fed diets supplemented with γ-linolenic acid. The chow group represents a reference group fed standard laboratory chow. GLA increased activity in the dark (active) phase (B) and decreased activity in the light (inactive) phase (A), ($P < 0.05$). (Note change of scale between light and dark.) Source: Ref. 64.

was no evidence of effects of chronic GLA treatment on swimming activity as measured in the Porsolt test, either alone or in combination with an antidepressant. These findings do not support the hypothesis that GLA will be an effective agent in the prevention of Fetal Alcohol Syndrome or in the treatment of affective disorders.

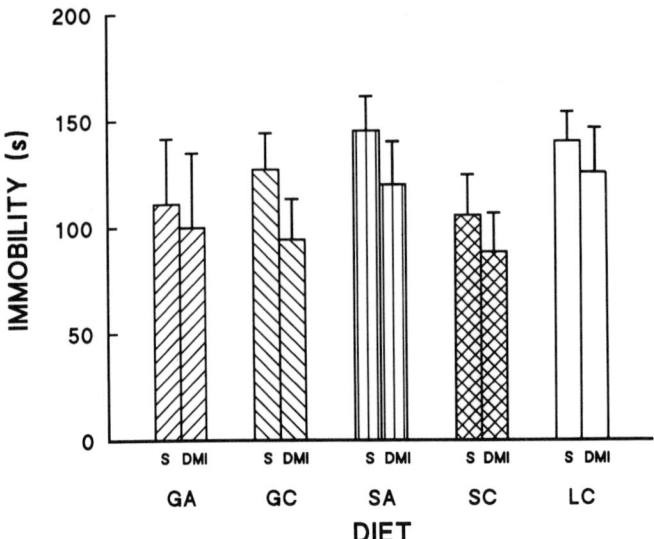

Fig. 18.4. Time spent immobile during the last 4 min of a 6-min forced swimming test in adult B6D2F$_2$ male mice treated with ethanol during gestation and fed diets supplemented with g-linolenic acid. Animals were tested twice, once after saline injection (control) and once after desmethylimipramine (DMI) 7.5mg/kg. The chow group represents a reference group fed standard laboratory chow. *Source:* Ref. 64.

Acknowledgments

The work described in this chapter was supported by a grant from the Natural Sciences and Engineering Research Council of Canada to P. Wainwright. During the conduct of the work, Y.-S. Huang was employed by Efamol Research Laboratories, Annapolis Valley, Nova Scotia, who also provided the experimental oils. The authors are grateful to Dr. R. Bell, Dr. G.R. Ward, and Dr. R. Cantrill for helpful comments on the manuscript.

References

1. Cook, H.W. Fatty Acid Desaturation and Chain Elongation in Eucaryotes (1991) in *Biochemistry of Lipids, Lipoproteins and Membranes,* Vance, D.E., and Vance, J., eds., Elsevier, Amsterdam, pp. 141–169.
2. Kinsella, J.E., Broughton, K.S., and Whelan, J.W. Dietary Unsaturated Fatty Acids: Interactions and Possible Needs in Relation to Eicosanoid Synthesis (1990) *J. Nutr. Biochem. 1,* 123–141.
3. Clandinin, M.T., Field, C.J., Hargreaves, K., Morson, L., and Zsigsmond, E. Role of Diet Fat in Subcellular Structure and Function (1985) *Can. J. Physiol. Pharmacol. 63,* 546–556.
4. Murphy, M. Dietary Fatty Acids and Membrane Protein Function (1990) *J. Nutr. Biochem. 1,* 68–79.

5. Burr, G.O., and Burr, M.M. On the Nature and Role of the Fatty Acids Essential in Nutrition (1930) *J. Biol. Chem.* 86, 587–621.
6. Neuringer, M. The Relationship of Fatty Acid Composition to Function in the Retina and Visual System (1992) in *Lipids, Learning and the Brain: Fats in Infant Formulas,* Dobbing, J., ed., Report of the 103rd Ross Conference on Pediatric Research, Ross Laboratories, Columbus, Ohio, pp. 134–163.
7. Uauy, R., Birch, D.G., Birch, E.E., Hoffman, D., and Tyson, J. Visual and Brain Development in Infants as a Function of Essential Fatty Acid Supply Provided by the Early Diet (1992) in *Lipids, Learning and the Brain: Fats in Infant Formulas,* Dobbing, J., ed., Report of the 103rd Ross Conference on Pediatric Research, Ross Laboratories, Columbus, Ohio, pp. 215–238.
8. Wainwright, P.E. Do Essential Fatty Acids Play a Role in Brain and Behavioral Development? (1992) *Neurosci. Biobehav. Rev.* 16, 193–205.
9. Gunstone, F.D. Gamma Linolenic Acid: Occurrence and Physical and Chemical Properties (1992) *Prog. Lipid Res.* 31, 145–161.
10. Willis, A.L., and Smith, D.L. Dihomo-Gamma-Linolenic and Gamma-Linolenic Acids in Health and Disease (1989) in *New Protective Roles for Selected Nutrients,* Spiller, G.A., and Scala, J., eds., Alan Liss Inc., New York, pp. 39–108.
11. Horrobin. D. F. Nutritional and Medical Importance of Gamma-Linolenic Acid (1992) *Prog. Lipid Res.* 31, 163–194.
12. Sastry, P. Lipids of Nervous Tissue: Composition and Metabolism (1985) *Prog. Lipid Res.* 24, 69–176.
13. Bourre J.M., Bonneil M., Chaudiere J., Clement M., Dumont O., Durand G., Lafont H., Nalbone G., Pascal G., and Piciotti M. Structural and Functional Importance of Dietary Polyunsaturated Fatty Acids in the Nervous System (1992) in *Neurobiology of Essential Fatty Acids,* Bazan, N.G., Murphy, M., and Toffano, G. eds., Plenum Press, New York, pp. 211–229.
14. Menon, N.K., and Dhopeshwarkar, G.A. Essential Fatty Acid Deficiency and Brain Development (1982) *Prog. Lipid Res.* 21, 309–326.
15. Tinoco, J. Dietary Requirements and Functions of Alpha-Linolenic Acid in Animals (1982) *Prog. Lipid Res.* 21, 1–45.
16. Innis, S.M. Essential Fatty Acids in Growth and Development (1991) *Prog. Lipid Res.* 30, 39–103.
17. Carlson, S. (1992) Lipid Requirements of Very-Low-Birth-Weight Infants for Optimal Growth and Development (1992) in *Lipids, Learning and the Brain: Fats in Infant Formulas,* Dobbing, J., ed., Report of the 103rd Ross Conference on Pediatric Research, Ross Laboratories, Columbus, Ohio, pp. 188–207.
18. Wainwright, P.E., Huang, Y.-S., Bulman-Fleming, B., Dalby, D., Mills, D.E., Redden, P., and McCutcheon, D. The Effects of Dietary n-3/n-6 Ratio on Brain Development in the Mouse: A Dose-Response Study with Long-Chain n-3 Fatty Acids (1992) *Lipids* 27, 98–103.
19. Huang, Y.-S., Wainwright, P.E., Redden, P.R., Mills, D.E., Bulman-Fleming, B., and Horrobin, D. Effect of Maternal Dietary Fats with Variable n-3:n-6 Ratios on Tissue Fatty Acid Composition in Suckling Mice (1992) *Lipids* 27, 104–110.
20. Huang, Y.-S., Wainwright, P.E., Mills, D.E., Lin, X., and Horrobin, D.F. Effects of Maternal Dietary n-3 and n-6 Fatty Acids (Pre- and Post- Delta-6 Desaturation) on Tissue Glycerophospholipid Fatty Acid Composition in Dams and Suckling Mice (1993) *Proc. Soc. Exp. Biol. Med.* 204, 54–64.

21. Smith, W.L., Borgeat, P., and Fitzpatrick, F.A. (1991) The Eicosanoids: Cycloxygenase, Lipoxygenase, and Epoxygenase Pathways in *Biochemistry of Lipids, Lipoproteins and Membranes,* Vance, D.E., and Vance, J., eds., Elsevier, Amsterdam, pp. 297–325.
22. Weber, P.C. (1988) Membrane Phospholipid Modification by Dietary n-3 Fatty Acids: Effects on Eicosanoid Formation and Cell Function in *Biological Membranes: Aberrations in Membrane Structure and Function,* Karnovsky, M.L., Leaf, A., and Bolls, L.C., eds., Alan R. Liss, New York, pp. 263–274.
23. Nassar, B.A., Manku, M.S., Huang. Y.-S., Jenkins, D.K., and Horrobin, D.F. The Influence of Dietary Marine Oil (Polepa) and Evening Primrose Oil (Efamol) on Prostaglandin Production by the Rat Mesenteric Vasculature (1987) *Prostaglandins Leukotrienes Med. 26,* 253–263.
24. Chapkin, R.S., Somers, S.D., and Erickson, K.L. Dietary Manipulation of Macrophage Phospholipid Classes: Selective Increase of Dihomogammalinolenic Acid (1988) *Lipids 23,* 766–770.
25. Chapkin, R.S., and Coble, K.J. Utilization of Gammalinolenic Acid by Mouse Perotoneal Macrophages (1991) *Biochim. Biophys. Acta 1085,* 365–370.
26, Brown, M.L., Marshall, L.A., and Johnston, P.V. Alterations in Cerebral and Microvascular Prostaglandin Synthesis by Manipulation of Dietary Essential Fatty Acids (1984) *J. Neurochem. 43,* 1392–1400.
27. Galli, C., Galli, G., Spagnuolo, C., Bosisio, E., Tosi, L., Folco, G.C., and Longiave, D. (1977) Dietary Essential Fatty Acids, Brain Polyunsaturated Fatty Acids, and Prostaglandin Biosynthesis in *Function and Biosynthesis of Lipids: Advances in Experimental Medicine and Biology,* vol. 88, Plenum Press, New York, pp. 561–573.
28. Vance, D. E. Phospholipid Metabolism and Cell Signalling in Eucaryotes (1991) in *Biochemistry of Lipids, Lipoproteins and Membranes,* Vance, D.E., and Vance, J., eds., Elsevier, Amsterdam, pp. 205–239.
29. Wolfe L.S, and Horrocks, L.A. Eicosanoids (1994) in *Basic Neurochemistry: Molecular, Cellular and Medical Aspects,* 5th Ed, Siegel, G.J., Agranoff, B.W., Albers, R.W., and Molinoff, P.B., eds., Raven Press, New York, pp. 475–490.
30. Templeton, W.W. Prostanoid Actions on Transmitter Release (1988) in *Prostaglandins: Biology and Chemistry of Prostaglandins and Related Eicosanoids,* Curtis-Prior, P.B., ed., Churchill Livingstone, Edinburgh, pp. 402–410.
31. Murphy, S., and Pearce, B. Eicosanoids in the CNS: Sources and Effects (1988) *Prostaglandins, Leukotrienes Essen. Fatty Acids: Reviews 31,* 165–170.
32. Kim, H.-Y., Sawazaki, S., and Salem, N., Jr., Lipoxygenation in Rat Brain? (1991) *Biochem. Biophys. Res. Commun. 174,* 729–734.
33. Piomelli, D., and Greengard, P. Lipoxygenase Metabolites of Arachidonic Acid in Neuronal Transmembrane Signalling (1990) *Trends Pharmacol. Sci. 11,* 367–373.
34. Simmet, T., and Peskar, B.A. Lipoxygenase Products of Polyunsaturated Fatty Acid Metabolism in the Central Nervous System: Biosynthesis and Putative Function (1990) *Pharmacol. Res. 22,* 667–682.
35. Chiu, E.K.Y, and Richardson, J.S. Behavioral and Neurochemical Aspects of Prostaglandins in Brain Function (1985) *Gen. Pharmacol. 16,* 163–175.
36. Rothwell, N.J. Eicosanoids: Thermogenesis and Thermoregulation (1992) *Prostaglandins, Leukotrienes Essen. Fatty Acids 46,* 1–7.
37. Hayaishi, O. Molecular Mechanisms of Sleep-Wake Regulation: Roles of Prostaglandins D_2 and E_2 (1991) *FASEB J. 5,* 2575–2581

38. Onoe H., Ueno, R., Fujita, I., Nishino, H., Oomura, Y., and Hayaishi, O. Prostaglandin D_2, a Cerebral Sleep-Inducing Substance in Monkeys (1988) *Proc. Natl. Acad. Sci. U.S.A. 5*, 4082–4086.
39. Mutsumura, H., Honda, K., Goh, Y., Ueno, R., Sakai, T., Inoue, S., and Hayaishi, O. Awaking Effect of Prostaglandin E_2 in Freely Moving Rats (1989) *Brain Res. 481*, 242–249.
40. Forstermann, U., Heldt R., and Hertting G. Effects of Intracerebroventricular Administration of Prostaglandin D_2 on Behavior, Blood Pressure and Body Temperature Compared to Prostaglandins E_2 and $F_{2\alpha}$ (1983) *Psychpharmacol. 80*, 365–370.
41. Poddubiuk, Z.M., and Kleinrok, Z. A Comparison of the Central Actions of Prostaglandins A_1, E_1, E_2, $F_{1\alpha}$, and $F_{2\alpha}$ in the Rat. II. The Effect of Intraventricular Prostaglandins on the Action of Some Drugs and on the Level and Turnover of Biogenic Amines in the Rat Brain (1976) *Psychopharmacology 50*, 95–102.
42. Poddubiuk, Z.M. A Comparison of the Central Actions of Prostaglandins A_1, E_1, E_2, $F_{1\alpha}$, and $F_{2\alpha}$ in the Rat. I. Behavioural, Antinociceptive and Anticonvulsant Actions of Intraventricular Prostaglandins in the Rat (1976) *Psychopharmacology 50*, 89–94.
43. Potts, W.J., East, P.F., Landry, D., and Dixon, J.P. The Effect of PGE_2 on Conditioned Avoidance Response Behavior and the Electroencephalogram (1973) *Adv. Biosci. 9*, 489–494.
44. Singer, P., Naumann, E., Hoffmann, P., *et al*. Attenuation of High Blood Pressure by Primrose Oil, Linseed Oil, and Sunflowerseed Oil in Spontaneously Hypertensive Rats (1984) *Biomed. Biochim. Acta 43*, S243–S246.
45. Mills, D.E., and Ward, R.P. Attenuation of Stress-induced Hypertension by Gamma Linolenic Acid in Rats (1984) *Proc. Soc. Exp. Biol. Med. 176*, 32–37.
46. Mills, D.E., and Ward, R.P. Effects of Essential Fatty Acid Administration on Cardiovascular Responses to Stress in Rats (1986) *Lipids 21*, 139–142.
47. Mills, D.E., and Ward, R.P. Effects of Eicosapentaenoic Acid on Cardiovascular Responses to Stress (1986) *Proc. Soc. Exp. Biol. Med. 182*, 127–131.
48. Mills, D.E., Prkachin, K.M., Harvey, K.A., and Ward, R.P. Dietary Fatty Acid Supplementation Alters Stress Reactivity and Performance in Man (1989) *J. Hum. Hypertens. 3*, 111–116.
49. Horrobin, D.F. Essential Fatty Acids, Prostaglandins, and Alcoholism: An Overview (1987) *Alcohol: Clin. Exp. Res. 11*, 2–9.
50. Anton, R.F., and Randall, C.L. Central Nervous System Prostaglandins and Ethanol (1987) *Alcohol: Clin. Exp. Res. 11*, 10–18.
51. Reitz, R.C. Dietary Fatty Acids and Alcohol: Effects on Cellular Membranes (1993) *Alcohol Alcoholism 28*, 59–71.
52. Salem, N., Jr., and Ward, G. The Effects of Ethanol on Polyunsaturated Fatty Acid Composition (1993) in *Alcohol, Cell Membranes and Signal Transduction in Brain*, Alling, C., and Sun, G., eds., Plenum Press, New York, pp. 33–46.
53. Alling, C., Becker, W., Jones, A.W., and Anggard, E. Effect of Chronic Ethanol Treatment on Lipid Composition and Prostaglandins in Rats Fed Essential Fatty Acid Deficient Diets (1984) *Alcohol: Clin. Exp. Res. 8*, 238–242.
54. Manku, M.S., Oka, M., and Horrobin, D.F. Differential Regulation of the Formation of Prostaglandins and Related Substances from Arachidonic Acid and from Dihomogammalinolenic Acid. I. Effects of Ethyl Alcohol (1979) *Prostaglandins Med. 3*, 119–128.

55. Rotrosen, J., Mandio, D., Segarnick, L., Traficante, L.J., and Gershon, S. Ethanol and Prostaglandin E_1: Biochemical and Behavioral Interactions (1980) *Life Sci. 26*, 1867–1876.
56. Segarnick, D.J., Mandio Cordasco, D., and Rotrosen, J. Biochemical and Behavioral Interactions between Prostaglandin E_1 and Alcohol (1983) in *Clinical Uses of Essential Fatty Acids*, Horrobin, D.F., ed., Eden Press, Montreal, pp. 175–189.
57. George, F.R., Jackson, S.J., and Collins, A.C. Prostaglandin Synthetase Inhibitors Antagonize the Sedative Hypnotic-Induced Hypothermia (1981) *Psychopharmacology 74*, 241–244.
58. George, F.R., and Collins, A.C. Prostaglandin Synthetase Inhibitors Antagonize the Depressant Effects of Ethanol (1979) *Pharmacol. Biochem. Behav. 10*, 865–869.
59. Ritz, M.C., George, F.R., and Collins, A.C. Indomethacin Antagonizes Ethanol-Induced but Not Pentobarbital-Induced Behavioral Activation (1981) *Subst. Alcohol Actions Misuse 2*, 289–299.
60. Horrobin, D.F, and Manku, M.S. Possible Role of Prostaglandin E_1 in the Affective Disorders and in Alcoholism (1980) *Br. Med. J. 280*, 1363–1366.
61. Horrobin, D. F. A Biochemical Basis for Alcoholism and Alcohol-induced Damage Including the Fetal Alcohol Syndrome and Cirrhosis: Interference with Essential Fatty Acid and Prostaglandin Metabolism (1980) *Med. Hypotheses 6*, 929–942.
62. Abel, E.L. (1984) *Fetal Alcohol Syndrome and Fetal Alcohol Effects*, Plenum Press, New York.
63. Wainwright, P.E., Ward, G.R., and Molnar, J.D. Gamma-Linolenic Acid Fails to Prevent the Effects of Prenatal Ethanol Exposure on Brain and Behavioral Development in $B6D2F_2$ Mice (1985) *Alcohol: Clin. Exp. Res. 9*, 377–383.
64. Wainwright, P.E., Huang, Y.-S., Lévesque, S., Mutsaers, L., McCutcheon, D., Balcaen, P., and Hammond, J. Effects of Dietary Gamma-Linolenic Acid and Prenatal Ethanol on Mouse Brain and Behavior (1996) *Pharmacol. Biochem. Behav. 54*, in press.
65. Duffy, O., Menez, J.-F., and Leonard, B.E. Effects of an Oil Enriched in Gamma-Linolenic Acid on Locomotor Activity and Behavior in the Morris Maze, Following in Utero Ethanol Exposure in Rats (1992) *Drug Alcohol Dep. 30*, 65–70.
66. Abbey, H., and Howard, E. Statistical Procedure in Developmental Studies on Species with Multiple Offspring (1973) *Dev. Psychobiol. 6*, 329–335.
67. Duffy, O., Ménez, J.F., and Leonard, B.E. Attenuation of the Effects of Chronic Ethanol Administration in the Brain Lipid Content of the Developing Rat by an Oil Enriched in Gamma Linolenic Acid (1992) *Drug Alcohol Depend. 31*, 85–89.
68. Scales, W.E., and Kluger, M.J. Effect of Antipyretic Drugs on Circadian Rhythm in Body Temperature of Rats (1987) *Am. J. Physiol. 253*, R306–R313.
69. Cooper, A.L., and Rothwell, N.J. Inhibition of the Thermogenic and Pyrogenic Responses to Interleukin-1-Beta in the Rat by Dietary n-3 Fatty Acid Supplementation (1993) *Prostaglandins Leukotrienes Essen. Fatty Acids 49*, 615–626.
70. Diagnostic and Statistical Manual of Mental Disorders (4th ed.), (1994) American Psychiatric Association, Washington, D.C.
71. Georgotis, A. Affective Disorders: Pharmacotherapy (1985) in *Comprehensive Textbook of Psychiatry/IV*, vol. 1, Kaplan, H.I., and Sadock, M.D., eds., Williams and Williams, Baltimore.
72. Stockert, M., Zieher, L.M., and Medina, J.H. Interactions of Phospholipids and Free Fatty Acids with Antidepressant Recognition Binding Sites in Rat Brain (1992) in *Neurobiology of Essential Fatty Acids*, Bazan, N., Murphy, M., and Toffano, G., eds., Plenum Press, New York, 325–330.

73. Porsolt, R.D., Bertin, A., and Jalfe, M. Behavioral Despair in Mice: A Primary Screening Test for Antidepressants (1977) *Arch. Int. Pharmacol. 229,* 327–336.
74. Wainwright, P.E., Huang, Y.-S., Simmons, V., Mills, D.E., Ward, R.P., Ward, G.R., Winfield, D., and McCutcheon, D. Effects of Prenatal Ethanol and Long-Chain n-3 Fatty Acid Supplementation on Development in Mice. 2. Fatty Acid Composition of Brain Membrane Phospholipids (1990) *Alcohol: Clin. Exp. Res. 14,* 413–420.

Chapter 19

γ-Linolenic Acid in Infant Formula

G.L. Crozier, M. Fleith, and M.-C. Secretin

Nestec Ltd. Research Centre, Vers-chez-les-Blanc, Post Office Box 44, CH 1000-Lausanne-26, Switzerland

There is evidence that the infant, especially the premature infant, may require dietary sources of preformed long-chain polyunsaturated fatty acids (LCPUFA) for optimal growth and development. One of these is arachidonic acid (AA, 20:4n-6). γ-Linolenic acid (GLA, 18:3n-6) is a metabolic precursor of this fatty acid and thus can serve as an indirect source of AA for the infant.

The Importance of Arachidonic Acid

Arachidonic acid plays important roles in cell structure and is a substrate for the synthesis of highly bioactive compounds such as prostaglandins and leukotrienes. It is therefore an important molecule in the regulation of communications between cells and thus of many physiological functions.

AA is a major component of all cell membranes. It is the major LCPUFA in most peripheral tissues (e.g., heart and liver) and is present in large amounts in nervous tissues. In brain tissue of many species, it is quantitatively the most important n-6 fatty acid present in phosphatidyl ethanolamine (1). The infant's brain grows rapidly in late gestation and during the first few years of life (2), and the accretion of AA is rapid. This accretion has been calculated at 18.8 mg/wk from 26 wks of gestation to term (3).

Metabolism of Arachidonic Acid

In the body, particularly in liver tissue, AA is synthesized from linoleic acid (LA, 18:2n-6) by sequential reactions involving three enzymes. First, the Δ6-desaturase inserts a double bond at the Δ6-position of the molecule to form GLA. An elongase then adds two carbons and the Δ5-desaturase inserts another double bond to form AA (Fig. 19.1). Of these enzymes, the desaturases are slower than the elongase, and the Δ6-desaturase has been shown to be the slowest and most limiting (4). GLA which by-passes the slow Δ6-desaturase step, is almost a direct precursor to AA and is therefore more easily transformed into AA than is LA. Work with stable isotope-labeled GLA in rats fed low-fat diets has demonstrated that GLA readily contributes to the pool of labeled arachidonic acid (5).

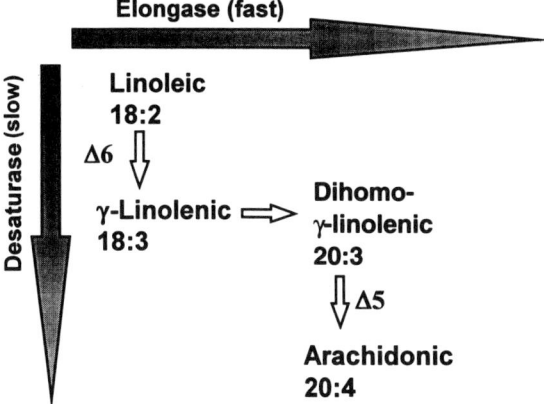

Fig. 19.1. Pathway of metabolism of n-6 fatty acids. The Δ6-desaturase is the slowest enzyme, followed by the Δ5-desaturase. Elongase activity is rapid.

The human neonate has the ability to synthesize arachidonic acid from precursor fatty acids (6). Poisson et al. demonstrated in liver tissue of infants who had died for reasons unrelated to liver disease that the relevant enzymes are active and thus the conversions can occur. Nevertheless it is not known whether this metabolism is fast enough to provide the infant with adequate supplies of AA. This is of particular concern when the infant is premature and in a more compromised developmental state.

Human milk, like other animal products, is a source of preformed AA. It contains low levels of AA in the range of 0.4–0.6 % of fatty acids (Table 19.1). This finding is consistent across many different populations and dietary groups (7). On the other hand, AA is not present in most infant formulas (8).

Carlson et al. (9) have shown that when premature infants are fed standard formula, AA in phosphatidyl choline of red blood cells drops significantly over 28 d. Other authors (10–14) have confirmed this finding in plasma phospholipids.

TABLE 19.1 Partial Fatty Acid Composition of Human Milk from Several Countries and Groups

Country/Group	Linoleic	α-Linolenic	AA	DHA
North America	14.2	0.9	0.5	0.2
Australia	10.8	0.6	0.4	0.3
Sweden	12.9	0.7	0.4	0.3
Sweden	12.9	0.7	0.4	0.3
United Kingdom	8.7	0.8	0.4	0.4
West Germany	10.4	0.8	0.4	0.2
Vegetarians	24.4	1.7	0.5	0.2
Inuit	10.1	0.5	0.6	2.4

Source: British Nutrition Foundation (7).

Eicosapentaenoic Acid-Rich Oils Increase the Requirement for Arachidonic Acid

There is now strong evidence that the premature infant requires a dietary source of another LCPUFA, docosahexaenoic acid (DHA, 22:6n-3). DHA is found in high levels in brain and retina and is important for optimal neural function. If preterm infants are fed standard infant formula, DHA decreases significantly in plasma phospholipids, red blood cell phospholipids (11-14) and even in brain tissue (15). Experiments in which formulas containing DHA have been fed to premature infants have shown successful normalization of this fatty acid in blood cells and plasma (16,17). These supplemented formulas have also been shown to improve retinal function as assessed by electroretinogram (16). Most of these studies have used formulas supplemented with fish oil rich in eicosapentaenoic acid (EPA, 20:5n-3) as a source of DHA. Feeding these fish oils has been shown to result in increased EPA and decreased AA in plasma and red blood cells (13). This response is proportional to the length of time of feeding and there is a dose effect (17). Functionally, these two changes have been associated with significantly diminished growth rates of premature infants (18).

Nutritional Recommendations

Results from these experiments and others have led to the recommendation that dietary sources of both AA and DHA be included in premature infant formulas. The European Society for Pediatric Gastroenterology and Nutrition (ESPGAN) recommends that formulas destined for low birth weight infants contain metabolites of linoleic acid not exceeding 2% of total fatty acids (19). The British Nutrition Foundation suggests that the long-chain fatty acids in infant formula should approximate the levels in human milk (7).

Sources of Arachidonic Acid

Preformed arachidonic acid is found in animal sources such as human milk, egg yolk, and offal. In addition, there are microalgae which can synthesize oils enriched in AA. Offal, such as brain and other internal organs, is not acceptable for use in infant feeding and, until now, use of the microalgal oils has not been considered acceptable by most health authorities. Lecithin, derived from egg yolk, is a valued source of AA because eggs are widely consumed as a food source. However, if lecithin is the sole source of arachidonic acid in infant formula, the phosphate levels are higher than believed desirable. In addition, unless highly purified, lecithin may be contaminated with residual ovalbumin which is a strong allergen. Therefore, egg lecithin is appropriate for use only after extensive purification.

GLA-containing oils, when supplemented in infant formula, can be considered as aids to the baby's own metabolism for synthesizing its own arachidonic acid. In term infants, formula supplemented with GLA alone has been shown to increase serum cholesteryl arachidonate to levels which are higher than those that occur with unsupplemented formula and which are more similar to levels found in human milk fed infants (20). Because AA is a highly bioactive fatty acid, it may even be safer to permit the baby's body to make its own decisions in this way about the appropriate level of AA required.

γ-Linolenic Acid-Containing Formulas in Europe: Results of Clinical Studies

In Europe, several companies are producing infant formulas that are enriched in LCPUFA, including GLA (Table 19.2). In these formulas, the content of GLA ranges from 0.2–0.9% of total fatty acids. The Nestle formula is based on a mixture of three different sources of the essential fatty acids: high DHA /low EPA fish oil, blackcurrant seed oil and highly purified egg yolk lecithin. The content of GLA is moderate, approximately 0.4% of fatty acids. Results of several clinical trials in preterm infants fed the LCPUFA formula have shown no differences in DHA nor AA levels in the plasma phospholipids and red blood cells when compared with the group of infants fed human milk (Fig. 19.2).

Conclusions

There is evidence that the premature infant may need a source of n-6 LCPUFA for optimal growth and health. This appears to be particularly true if the infant is fed a source of fish oil. GLA has been shown to be an effective precursor of AA in studies with stable isotopes. In clinical studies with preterm babies, GLA-supplemented formula supported plasma and red blood cell AA status. GLA-supplemented formulas are being used in Europe. They have demonstrated safety, and have been shown to be effective in supporting the essential fatty acid status of the premature infant.

TABLE 19.2 GLA-Supplemented Formulas for Low Birthweight Infants in Europe

Company	n-6	n-3	Source
Nestle	GLA	0.5% DHA	Blackcurrant seed oil
	AA	0.1% EPA	Egg lecithin
			High DHA fish oil
Cow and Gate	GLA	0.3% DHA	Borage oil
		0.1% EPA	Fish oil
Friesche Flag	0.35% GLA	0.3% DHA	Borage oil
		0.2% EPA	Fish oil
Farley	0.9% GLA	0.5% DHA	Borage oil
		0.1% EPA	Fish oil
Milupa	0.2% GLA	0.2% DHA	Evening primrose oil
	0.4% AA		Egg lipid

Source: B. Koletzko (21).

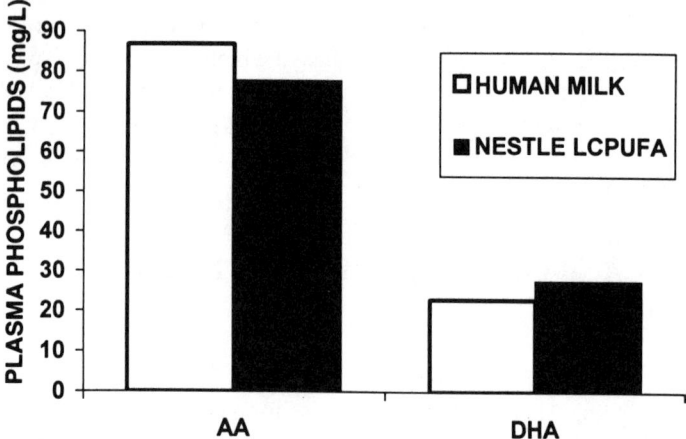

Fig. 19.2. Arachidonic acid and docosahexaenoic acid composition of plasma phospholipids in premature infants fed the formula supplemented with long-chain polyunsaturated fatty acids compared with infants fed human milk. There were no differences.
Source: B. Koletzko (in preparation).

References

1. Crawford, M.A., Doyle, W., Drury, P., Lennon, A., Costeloe, K., and Leighfield, M. n-6 and n-3 Fatty Acids During Early Human Development (1989) *J. Int. Med. 225*, 159–169.
2. Martinez, M. Tissue Levels of Polyunsaturated Fatty Acids During Early Human Development (1992) *J. Pediatr. 120*, S129–S138.
3. Clandinin, M.T., Chappell, J.E., Leong, S., Heim, T., Swyer, P.R., and Chance, G.W. Intrauterine Fatty Acid Accretion Rates in Human Brain: Implications for Fatty Acid Requirements (1980) *Early Human Dev. 4*, 121–129.
4. Hassam, A.G., Sinclair, A.J., and Crawford, M.A. The Incorporation of Orally Fed Radioactive γ-Linolenic Acid and Linoleic Acid into Liver and Brain Lipids of Suckling Rats (1975) *Lipids 10*, 417–420.
5. Sprecher, H., Luthria, D., Geiger, M., Mohammed, B.S., and Reinhart, M. Intercellular Communication in Fatty Acid Metabolism (1994) in *Fatty Acids and Lipids: Biological Aspects.* World Rev. Nutr. Diet. (Galli, C., Simopoulos, A.P., Tremoli, E., eds.), vol. 75, 1–7.
6. Poisson, J.-P., Dupuy, R.-P., Sarda, P., Descomps, B., Narce, M., Rieu, D., and Crastes de Paulet, A. Evidence That Liver Microsomes of Human Neonates Desaturate Essential Fatty Acids (1993) *Biochim. Biophys. Acta 1167*, 109–113.
7. British Nutrition Foundation (1992) *Unsaturated Fatty Acids: Nutritional and Physiological Significance.* Chapman and Hall, London.
8. Koletzko, B., and Bremer, H.J. Fat Content and Fatty Acid Composition of Infant Formulas (1989) *Acta Paediatr. Scand. 78*, 513–521.
9. Carlson, S.E., Rhodes, P.G., and Ferguson, M.G. Docosahexaenoic Acid Status of Preterm Infants at Birth and Following Feeding with Human Milk or Formula (1986) *Am. J. Clin. Nutr. 44*, 798–804.

10. Koletzko, B., Schmidt, E., Bremer, H.J., Haug, M., and Harzer, G. Effects of Dietary Long Chain Polyunsaturated Fatty Acids on the Essential Fatty Acid Status of Premature Infants (1989) *Eur. J. Pediatr. 148,* 669–675.
11. Koletzko, B. Long Chain Polyunsaturated Fatty Acids in the Diets of Premature Infants (1992) in *Polyunsaturated Fatty Acids in Human Nutrition,* Bracco, U., and Deckelbaum, R.J., eds., Nestle Nutrition Workshop Series, vol. 28, Raven Press Ltd., New York.
12. Pita, M.L., Giron, M.D., Perez-Ayala, M., Delucci, C., Martinez Valverde, A., and Gil, A. Effects of Postnatal Age and Diet on the Fatty Acid Composition of Plasma Lipid Fraction in Preterm Infants (1989) *Clin. Physiol. Biochem. 7,* 238–48.
13. Carlson, S.E., Cooke, R.J., Peeples, J.M., Werkman, S.H., and Tolley, E.A. Longterm Feeding of Formulas High in Linolenic Acid and Marine Oil to Very Low Birth Weight Infants: Phospholipid Fatty Acids (1991) *Pediatr. Res. 30,* 404–412.
14. Luukainen, P., Salo, M.K., Janas, M., and Nikkari, T. Fatty Acid Composition of Plasma and Red Blood Cell Phospholipids in Preterm Infants from 2 Weeks to 6 Months Postpartum (1995) *J. Ped. Gastroent. Nutr. 20,* 310–315.
15. Farquharson, J., Cockburn, F., Patrick, W.A., Jamieson, E.C., and Logan, R.W. Infant Cerebral Cortex Phospholipid Fatty Acid Composition and Diet (1992) *Lancet 340,* 810–813.
16. Uauy, R., Birch, D.G., Birch, E.E., Tyson, J.E., and Hoffman, D.R. Effect of Dietary Omega 3 Fatty Acids on Retinal Function of Very Low Birthweight Neonates (1990) *Pediatr. Res. 28,* 485–492.
17. Carlson, S., Cooke, R.J., Werkman, S.H., and Tolley, E.A. First Year Growth of Preterm Infants Fed Standard Compared to Marine Oil n-3 Supplemented Formula (1992) *Lipids 27,* 901–907.
18. Carlson, S.E., Werkman, S.H., Peeples, J.M., Cooke, R.J., and Toolley, E.A. Arachidonic Acid Status Correlates with First Year Growth in Preterm Infants (1993) *Proc. Natl. Acad. Sci. U.S.A. 90,* 1073–1077.
19. ESPGAN Committee on Nutrition. Comment on the Content and Composition of Lipids in Infant Formulas (1991) *Acta. Paediatr. Scand. 80,* 887–896.
20. Van Biervliet, J.-P., Vinaimont, N., Vercaemst, R., and Rosseneu, M. Serum Cholesterol, Cholesteryl Ester, and High Density Lipoprotein Development in Newborn Infants: Response to Formulas Supplemented with Cholesterol and γ-Linolenic Acid (1992) *J. Pediatr. 120,* S101–S208.
21. Koletzko, B. Long-Chain Polyunsaturated Fatty Acids in Infant Formulas in Europe (1995) *ISSFAL Newsletter 2,* 3–5.

Chapter 20

γ-Linolenic Acid Biosynthesis and Chain Elongation in Fasting and Diabetes Mellitus

Jean-Pierre Poisson,[a] Michel Narce,[a] Yung-Sheng Huang,[b] and David Mills[c]

[a]Unité de Nutrition Cellulaire et Métabolique, Université de Bourgogne, Faculté des Sciences Mirande, B.P. 1381, 21004 Dijon Cedex, France
[b]Ross Products, Abbott Laboratories, Cleveland Avenue, Columbus, OH 43215
[c]Scientific Laboratory Division, P.O. Box 4700, Albuquerque, NM 87196

Introduction

Long-chain polyunsaturated fatty acids (LC-PUFAs) are vital components of mammalian cells, providing an important store of energy and also playing a leading role in membrane structure and function. Genetically induced diabetes in humans and animals or experimentally induced diabetes in animals is associated with a variety of derangements manifested by defects in the utilization of carbohydrates, the synthesis and catabolism of proteins, and the metabolism of lipids, as well as by acid-base disturbances. Administration of appropriate doses of insulin generally restores these metabolic functions to within normal limits. In diabetes, essential fatty acid (EFA) metabolism is disrupted, and this is superimposed on all of the complex abnormalities of carbohydrate and lipid metabolism characteristic of the disease. Research on lipid metabolism in diabetes has provided a wealth of information on changes in fatty acid (FA) composition and metabolism as well as the importance of insulin in these processes.

The FA composition of membranes and whole organs is dependent on desaturation/chain elongation. Furthermore, factors that alter desaturation and elongation, e.g., fasting and diabetes, also affect FA composition. However, it is not clear that one necessarily sees a similar change in enzyme activity and FA composition simultaneously. Changes in desaturase/elongase activities are only two factors governing membrane or tissue FA composition.

This review addresses the relation between γ-linolenic acid (18:3n-6; GLA) biosynthesis and chain elongation and fasting and diabetes as influenced by factors such as glucagon and insulin.

Desaturation/Chain Elongation

While some LC-PUFAs can be synthesized *de novo* in animals, others have to be obtained from plant sources. Linoleic acid (18:2n-6; LA) originates from the diet, i.e., it must be ingested and then converted endogenously by the animal to longer-chain fatty acids with higher unsaturation such as GLA and then to other substances. Thus LA might be regarded in a sense as an analogue to a provitamin (1). All of the PUFAs derived from LA constitute the "n-6" EFAs, based on the position of their double bond, starting from the methyl end of the chain. Biosynthesis of 18:3n-6, which has been extensively studied in rat liver, is controlled by a $\Delta 6$-desaturation. For LA to exert its full range of biological activity, it must be metabolized to other substances. Thus, $\Delta 6$-desaturation plays a crucial role in ensuring the normal function of animals. It is followed by chain elongation to dihomo-γ-linolenic acid (20:3n-6; DGLA) that takes place in the microsomal fraction of the cell (2). $\Delta 6$-desaturation is the rate-limiting step in the biosynthesis of polyunsaturated fatty acids (PUFAs) of the n-6 series. $\Delta 6$-desaturase requires ATP and acts on acyl-CoA esters under aerobic conditions (3); it is the integral protein of the microsomal membrane and receives reducing equivalents from NADH via the NADH-cytochrome c reductase system (4) or from NADPH through cytochrome P450 reductase and cytochrome b_5 (5). LA and GLA have an indispensable structural function as integral parts of biomembrane phospholipids (PL) that cannot be entirely fulfilled by unsaturated fatty acids of another type (6). In addition to its structural function, DGLA can give rise to a short-lived eicosanoid metabolite, PGE_1 (7).

Fatty acid chain elongation, which has been detected in microsomal fractions from several mammalian organs and extensively studied in liver and brain, proceeds by incorporation of malonyl-CoA into acyl-CoA chains. The liver endoplasmic reticulum elongates FAs in four reaction steps: (1) the initial reaction involves the condensation of an activated fatty acid (acyl CoA) with malonyl-CoA to form 13-ketoacyl CoA; this reaction is catalyzed by the condensing enzyme; (2) NAD(P)H-dependent reduction of the 13-ketoacyl CoA to the secondary alcohol by the 13-ketoacyl CoA reductase; (3) dehydratation of the secondary alcohol to *trans*-2-enoyl CoA by 13-hydroxyacyl CoA dehydrase; and (4) NAD(P)H-dependent reduction of the *trans*-2-enoyl CoA catalyzed by the enoyl CoA reductase to form the elongated product. In the first reduction step, there was evidence of the involvement of cytochrome b5 and NADPH-cytochrome c reductase in the transfer of reducing equivalents to the 13-ketoacyl CoA reductase (5). It is assumed that the malonyl-CoA-dependent condensation step is rate limiting of overall elongation activity of long-chain acyl-CoA (8). With unsaturated FAs, the rate of elongation is more rapid than the rate of desaturation, especially if the first double bond is between carbons 6 and 7, as in GLA. Hence, there are usually low levels of elongase substrates in most organs, indicating that the elongation reaction is not the rate-limiting step. The physiological regulation of the elongation system has not been extensively studied (4).

It should also be mentioned that LA, instead of being desaturated first by the $\Delta 6$-desaturase, may also first be elongated to the corresponding 20-carbon unsaturated acid. This acid may then be desaturated by a $\Delta 5$-desaturase, producing a fatty acid that, as far as is known, can be further desaturated only in rat testes ($\Delta 8$-desaturase) (4).

The $\Delta 6$-desaturase is specifically distributed in animals (protista, protozoan, fish, birds and mammals such as rat, mouse, rabbit, guinea pig, dog and human) but absent in bacteria and insects, and rather lacking or scarcely active in mollusks. It is also specifically localized, present in many tissues (liver, adrenals, testes, brain, kidney, and heart) but not in all (lung, adipose tissue, and probably prostate gland) (4). Its presence in mammals is not ubiquitous, and its activity varies broadly with the kind of tissue and species considered. Strictly carnivorous animals such as cat and lion have little or no Δ6-desaturase activity, and LA has correspondingly little EFA activity; GLA, by-passing the Δ6-desaturation step, is an effective EFA in the cat (9).

In addition to chain desaturation and elongation reactions involved in LA transformation in animals, retroconversion may play a role in the conversion of unsaturated FAs to acids of shorter chain length. Oxidative degradation, produced by mitochondria and peroxisomes of ingested FAs, may also play an important role in the selection of tissue FAs. Because FAs are esterified primarily to lipid molecules, the existence, activity and specificity of FA esterification and hydrolyzing reactions also play a noticeable role in determining the final composition of tissues (4,10).

The possibility that inadequate GLA biosynthesis and/or chain elongation may play a role in some animal diseases, including human diseases, as opposed to normal development, will now be discussed in relation to fasting and diabetes mellitus.

Fasting

Fasting involves an imbalance between caloric availability and requirement. It appears to have effects similar to those of experimental diabetes on enzyme synthesis and several aspects of lipid metabolism—including desaturation and elongation. The major stimulus for these changes is an absolute or relative deficiency of insulin, but exogenous factors such as diet also play a role (2,10).

Several studies have demonstrated that fasting decreases Δ6-desaturation. Liver microsomal desaturation of LA is largely recovered by simply refeeding animals for 12 h with 10% glucose in the drinking water after starvation for 48 h. Furthermore, refeeding rats a 50% solution of glucose after a 96-h fast evoked a significant increase in the linoleic acid-1-^{14}C conversion rate that reached a maximum at 12 h; this maximum value was the same as that of the control rats (11). A long-term administration of glucose to fasted animals produced a significant decrease in the Δ6-desaturation of LA to GLA: after 12 h, the desaturation rate decreased abruptly; thus, 48 h after refeeding, the conversion of LA to GLA was only 50% of the control value (12). The transient increase has been interpreted as the effect of insulin secretion followed by active glycolysis (13).

Under the same conditions, a 12-h casein refeeding evoked a 50% increase in the LA desaturating capacity compared with the controls and remained constant for the following 36 h (11). Further, it is important to add that the activation of LA desaturation evoked by dietary casein is maintained, in spite of the fasting of the animals during 24 h, and only then does the conversion begin to decrease (11). It is definitively confirmed that a high protein diet produces stimulation of LA desaturation to GLA not only in normal but also in fasted rats (11). These results agree with the work of Inkpen et al. (14), who studied the Δ6-desaturation of α-linolenic acid (18:3n-3; ALA) and found that when casein was the only source of calories in the diet the conversion of ALA to octadecatetraenoic acid (18:4n-3) was also stimulated compared with the nonfasted state. Therefore, dietary protein would be a key factor in the cellular control mechanism for EFA desaturation (11). Fasting and refeeding evoke their deactivation-activation effects upon the microsomal desaturase enzyme system itself and not upon a cytosolic protein factor (15). Fasting depresses the activity of microsomal chain elongation; the reaction is reactivated when feeding commences (16).

Based on the different fasting periods, it was observed that LA increased in total lipids of fasted HTC cells as well as in microsomes of fasted rats (17). De Alaniz et al. (17) suggested that the relative increase of LA could be responsible for the increased $\Delta 5$-desaturation of DGLA that led to the increased synthesis of arachidonic acid (20:4n-6; AA), thus avoiding the accumulation of intermediate acids.

Glucagon, Insulin, and Chemically-Induced Diabetes

Glucagon

Glucagon is antagonistic to insulin, which is clearly seen by its inhibition of $\Delta 6$-desaturation in rat liver microsomal preparations: administration of glucagon to rats *in vivo* reduced the liver microsomal $\Delta 6$-desaturase activity; the addition of glucagon to isolated liver cells markedly reduced the conversion of LA to AA, suggesting an inhibitory effect on $\Delta 6$-desaturase (18,19).

Glucagon also prevents the refeeding-induced activation of $\Delta 6$-desaturation in previously fasted rats (20). The mechanism of the glucagon inhibitory effect is thought to occur through stimulation of adenyl cyclase and increased intracellular cyclic AMP because dibutyryl cyclic AMP induces the same effect as glucagon (21). The effects of glucagon on FA composition are not known.

Insulin

Insulin, among other hormonal factors, has been extensively studied in this model. Although diabetes causes increased energy expenditure and increased appetite, reducing food availability to diabetics actually reduces the diabetes-induced changes in LA and AA composition. Hence, it is clearly important to distinguish the roles of food intake and diabetes itself on changes in both desaturation/elongation and FA composition.

Linoleic Acid $\Delta 6$-Desaturation

Lyman (22) reported that Stetten and Boxer were the first to point out an impaired synthesis of LC-PUFAs in the alloxan-diabetic rat. It was then reported that diabetic animals required much more LA than did normal animals. Subsequent studies have clearly shown that PUFA synthesis is severely depressed in alloxan-diabetes and that the defect is reversible by administration of insulin (22). Because LA exerts most of its biological effects by being converted to GLA and beyond, this means that in diabetes the proportion of biologically effective dietary LA is reduced. The need for an increased intake is therefore not surprising.

The fatty acid composition of plasma and liver PL and triglycerides (TG) of lean diabetic rats has a higher content of PUFAs, especially LA (22–26). In addition to altered LA content, abundant evidence also exists for altered LA metabolism in experimental diabetes. Decreased incorporation of [1-^{14}C]acetate into PUFAs suggests an impairment of AA synthesis in the epididymal fat pad of alloxan-diabetic rats, leading to an accumulation of LA (27). However, multiple metabolic pathways from acetate metabolism make it difficult to interpret these results.

Evidence then became available from several sources to support the hypothesis that insulin induces or enhances the desaturation of many PUFAs including LA *in vivo* (28): after 48 h, insulin corrects partial inhibition of linoleic acid Δ6-desaturation induced by alloxan-diabetes (29). Mercuri et al. (30) have shown that the desaturation of LA to GLA is significantly depressed in liver microsomes from alloxan-diabetic rats; further, it has also been shown that insulin increases glycolytic activity.

Therefore, because either dietary protein or insulin enhances LA conversion to GLA, a new series of experiments were carried out to investigate both effects simultaneously. Not only do insulin administration and protein feeding not show a nonadditive effect, but insulin appears to be acting as an antagonist of the protein-induced stimulation of LA desaturation in the normal rat (11). According to Peluffo et al. (11), restoration of LA desaturation to normal values is not proportional to insulin dose; hypoglycemic injection of insulin does not increase the Δ6-desaturation in the alloxan-diabetic rat. Casein administration without insulin treatment also restored LA desaturation to a normal level, and this value was not statistically different than those obtained by the simultaneous administration of protein and insulin. Although LA desaturation was restored by either insulin or protein administration, no significant additive effect was demonstrated. The defect in this instance appeared localized at the terminal desaturase protein and was corrected by the treatment of the animals with insulin (30, 31).

Friedman et al. (28) also showed decreased desaturation in liver and lung of alloxan-diabetic rats. However, liver AA levels were unchanged in this study. Furthermore, incorporation of radiolabeled LA into liver and lung was decreased in the diabetic group. Thus, LA oxidation may be increased in diabetes affecting its availability for desaturation.

Eck et al. (25) showed that at least 24 h of insulin treatment, given a dose sufficient to transiently lower blood glucose, is required to correct the defect in linoleic acid Δ6-desaturase activity of streptozotocin-diabetic rats. Faas and Carter (32) brought to light a "super" repair of the Δ6-desaturation. The 17 h required to normalize desaturation after insulin was given to diabetic rats (25) is consistent with a reported peak in desaturase activity (33) and is also attributable to an effect on synthesis of terminal desaturase protein, rather than to an effect on the prior components of the microsomal electron transport system which is responsible for FA desaturation (25). The effect is apparently caused by enzyme induction, because inhibitors of protein synthesis impair the recovery of enzyme activity produced by insulin injection (2,4,10,11,13,23,27,28,31,34). However, insulin does not increase Δ6-desaturase activity when injected into nondiabetic animals (33,35); in fact, it promoted a small increase in linoleate desaturation 3 hours after the injection (34).

Fatty Acid Composition

Although the findings have not been uniform, it has been generally concluded that alterations in FA composition may be at least partly attributable to the impairment of fatty acid desaturation (26–28,31). The interpretation of these experiments has been made difficult by the presence of factors others than diabetes and by the failure to study specific subcellular components, whose composition varies considerably (36).

Some of the previous studies have been carried out in animals fed diets deficient in EFAs (26,28,36,37), which normally accelerate FA desaturation (13). If the dietary supply of LA is limited, e.g., by dietary deficiency, AA cannot be adequately synthesized due to the lack of substrate. However, oleic acid (18:1n-9) is synthesized in abundance, and its longer-chain product, eicosatrienoic acid (20:3n-9), is also synthesized from oleic acid. Because streptozotocin- or alloxan-induced diabetes impairs Δ6-desaturation, diabetes actually lowers the 20:3n-9/20:4n-6 ratio in PL of the LA-deficient rat liver despite decreasing the AA/LA ratio. Thus, a low 20:3n-9/20:4n-6 ratio of this tissue PL is not a reliable index of adequate LA intake or normal synthesis of AA in diabetes (38).

Mercuri et al. (39) observed a decrease in AA and an increase in LA content in the fatty acid composition of the total liver lipids of alloxan-diabetic rats after 2 wk of alloxan injection, an effect consistent with impaired Δ6-desaturase activity. Comparing the distribution of the fatty acids in liver PL of normal and diabetic rats fed a normal or EFA-deficient diet, Friedman et al. (28) reported a similar fatty acid composition whatever the diet. In both rat testes and epididymal fat, Brenner et al. (31) found a significant increase in the percentage of LA and a decrease in the AA/LA ratio in the tissues of diabetic rats compared with controls.

The major alterations in liver microsomal fatty acid composition found in streptozotocin-diabetic rats were decreased proportions of AA and increased proportions of LA (32), probably related to, but not necessarily resulting from, impaired Δ6-desaturase activity. A decrease in LA following insulin injection was consistent with the marked stimulation of Δ6-desaturation; however, the expected increase in AA did not occur (32,40). These changes were present in phosphatidylethanolamine (PE), with very little change in FA composition in the phosphatidylserine (PS)/phosphatidylinositol (PI) fraction (40).

In short-term streptozotocin-diabetic rats, the FA composition of red blood cells and plasma cholesterol esters (CE) and PL were altered similarly to that previously found in the diabetic liver but remained unchanged in platelet and aorta PL (41). However, in long-term diabetes, the PL fatty acid composition of the platelet and aorta became significantly altered, i.e., an increase in LA and DGLA and a decrease in AA occurred. Insulin treatment of the diabetic rats decreased the levels of LA in platelet and aorta lipids, suggesting an overcorrection of diminished Δ6-desaturation, compared with the nondiabetic controls. In platelet-poor plasma from streptozotocin-diabetic rats, Dang et al. (42) evidenced a significant increase of free LA and DGLA, when AA was decreased and LA increased in erythrocytes PL. Insulin treatment of the diabetic rats resulted in normalization of AA and LA levels in erythrocytes PL. The incorporation of AA into diabetic erythrocytes PL was significantly decreased, but not specific for arachidonate, because the incorporation of other LC-PUFAs such as DGLA and LA was also decreased comparably. More important, the decreased incorporations were reversed by insulin treatment of the diabetic rat. Okumura et al. (43) showed that the percentage of AA 1,2-diacylglycerol (DAG) in isolated thoracic aortas of streptozotocin-diabetic rats is decreased, when compared with age-matched controls; such alteration was inhibited by insulin treatment.

In total PL of liver, plasma, and heart of steptozotocin-diabetic rats, the main FA differences compared with controls are an increased proportion of LA and DGLA and a decreased proportion of AA (38,44). This was confirmed in the myocardium of alloxan-diabetic rats by Chattopadhyay et al. (45). However, in several tissues, AA is not significantly changed in the diabetic rats. On the contrary, an increase in the proportion of AA and a reduction in the proportion of LA were observed in the skin of diabetic rats (44).

The higher levels of LA and lower levels of AA observed in adipose tissue of streptozotocin-induced diabetic rats, consistent with altered Δ6-desaturase activity, may alter the total body pool of available FAs for the synthesis of other lipids such as PL (46,47).

Alloxan- and streptozotocin-diabetic Sprague-Dawley rats showed a consistent reduction of AA content in PC and PE in whole renal cortex plasma membranes purified from renal cortex, and in isolated glomeruli. Associated with this fall was a rise in LA. Insulin therapy returned the fatty acid profile to normal. These results are similar to patterns observed in other diabetic tissues and suggest that diabetes is associated with generalized changes in cell membranes (48). Examination of LC-PUFAs of kidney cortex TG revealed that LA fell in hyperglycemic nonacidotic, ketoacidotic and insulin-treated normoglycemic streptozotocin rats (49).

The major alterations in pancreas phospholipid-fatty acid composition of streptozotocin-induced diabetic rats were characterized by an increase of linoleate coupled with a decrease of arachidonate, suggesting defective metabolism of linoleate. This was further supported by fatty acid ratios that suggested low desaturation. Daily administration of insulin restored and overcorrected the various fatty acid alterations (50).

Studies carried out on the adrenal gland of streptozotocin-diabetic rats have shown an important inhibition in polyenoic fatty acid biosynthesis, the Δ6 n-6 desaturation being depressed in the insulin-deprived animals and partially restored after insulin injections. This effect could result from direct action by the hormone because the restoration was reproduced when AA biosynthesis was measured after insulin was added to the incubation medium of adrenocortical cells isolated from diabetic animals (51).

A substantial decrease in the proportion of AA and increase in the relative content of LA occurred in the phosphoglycerides of visceral tissues from diabetic animals when, in contrast, only a small rise in the percentage of LA was detected in PC, PE, ethanolamine plasmalogen, PI and PS from brain or nerve. The differences which developed as a result of diabetes were completely prevented if animals were maintained continuously on insulin commencing shortly after administration of streptozotocin (52).

These studies of alloxan- or streptozotocin-induced diabetes in the rat clearly show that insulin deficiency is associated with impaired Δ6-desaturation. What is not clear is the extent to which impaired desaturation is reflected by appropriate changes in FA composition, e.g., increased LA/AA. Some composition data are consistent with the desaturation data, some are not. Therefore, it seems that different models, different degrees of insulin depletion, and different organs are affected differently in experimental diabetes. In addition, the degree of LA that may be required for oxidation in diabetes could also affect its availability for desaturation and its depletion from tissues relative to AA (28). This is especially evident when the quantitative whole-body losses of PUFAs from the diabetic rat are calculated because these losses are accounted for mainly by lower LA and little quantitative change in AA (44).

In view of some of the inconsistencies we have reviewed here in streptozotocin- or alloxan-induced diabetes with respect to changes in fatty acid composition compared with changes in desaturase data, it may be worth bearing in mind that these diabetes-inducing agents may alter tissue fatty acid composition through effects not initially or directly related to desaturation, e.g., LA oxidation, acyl exchange, or PL synthesis. Because diabetic rats have an increased energy requirement that is responded to in part by LA oxidation leading to whole-body LA depletion (28,44,46), this may directly affect microsomal lipid composition, thereby impairing desaturation. The time course of these effects on desaturation and microsomal lipid composition may be different, which might then account for apparent inconsistencies in fatty acid compositional and desaturase data when only one data point is collected.

Genetic Diabetes

The Bio-Breeding (BB) genetically diabetic Wistar rat is a well-characterized spontaneous model of insulin-dependent diabetes, with destructive insulitis resembling the lesions described in human type I diabetes (53).

We have shown (53) that liver microsomal Δ6-desaturase activity is unchanged compared with the controls in 21-wk-old female BB-diabetic rats, killed 20 h after insulin injection while still hyperglycemic, 28 d after the onset of the disease. However, LA levels in hepatic microsomes of BB-diabetic rats were increased compared with control rats, whereas AA was decreased. Thus, the altered liver FA composition of the BB-diabetic rats was inconsistent with apparently normal desaturase activity in the same animals. The daily treatment with insulin may explain why Δ6-desaturase activity of BB-diabetic rats was not different than control rats but it does not explain why the LA/AA ratio was increased. The experimental conditions for insulin injections were sufficient to normalize desaturase activity in the BB-diabetic rats and required similar amounts of insulin and time treatment as for chemical diabetes (35). Insulin has been shown to stimulate FA desaturation, probably via an effect on enzyme protein synthesis (25). On the other hand, a decrease in the level of desaturation through insulin-deficiency-induced glycolysis has also been reported (39). The activation of acyl-CoA desaturase by soluble proteins has been reported (15,54). We are inclined to attribute these opposing effects of diabetes and insulin to their effects on such protein factors. In BB-diabetic rats, the amount of FAs in liver microsomal total lipids suggests an inhibition of Δ6-desaturation, but this is inconsistent with the measured desaturase activities, e.g., the decreased ratio of AA to LA would have suggested a decreased synthesis of AA.

Mimouni and Poisson (55,56) have shown that Δ6-desaturase activity was defective in BB-diabetic rats during the hyper- and normoglycemic periods that followed insulin injection. Correction of the enzyme activity occurred rapidly and completely, either 3 h after the insulin injection [1 IU insulin/(100 g body weight·d)] to BB-diabetic rats that had not received insulin during the previous 48 h, or when the BB-diabetic rats received insulin twice a day, for 2 d, at a dose of 1 IU/100 g body weight. The restoration was not paralleled by reduced glycemia, e.g., the desaturase activities had normalized when the BB-diabetic rats were still hypoglycemic but decreased when they were normoglycemic. Inhibition of the desaturase activity increased from the normo- to the hyperglycemic period (56).

Few significant differences from controls have been apparent in the FA composition of liver total lipids and PL (55–57). During the hyper- and normoglycemic periods, but not during the hypoglycemic period, LA of BB-diabetic rat liver PL increased while AA decreased, which is consistent with previously reported results on streptozotocin- and alloxan-diabetes (38) and also consistent with defective Δ6-desaturation. Insulin treatment of BB-diabetic rats was sufficient to maintain a relatively normal FA composition of liver microsomal total lipids. However, this was not consistent with the altered desaturase activity at the different periods of glycemia. The decreased AA/LA ratio after insulin treatment suggested decreased synthesis of AA compensated for by an increased synthesis following the insulin-deficient state, consistent with impaired Δ6-desaturase activity. As discussed with respect to alloxan- or streptozotocin-induced diabetes, the poor agreement between the effect of a change in glycemia (induced by different quantities of insulin injected or by a different time period from the last insulin injection) on microsomal or whole liver lipids and Δ6-desaturase activity implies that they are not closely linked in a direct cause–effect relationship (10).

EFA deprivation reduced the frequency of diabetes in both diabetes-prone and diabetes-resistant BB rats. This protective effect was strongly associated with depletion of n-6 fatty acids, particularly AA, but not with accumulation of the abnormal 20:3n-9, which is considered a sign of EFA deficiency. Conjecturally, AA and/or a metabolite may play a role in mediating inflammatory injury in this animal model of autoimmune diabetes (58).

γ-Linolenic Acid Chain Elongation

Acetyl-CoA carboxylase, and thereby malonyl-CoA biosynthesis and fatty acid chain elongation, are stimulated by insulin (27). Streptozotocin-induced diabetic rats have decreased linoleoyl-CoA chain elongation activity, which is not influenced by administration of insulin (59).

Poisson et al. (60) demonstrated that with GLA as the radioactive precursor, alloxan-diabetes causes a decreased synthesis of AA in the liver, kidney and whole rat, leading to the hypothesis that diabetes also causes a decrease in GLA elongation in rats. In streptozotocin-diabetic rats that received the same tracer dose of ^{14}C GLA by stomach tube, the ^{14}C radioactivity incorporated into AA was considerably lower compared with control rats (61,62).

Suneja et al. (63) reported that hepatic microsomal chain elongation of γ-linolenoyl-CoA was decreased in streptozotocin-diabetic rats and was not restored following insulin administration to these rats. Mimouni et al. reported a decreased hepatic microsomal fatty acid chain elongation of γ-linolenoyl-CoA in the diabetic Wistar BB rat, compared with the nondiabetic Wistar BB rat (64). This decline is noted in diabetic Wistar BB rats during both hyper- and normoglycemic states. During the hypoglycemic period, a high insulin dose (1 IU/100 g body weight twice a day for 2 d) restores the diminished γ-linolenoyl-CoA elongation to normal, supporting the nonparallel relationship between the chain elongation system and the glycemia.

The fatty acid composition of liver microsomal total lipids is only partially consistent with changes in elongase activity at the different periods of glycemia, probably because factors other than elongation impairments were involved in the evolution of FA composition, but is in agreement with previously reported data on the evolution of Δ6-desaturase activity (55).

Effects of Dietary Linoleic and γ-Linolenic Acids on γ-Linolenic Acid Biosynthesis and Elongation

Feeding a high polyunsaturated to saturated fatty acid (P/S) ratio to diabetic animals increased adipocyte plasma membrane LA content and prevented the decrease observed in the AA content of membrane PL. The high P/S diet was associated with increased insulin binding in nondiabetic animals but did not change the amount of insulin bound by cells from diabetic animals. Diet-induced alterations in membrane composition may provide a mechanism for improving the cellular response to insulin in cells from diabetic animals (47).

Streptozotocin-diabetic rats fed 11% evening primrose oil (EPO; rich in LA and GLA) or safflower oil (SO; rich in LA) for 38 wk showed a clear beneficial effect on proteinuria, glomerular sclerosis, and tubular abnormalities compared with rats fed a beef tallow (rich in saturated FAs) diet. The high LA diets also increased the ratio of renal cortical production of 6-keto-$PGF_{1\alpha}$ to thromboxane B_2 (TXB_2), the stable metabolites of PGI_2 and TXA_2, respectively. They did not induce significant changes in plasma lipid composition. Barcelli et al. (65) concluded that diets rich in LA are protective in this model of diabetic nephropathy. The effect may be secondary to modifications of the eicosanoid balance.

T-Lymphocytes play a central role in the initiation, regulation and effector functions of immune responses. Altered immune response in the diabetic state may be attributed in part to diabetes-induced alterations in the metabolism of EFA. Feeding streptozotocin-induced diabetic rats a diet low in LA was found by Singh et al. (66) to lower LA in the membrane PL of T cells. Levels of AA were altered as a result of diabetes and diet composition. It was concluded that diabetes results in significant alterations in T cell membrane composition and function in a manner that can be manipulated by modifications of the FA composition of the diet, DGLA and AA being the precursors of PGs which are known to influence immune response.

The possibility that an increased requirement for EFAs is an important factor in the development of diabetic complications has been tested by Patterson (67) and confirmed by other investigators (68,69): diabetic cataract in rats could be completely prevented by raising the LA content of the diet.

Ikeda et al. (70) showed that in normal rats fed a diet containing perilla oil (rich in α-linolenic acid; ALA; 18:3n-3), the LA desaturation index in liver microsomal PL was significantly higher in casein (CAS)-fed animals than in a soybean protein (SOY)-fed group, whereas it was reversed in streptozotocin-diabetic rats. The proportion of AA increased in diabetic rats, in particular those fed SOY. The ratio of aortic prostacyclin production to platelet TXA_2 production decreased only in diabetic rats fed SOY. Thus dietary protein modified the PUFA composition and eicosanoid balance differently even in the diabetic rat.

An alternative approach to LA-enriched diets, which might be successful because of the much lower amounts required to achieve a response, would be to supplement the diet with GLA directly. Because EFAs and their metabolites are exceptionally important in both the structure and function of nerves, its seems possible that diabetic nerve damage (neuropathy) might be particularly responsive to this approach (1). A range of animal experiments provided interesting results. In streptozotocin-diabetic rats receiving a 5-wk dietary supplementation of GLA alone, the cutaneous nerve conduction velocity (sural and sciatic nerves) increased by 5–7%, which was significantly faster than in those without EFA supplementation (71). There was no effect on blood glucose, thus the effect could not be attributed to improved diabetic control. Tomlinson et al. (72) and Cameron et al. (73) obtained similar results, with LA having no effect.

Arachidonic acid in plasma PL seems to be kept constant, regardless of the presence of diabetes of the NIDDM Type, whereas in aorta PL, arachidonic acid was reduced; this may be compensated by GLA supplementation, which may lead to an increase of DGLA and AA levels (74). Nevertheless, LA, GLA, and DGLA were less active than AA in promoting insulin release from intact or permeabilized rat pancreatic islets, indicating a structure-function relationship (75).

Diabetes in Humans and γ-Linolenic Acid Biosynthesis and Chain Elongation

In humans, diabetes mellitus is characterized by the level of dependence on exogenous insulin, e.g., insulin dependent or insulin independent. In humans, direct evidence of impaired conversion of LA to GLA and/or of GLA to DGLA is difficult to obtain for ethical reasons. However, there is much indirect evidence. As in the animal models, data from human diabetes suggest that desaturation of LA is quite sensitive to insulin status without fatty acid composition necessarily being affected. Diabetics appear to have an abnormality of EFA and prostanoid metabolism that may lead to an increased requirement for the fatty acids such as LA that are dietarily essential. However, these fatty acids may not be metabolized normally in diabetes, e.g., increased LA oxidation may occur as observed in streptozotocin-induced diabetes (28,44,46). Studies with close control of energy metabolism and assessement of LC-PUFA oxidation in human diabetes should provide the link between these apparently inconsistent data.

The pattern of changes of fatty acid composition of amniotic fluid lecithin is essentially the same in pregnancies complicated by diabetes as in nondiabetic controls in the 34th–39th wk of pregnancy (76). High concentrations of PUFAs in milk of a diabetic mother on d 3–7 postpartum suggest increased chain elongation, with diabetes producing changes in lipid metabolism in the mammary gland that alter the milk composition (77).

Studies on FA composition of both types of diabetes have yielded inconsistent data: some suggest that LA/AA is increased in plasma lipids (78–81), but others have found no such effect (82,83). Nevertheless, LA concentrations are almost always normal or slightly above normal in diabetic patients, whereas the concentrations of LA metabolites are consistently below normal. When diabetics are treated with continuous subcutaneous insulin therapy, the concentrations of the major LA metabolites rise significantly (79,80). The main problem of the management of diabetes is the development of long-term damage to the retina, kidneys, cardiovascular system, and peripheral nerves. Although there are many hypotheses, none has found universal acceptance and treatment is generally unsatisfactory. Good control of blood glucose may be beneficial, but many well-controlled diabetics develop severe complications whereas some poorly controlled diabetics do not (1).

Different data have been reported concerning modifications of the erythrocyte lipid composition in the different types of diabetes. The heterogeneity of diabetes could be a cause for such differences. Analysis of the plasma and erythrocyte FA composition of poorly controlled insulin-dependent diabetic patients revealed a low level of GLA and DGLA; improvement of diabetic control, achieved by treatment with continuous subcutaneous insulin, infusion coincided with an increase of AA (84). Schimke et al. (85) showed that in long-term IDDM patients (about 40 y), the percentage of AA in both serum CE and PL was decreased in comparison with control subjects, indicating a disturbed FA metabolism. Taylor et al. (86) also observed a significant decrease in AA and AA/LA ratio in erythrocytes from IDDM subjects, compared with controls.

Ruiz-Gutierrez et al. (87), win a study of the FA composition of erythrocyte membrane PL in IDDM patients, evidenced a marked decrease in the total amount of PUFAs, mainly at the expense of AA, and related to sodium transport systems and to poor metabolic control of either diet or the diabetic state, being responsible for these observed cell membrane abnormalities. The LA content of serum TG, CE, and PL and of red cells and platelets was elevated in insulin-dependent diabetic women with IDDM, in proportion to their dietary linoleate intake. However, the serum lipid content of AA was decreased in IDDM patients, but was normal or increased in their cell membranes. These results suggest that desaturation and elongation of LA are decreased in women with IDDM (88). Insulin deficiency and high blood sugar in diabetic children may disturb the supply of DGLA from LA, decreasing PG formation in series 1, with altered PG metabolism possibly being responsible for the occurrence and progression of vascular complications in these children (89). Levels of DGLA and AA in serum lipids decreased in association with increased plasma levels of PGE_2 and $PGF_{2\alpha}$ in patients with IDDM.

Platelet function, estimated from B-thromboglobulin (B-TG), is frequently altered in IDDM patients: the plasma B-TG correlated negatively with the percentage of LA in plama lipids, but no correlation was found between B-TG and the percentages of GLA, DGLA, and AA (90).

A significant inverse correlation between LA and AA occurred in normal subjects but was not seen in Type I and Type II diabetics, suggesting that a functional impairment of platelet $\Delta 6$- and/or $\Delta 5$-desaturase may occur in diabetes which disrupts the normal equilibrium between LA and AA (91). Nevertheless, IDDM platelets may have a specific defect of PGE_1 synthesis, quite distinct from the $\Delta 6$-desaturase defects, which may contribute to platelet hyperaggregability in diabetes (83). Myrup et al. (92) found a raised content of AA in platelets from IDDM patients with retinopathy, without differences in platelet aggregation; platelet aggregability was not related to platelet fatty acid composition. Variations in levels of nonesterified FAs in plasma might interfere with platelet aggregation.

Before insulin treatment, but less strongly during it, the content of LA, DGLA, and AA and the AA/LA ratios of plasma and erythrocyte membrane lipids suggest that the conversion of LA to prostanoid precursor fatty acids is affected by a poor glycemic control in Type II diabetic patients (93). Dobrev et al. (94) found a decrease of AA and an increase of LA in the serum and in the HDL of decompensates NIDDM patients, suggesting that the contents of HDL depend on the serum FAs playing a role in the complex mechanism of vascular lesions in diabetes mellitus. Salomaa et al. (95) evidenced that the proportion of LA was lower in serum CE of NIDDM subjects than in the subjects with impaired glucose tolerance (IGT) or normal glucose tolerance (NGT). The proportions of GLA, DGLA, and AA were highest in diabetic patients and lowest in NGT subjects. These authors concluded that both serum insulin and blood glucose concentrations probably have an effect on the elongation and desaturation of FAs, but that the metabolism of LA to PG precursors seems to be different in different types of diabetes, with NIDDM patients showing no abnormalities.

Because platelet abnormalities are linked with vascular disease and diabetes has a high incidence of vascular complications, the fatty acid composition in platelet PL of NIDDM patients was investigated by Morita et al. (96). AA levels increased significantly in diabetes mellitus, compared with age-matched control subjects and were disproportionately high compared with those in plasma total lipids. The AA uptake activity of platelets is significantly higher in diabetic patients with proliferative retinopathy than in those with little or no background retinopathy, in addition, there were no significant differences between control and diabetic subjects in the uptake activity of platelets for LA (74).

Attempts to overcome impaired desaturation by giving large amounts of dietary LA or by by-passing the blocked $\Delta 6$-desaturase by giving longer-chain metabolites such as GLA have provided clinically positive results (78).

Piper et al. (97) reported a case of symptomatic EFA deficiency in a free-living individual with Type I diabetes mellitus, without chronic complications. Biochemical studies revealed abnormally low levels of LA and AA. Treatment with LA supplementation in the diet corrected the FA profile.

Poorly controlled patients with low levels of LA in CE had a significantly greater frequency of retinopathy than well-controlled patients or patients with similarly unsatisfactory control but higher levels of LA, suggesting that LA might protect against diabetic retinopathy (98). Kinsell et al. (99), followed by King et al. (100) and Houtsmuller et al. (101) reported that increased LA could reverse the development of diabetic retinopathy, with large amounts of LA (30–50 g) being required for this effect. But, because many patients find the diets unpalatable and compliance is poor, high LA diets are not often recommended to such patients. A pilot placebo-controlled study indicated that the retinopathy may also respond to GLA (102).

A lowering effect of GLA on serum TG, cholesterol and plasma B-TG occurs with daily intake of only 2 g. Both continuous subcutaneous insulin infusion and optimized conventional insulin therapy were followed by a significant increase of arachidonate in plasma lipids of IDDM patients (103). The changes in fatty acid composition of serum lipids suggest that a GLA intake of 2 g may exert its beneficial effect through an increased incorporation of long-chain PUFAs (104).

In addition to their usual diet, Type I diabetic men and male control subjects took 20 g/d EPO (14.45 g/d LA and 1.73 g/d GLA). At the start, diabetic patients had more LA and less GLA, DGLA, and AA in plasma, erythrocytes, and/or platelets. Futhermore, they had a lower AA/DGLA ratio and a higher DGLA/GLA ratio. In both groups, the 1-wk oil intake changed the fatty acid profiles. Most markedly, DGLA increased, whereas the DGLA/GLA and AA/DGLA ratios decreased. Arachidonic acid increased in control subjects, but not in diabetic patients. Erythrocytes and platelets responded differently in their fatty acid profiles (105). At the end of a 2-mo intake of a GLA mixture (3 g/d) given to IDDM patients, favorable changes of HDL-cholesterol and platelet adhesiveness were observed, when no change was found in the control group (106).

After daily administration of 4 capsules of EPO (45 mg GLA plus 360 mg LA) for 4 mo to children with IDDM, the serum DGLA levels increased and the plasma PGE2 levels decreased significantly, when neither fatty acid nor PGE_2 or $PGF_{2\alpha}$ levels were altered by daily administration of 2 EPO capsules. This suggested that the altered EFA and PG metabolism in diabetes may be reversed by direct GLA supplementation (107).

Diabetic patients with distal diabetic polyneuropathy, who received 360 mg/d GLA as EPO for 6 mo, improved all of their tested clinical and neurophysiological variables; the placebo group remained more or less unchanged or deteriorated (108). In another 12-mo experiment, 13 of the 16 variables were statistically significant between the active and placebo treatments (109). Thus there can be no doubt that the neuropathy of diabetes can be both prevented and reversed by the administration of GLA (1).

Conclusions

Substantial evidence, from both animals and humans, indicates that LC-PUFA metabolism is abnormal in diabetes and leads to impaired formation of fatty acids dependent on Δ6-desaturation as well as on chain elongation. Because the control of membrane lipid composition is multifactorial, factors other than changes in desaturation-elongation, e.g., membrane lipid degradation and synthesis, fatty acid oxidation, PG synthesis, and altered hormonal status, may all be important in determining both fatty acid composition and desaturase/elongase activity. The influence of age, sex, duration of disease, diet, and/or fatty acids associated with insulin treatment, as well as type and duration of insulin administration, may also influence fatty acid metabolism during diabetes and insulin therapy. Further work is necessary to understand the insulin-dependent control of the biosynthesis and chain elongation of GLA. Extensive ongoing animal and clinical studies should allow definitive descriptions of the roles of linoleic acid Δ6-desaturation and of GLA elongation to emerge in future years. Because diabetes is a heterogeneous group of diseases, the effects of LA and GLA must be considered and addressed separately for patients with IDDM, NIDDM, and possibly other forms of diabetes. By-passing the rate-limiting step by using GLA may have further desirable effects. The direct measurement of actual enzyme levels by specific antibodies raised against the enzyme proteins also offers promising results. Such studies are necessary to elucidate the mechanisms controlling microsomal desaturation and chain elongation and their dependence vs. the effect on the fatty acid composition of the membranes surrounding the enzymes.

References

1. Horrobin, D.F. Fatty Acid Metabolism in Health and Disease: The Role of Δ6-Desaturase (1993) *Am. J. Clin. Nutr. 57 (Suppl.)*, 732S–737S.
2. Poisson, J.-P. Essential Fatty Acid Metabolism in Diabetes (1989) *Nutrition 5*, 263–266.
3. Nugteren, D.H. Conversion in Vitro of Linoleic Acid into Gamma-Linolenic Acid by Rat-Liver Enzymes (1962) *Biochim. Biophys. Acta 60*, 656–657.
4. Brenner, R.R. (1989) in *The Role of Fats in Human Nutrition*, Vergroesen, A.J., and Crawford, M., eds., Academic Press, London, pp. 45–79.
5. Laguna, J.C., Nagi, M.N., Cook, L., and Cinti, D.L. Action of Ebselen on Rat Hepatic Microsomal Enzyme-Catalyzed Fatty Acid Chain Elongation, Desaturations and Drug Biotransformation (1989) *Arch. Biochem. Biophys. 269*, 272–283.
6. Houtsmuller, U.M.T. (1975) in *The Role of Fats in Human Nutrition*, Vergroesen, A.J., ed., Academic Press, London, pp. 231–302.
7. Van Dorp, D.A., Beerthuis, R.K., and Nugteren, D.H. The Biosynthesis of Prostaglandins (1964) *Biochim. Biophys. Acta 90*, 204–207.
8. Yoshida, S., and Takeshita, M. Comparison Between Condensation and Overall Chain Elongation of Arachidonyl-CoA and Arachidonoyl-CoA in Swine Cerebral Microsomes (1987) *Arch. Biochem. Biophys. 254*, 180–187.
9. Frankel, T.L., and Rivers, J.P.W. The Nutritional and Metabolic Impact of Gamma-Linolenic Acid on Cats Deprived of Animal Lipid (1978) *Br. J. Nutr. 39*, 227–231.
10. Poisson, J.-P., and Cunnane, S.C. Long-Chain Fatty Acid Metabolism in Fasting and Diabetes: Relation Between Altered Desaturase Activity and Fatty Acid Composition (1991) *J. Nutr. Biochem. 2*, 60–70.
11. Peluffo, R.O., De Gomez Dumm, I.N.T., De Alaniz, M.J.T., and Brenner, R.R. Effect of Protein and Insulin on Linoleic Acid Desaturation of Normal and Diabetic Rats (1971) *J. Nutr. 101*, 1075–1084.

12. De Gomez Dumm, I.N.T., De Alaniz, M.J.T., and Brenner, R.R. Effect of Diet on Linoleic Acid Desaturation and Some Enzymes of Carbohydrate Metabolism (1970) *J. Lipid Res. 11,* 96–101.
13. Brenner, R.R. The Oxidative Desaturation of Unsaturated Fatty Acids in Animals (1974) *Mol. Cell. Biochem. 3,* 41–52.
14. Inkpen, C.A., Harris, R.R., Forrest, W., and Quackenbush, F.Q. Differential Responses to Fasting and Subsequent Feeding by Microsomal Systems of Rat Liver: $\Delta 6$ and $\Delta 9$ Desaturation of Fatty Acids (1969) *J. Lipid Res. 10,* 277–282.
15. Nervi, A.M., Catala, A., Brenner, R.R., and Peluffo, R.O. Dietary and Hormonal Effects upon the Activity of "Soluble" Protein and Particulate Fraction of Fatty Acid Desaturation System of Rat Liver Microsomes (1975) *Lipids 10,* 348–352.
16. Donaldson, W.E., Wit-Peeters, E.M., and Scholte, H.R. Fatty Acid Synthesis in Rat Liver: Relative Contribution of the Mitochondrial, Microsomal and Non-Particulate Systems (1970) *Biochim. Biophys. Acta 202,* 35–42.
17. De Alaniz, M.J.T., De Gomez Dumm, I.N.T., and Brenner, R.R. Effect of Fasting on $\Delta 5$-Desaturation Activity in Rat Liver Microsomes and HTC Cells (1980) *Mol. Cell. Biochem. 33,* 165–170.
18. De Gomez Dumm, I.N.T., De Alaniz, M.J.T., and Brenner, R.R. Effects of Glucagon and Dibutyryl Adenosine 3′, 5′-Cyclic Monophosphate on Oxidative Desaturation of Fatty Acids in the Rat (1975) *J. Lipid Res. 16,* 264–268.
19. De Gomez Dumm, I.N.T., De Alaniz, M.J.T., and Brenner, R.R. Comparative Effect of Glucagon, Dibutyryl Cyclic AMP, and Epinephrine on the Desaturation and Elongation of Linoleic Acid by Rat Liver Microsomes (1976) *Lipids 11,* 833–836.
20 Brenner, R.R. Nutritional and Hormonal Factors Influencing Desaturation of Essential Fatty Acids (1984) *Prog. Lipid Res. 23,* 41–47.
21. Brenner, R.R. (1977) in *Function and Biosynthesis of Lipids,* Bazan, N.G., Brenner, R.R., and Giusto, N.M., eds., Plenum Press, New York, pp. 85–101.
22. Lyman, R.L. (1971) in *Progress in the Chemistry of Fats and Other Lipids,* Holman, R.T., ed., Pergamon Press, Oxford, pp. 193–230.
23. Gellhorn, A., and Benjamin, W. The Effect of Insulin on Monounsaturated Fatty Acid Synthesis in Diabetic Rats. The Stability of the Informational RNA and of the Enzyme System Concerned with Fatty Acid Desaturation (1966) *Biochim. Biophys. Acta 116,* 460–466.
24. Mercuri, O., and De Tomas, M.E. (1977) in *Function and Biosynthesis of Lipids,* Bazan, N.G., Brenner, R.R., and Giusto, N.M., eds., Plenum Press, New York, pp. 75–83.
25. Eck, M.G., Wynn, J.O., Carter, W.J., and Fass, F.H. Fatty Acid Desaturation in Experimental Diabetes Mellitus (1979) *Diabetes 28,* 479–485.
26. Worcester, N.A., Bruckdorfer, K.R., Hallinan, T., Wilkins, A.J., Mann. J.A., and Yudkin, J. The Influence of Diet and Diabetes on Stearoyl Coenzyme A Desaturase (EC 1. 14. 99. 5) Activity and Fatty Acid Composition in Rat Tissues (1979) *Br. J. Nutr. 41,* 239–252.
27. Gellhorn, A., and Benjamin, W. Insulin Action in Alloxan Diabetes Modified by Actinomycin D (1964) *Science 146,* 1166–1168.
28. Friedmann, N., Gellhorn, A., and Benjamin, W. Synthesis of Arachidonic Acid from Linoleic Acid *in Vivo* in Diabetic Rats (1966) *Israel J. Med. Sci. 2,* 677–682.
29. Lee, T.C., Baker, R.C., Stephens, N., and Snyder, F. Evidence for Participation of Cytochrome B5 in Microsomal D6-Desaturation of Fatty Acids (1977) *Biochim. Biophys. Acta 489,* 25–31.

30. Mercuri, O., Peluffo, R.O., and Brenner, R.R. Depression of Microsomal Desaturation of Linoleic to Gamma-Linolenic Acid in the Alloxan-Diabetic Rat (1966) *Biochim. Biophys. Acta 116*, 409–411.
31. Brenner, R.R., Peluffo, R.O., Mercuri, O., and Restelli, M.A. Effect of Arachidonic Acid in the Alloxan-Diabetic Rat (1968) *Am. J. Physiol. 215*, 63–70.
32. Faas, F.H., and Carter, W.J. Altered Fatty Acid Desaturation and Microsomal Fatty Acid Composition in the Streptozotocin Diabetic Rat (1980) *Lipids 15*, 953–961.
33. Oshino, N., and Sato, R. The Dietary Control of the Microsomal Stearyl-CoA Desaturation Enzyme System in the Rat Liver (1972) *Arch. Biochem. Biophys. 149*, 369–377.
34. De Gomez Dumm, I.N.T., De Alaniz, M.J.T., and Brenner, R.R. Effect of Insulin on the Oxidative Desaturation of Fatty Acids in Non-Diabetic Rats and in Isolated Liver Cells (1985) *Acta Physiol. Pharmacol. Latinoam. 35*, 327–335.
35. Poisson, J.-P. Comparative *in Vivo* and *in Vitro* Study of the Influence of Experimental Diabetes on Rat Liver Linoleic Acid $\Delta 6$- and $\Delta 5$-Desaturation (1985) *Enzyme 34*, 1–14.
36. Colbeau, A., Nachbaur, J., and Vignais, P.M. Enzymic Characterization and Lipid Composition of Rat Liver Subcellular Membranes (1971) *Biochim. Biophys. Acta 249*, 462–464.
37. Riisom, T., Johnson, S., Hill, E.G., and Holman, R.T. Effect of Experimental Diabetes on Essential Fatty Acid Deficient Rat (1981) *J. Lab. Clin. Med. 98*, 764–775.
38. Holman, R.T., Johnson, S.B., Gerrard, J.M., Mauer, S.M., Kupcho-Sandberg, S., and Brown, D.M. Arachidonic Acid Deficiency in Streptozotocin-Induced Diabetes (1983) *Proc. Natl. Acad. Sci. U.S.A. 80*, 2375–2379.
39. Mercuri, O., Peluffo, R.O., and Brenner, R.R. Effect of Insulin on the Oxidative Desaturation of Alpha-Linolenic, Oleic and Palmitic Acids (1967) *Lipids 2*, 284–285.
40. Faas, F.H., and Carter, W.J. Altered Microsomal Phospholipid Composition in the Streptozotocin Diabetic Rat (1983) *Lipids 18*, 953–961.
41. Dang, A.Q., Faas, F.H., Lee, J.A., and Carter, W.J. Altered Fatty Acid Composition in the Plasma, Platelets, and Aorta of the Streptozotocin-Induced Diabetic Rat (1988) *Metabolism 37*, 1065–1072.
42. Dang, A.Q., Faas, F.H., Jethmalani, S.M., and Carter, W.J. Decreased Incorporation of Long-Chain Fatty Acid into Erythrocyte Phospholipids of Streptozotocin-Diabetic Rats (1991) *Diabetes 40*, 1645–1651.
43. Okumura, K., Nishiura, T., Awaji, Y., Kondo, J., Hashimoto, H., and Ito, T. 1,2-Diacylglycerol Content and Its Fatty Acid Composition in Thoracic Aorta of Diabetic Rats (1991) *Diabetes 40*, 820–824.
44. Huang, Y.-S., Horrobin, D.F., Manku, M.S., Mitchell, J., and Ryan, M.A. Tissue Phospholipid Fatty Acid Composition in the Diabetic Rat (1984) *Lipids 19*, 367–370.
45. Chattopadhyay, J., Thompson, E.W., and Schmid, H.H. Elevated Levels of Nonesterified Fatty Acids in the Myocardium of Alloxan Diabetic Rats (1990) *Lipids 25*, 307–310.
46. Field, C.J., Goruk, S.D., Wierzbicki, A.A., and Clandinin, M.T. The Effect of Dietary Content and Composition on Adipocyte Lipids in Normal and Diabetic States (1989) *Int. J. Obes. 13*, 747–756.
47. Field, C.J., Ryan, E.A., Thomson, A.B., and Clandinin, M.T. Diet Fat Composition Alters Membrane Phospholipid Composition, Insulin Binding, and Glucose Metabolism in Adipocytes from Control and Diabetic Animals (1990) *J. Biol. Chem. 265*, 11143–11150.
48. Clark, D.L., Hamel, F.G., and Queener, S.F. Changes in Renal Phospholipid Fatty Acids in Diabetes Mellitus: Correlation with Changes in Adenylate Cyclase Activity (1983) *Lipids 18*, 696–705.
49. Lemieux, G., Moulin, B., Davignon, J., and Huang, Y.-S. The Lipid Content of the Diabetic Kidney of the Rat (1984) *Can. J. Physiol. Pharmacol. 62*, 1274–1278.

50. Levy, E., Roy, C.C., Lepage, G., and Bendayan, M. Lipid Abnormalities in Pancreatic Tissue of Streptozotocin-Induced Diabetic Rats (1988) *Lipids 23*, 771–778.
51. Igal, R.A., Mandon, E.C., and De Gomez Dumm, I.N.T. Abnormal Metabolism of Polyunsaturated Fatty Acid Adrenal Glands of Diabetic Rats (1991) *Mol. Cell. Endocrinol. 77*, 217–227.
52. Lin, C.J., Peterson, R., and Eichberg, J. The Fatty Acid Composition of Glycerolipids in Nerve, Brain, and Other Tissues of the Streptozotocin Diabetic Rat (1985) *Neurochem. Res. 10*, 1453–1465.
53. Chanussot, B., Narce, M., and Poisson, J.-P. Liver Microsomal Delta-6 and Delta-5 Desaturation in Female BB Rats (1989) *Diabetologia 32*, 786–791.
54. Leikin, A.I., and Brenner, R.R. Regulation of Linoleic Acid Delta-6 Desaturation by a Cytosolic Lipoprotein-Like Fraction in Isolated Rat Liver Microsomes (1986) *Biochim. Biophys. Acta 876*, 300–308.
55. Mimouni, V., and Poisson, J.-P. Spontaneous Diabetes in BB Rats: Evidence for Insulin Dependent Liver Microsomal Delta-6 and Delta-5 Desaturase Activities (1990) *Horm. Metab. Res. 22*, 405–407.
56. Mimouni, V., and Poisson, J.-P. Altered Desaturase Activities and Fatty Acid Composition in Liver Microsomes of Spontaneously Diabetic Wistar BB Rat (1992) *Biochim. Biophys. Acta 1123*, 296–302.
57. Mimouni, V., and Poisson, J.-P. Liver Fatty Acid Composition in the Spontaneously Diabetic BB Rat (1991) *Arch. Intern. Physiol. Biochim. 99*, 111–121
58. Lefkowith, J., Schreiner, G., Cormier, J., Handler, E.S., Driscoll, H.K., Greiner, D., Mordes, J.P., and Rossini, A.A. Prevention of Diabetes in the BB Rat by Essential Fatty Acid Deficiency. Relationship Between Physiological and Biochemical Changes (1990) *J. Exp. Med. 171*, 729–743.
59. Kawashima, Y., Musoh, K., and Kosuka, H. Peroxisome Proliferators Enhance Linoleic Acid Metabolism in the Rat Liver. Increased Biosynthesis of Omega Polyunsaturated Fatty Acids (1990) *J. Biol. Chem. 265*, 9170–9175.
60. Poisson, J.-P., Lemarchal, P., Blond, J.P., Lecerf, J., and Mendy, F. Influence du Diabète Alloxanique sur la Conversion des Acides Linoléique et Gamma-Linolénique (I-^{14}C) en Acide Arachidonique chez le Rat *in Vivo* (1978) *Diabet. Metab. 4*, 39–45.
61. Poisson, J.-P., Blond, J.P., and Lemarchal, P. Influence du Diabete Streptozotocique sur la Conversion des Acides Gamma-Linolénique et Dihomogamma-Linolénique (1-^{14}C) en Acide Arachidonique chez le Rat *in Vivo* (1979) *Diabet. Metab. 5*, 43–46.
62. Poisson, J.-P., and Blond, J.P. Influence du Diabete Streptozotocique sur la Conversion *in Vivo* des Acides Gamma-Linolénique et Dihomo-Gammalinolénique (^{14}C) en Acide Arachidonique dans les Reins et le Rat Entier (1985) *Diabet. Metab. 11*, 289–294.
63. Suneja, S.K., Osei, P., Cook, L., Nagi, M.N., and Cinti, D.L. Enzyme Site Specific Changes in Hepatic Microsomal Fatty Acid Chain Elongation in Streptozotocin-Induced Diabetic Rats (1990) *Biochim. Biophys. Acta 1042*, 81–85.
64. Mimouni, V., Narce, M., and Poisson, J.-P. Evidence for Insulin-Dependent Hepatic Microsomal Gamma-Linolenic Acid Chain Elongation in Spontaneously Diabetic BB Rats (1992) *Biochim. Biophys. Acta 1133*, 187192.
65. Barcelli, U.O., Weiss, M., Beach, D., Motz, A., and Thompson, B. High Linoleic Acid Diets Ameliorate Diabetic Nephropathy in Rats (1990) *Am. J. Kidney Dis. 16*, 244–251.
66. Singh, B., Lauzon, J., Venkatraman, J., Thomson, A.B., Rajotte, R.V., and Clandinin, M.T. Effect of High/low Dietary Linoleic Acid Levels on the Function and Fatty Acid Composition of T-Lymphocytes of Normal and Diabetic Rats (1988) *Diabetes Res. 8*, 129–134.

67. Patterson, J.W. Effect of a High Fat Fructose and Casein Diet on Diabetic Cataracts (1955) *Proc. Soc. Exp. Biol. Med. 90*, 706–708.
68. Patterson, J.W., Patterson, M.E., Kinsey, V.E., and Reddy, D.V.N. Lens Assays on Diabetic and Galactosemic Rats Receiving Diets That Modify Cataract Development (1965) *Invest. Ophthalmol. 4*, 98–103.
69. Hutton, J.C., Schofield, P.J., Williams, J.F., Regtop, H.L., and Hollows, F.C. The Effect of an Unsaturated Fat Diet on Cataract Formulation in Streptozotocin-Induced Diabetic Rats (1976) *Br. J. Nutr. 36*, 161–177.
70. Ikeda, A., and Sugano, M. Interaction of Dietary Protein and Alphalinolenic Acid on Polyunsaturated Fatty Acid Composition of Liver Microsomal Phospholipids and Eicosanoid Production in Streptozotocin-Induced Diabetic Rats (1993) *Ann. Nutr. Metab. 37*, 101–109.
71. Julu, P.O.O. Essential Fatty Acids Prevent Slowed Nerve Conduction in Streptozotocin Diabetic Rats (1988) *J. Diabetic Complications 2*, 185–188.
72. Tomlinson, D.R., Robinson, J.P., and Compton, A.M. (1990) in *Omega-6 Essential Fatty Acids: Pathophysiology and Roles in Clinical Medecine*, Horrobin, D.F., ed., Alan Liss, New York, pp. 457–463.
73. Cameron, N.E., Cotter, M.A., and Robertson, S. Essential Fatty Acid Diet Supplementation. Effects on Peripheral Nerve and Skeletal Muscle Function and Capillarization in Streptozotocin-Induced Diabetic Rats (1991) *Diabetes 40*, 532–539.
74. Takahashi, R., Morse, N., and Horrobin, D.F. Plasma, Platelet, and Aorta Fatty Acids Composition in Response to Dietary n-6 and n-3 Fats Supplementation in a Rat Model of Non-Insulin Dependent Diabetes (1988) *J. Nutr. Sci. Vitaminol. 34*, 413–421.
75. Metz, S.A. Exogenous Arachidonic Acid Promotes Insulin Release from Intact or Permeabilized Rat Islets by Dual Mechanisms. Putative Activation of Ca^{++} Mobilization and Protein Kinase C (1988) *Diabetes 37*, 1453–1469.
76. Pschera, H., Persson, B., and Lunell, N.O. Fatty Acid Composition of Amniotic Fluid Lecithin and Its Relationship to Amniotic Fluid C-Peptide in Diabetic Pregnancy (1984) *Horm. Metab. Res. 16*, 186–189.
77. Bitman, J., Hamosh, M., Hamosh, P., Lutes, V., Neville, M.C., Seacat, J., and Wood, D.L. Milk Composition and Volume During the Onset of Lactation in a Diabetic Mother (1989) *Am. J. Clin. Nutr. 50*, 1364–1369.
78. Horrobin, D.F. Essential Fatty Acids and the Complications of Diabetes Mellitus (1989) *Wein. Klin. Wochenschr. 101*, 289–293.
79. El Boustani, S., Descomps, B., Monnier, L., Warnant, J., Mendy, F., and Crastes de Paulet, A. *In Vivo* Conversion of Dihomo-Gamma-Linolenic Acid into Arachidonic Acid in Man (1986) *Prog. Lipid Res. 25*, 67–71.
80. El Boustani, S., Causse, J.E., Descomps, B., Monnier, L., Mendy, F., and Crastes de Paulet, A. Direct *in Vivo* Characterization of Delta-5 Desaturase Activity in Humans by Deuterium Labelling: Effect of Insulin (1989) *Metabolism 38*, 315–321.
81. Lagarde, M., Berciaud, P., and Burtin, M. Refractoriness of Diabetic Platelets to Inhibitory Prostaglandins (1981) *Prostaglandins Med. 7*, 341–348.
82. Mikhailidis, D.P., Kirtland, S.J., Barradas, M.A., Mahadeviah, S., and Dandona, P. The Effect of Dihomo-Gamma-Linolenic Acid on Platelet Aggregation and Prostaglandin Release, Erythrocyte Membrane Fatty Acids and Serum Lipids: Evidence for Defects in Prostaglandin E_1 Synthesis and Delta-5 Desaturase Activity in Insulin-Dependent Diabetics (1986) *Diabetes Res. 3*, 7–12.
83. Freyburger, G., Gin, H., Heape, A., Juguelin, H., Boisseau, M.R., and Cassagne, C. Phospholipid and Fatty Acid Composition of Erythrocytes in Type I and Type II Diabetes (1989) *Metabolism 38*, 673–678.

84. Van-Doormaal, J.J., Muskiet, F.A., van Ballegooie, E., Sluiter, W.J., and Doorenbos, H. The Plasma and Erythrocyte Fatty Acid Composition of Poorly Controlled Insulin-Dependent (Type I) Diabetic Patients and the Effect of Improved Metabolic Control (1984) *Clin. Chim. Acta 144*, 203–212.
85. Schimke, E., Hildebrandt, R., and Grzeskowiak, B. Relationship Between Fatty Acid Pattern and Platelet Aggregation in Long-Term Insulin-Dependent Type I Diabetics (1988) *Biomed. Biochim. Acta 47*, S274–S277.
86. Taylor, A.J., Jennings, P.E., Barnett, A.H., Pandov, H.I., and Lawson, N. An Alternative Explanation for the Changes in Erythrocyte Fatty Acids Observed in Diabetes Mellitus (1987) *Clin. Chem. 33*, 2083–2085.
87. Ruiz-Gutierrez, V., Stiefel, P., Villar, J., Garcia-Donas, M.A., Acosta, D., and Carneado, J. Cell Membrane Fatty Acid Composition in Type 1 (Insulin-Dependent) Diabetic Patients: Relationship with Sodium Transport Abnormalities and Metabolic Control (1993) *Diabetologia 36*, 850–856.
88. Tilvis, R.S., and Miettinen, T.A. Fatty Acid Composition of Serum Lipids, Erythrocytes and Platelets in Insulin-Dependent Diabetic Women (1985) *J. Clin. Endocrinol. Metab. 61*, 741–745.
89. Arisaka, M., Arisaka, O., Fukuda, Y., and Yamashiro, Y. Prostaglandin Metabolism in Children with Diabetes Mellitus. I. Plasma Prostaglandin E_2, $F_{2\alpha}$, TXB_2, and Serum Fatty Acid Levels (1986) *J. Pediatr. Gastroenterol. Nutr. 5*, 878–882.
90. Monnier, L.H., Chaintreuil, J.S., Colette, C., Blotman, M.J., Crastes de Paulet, P., Orsetti, A., and Crastes de Paulet, A. Plasma Lipid Fatty Acids and Platelet Function in Insulin-Dependent Diabetic Patients (1983) *Diabet. Metab. 9*, 283–287.
91. Jones, D.B., Carter, R.D., and Mann, J.I. Indirect Evidence of Impairment of Platelet Desaturase Enzymes in Diabetes Mellitus (1986) *Horm. Metab. Res. 18*, 341–344.
92. Myrup, B., Bregengaard, C., Petersen, L.R., and Winther, K. Platelet Aggregation and Fatty Acid Composition of Platelets in Type I Diabetes Mellitus (1991) *Clin. Chim. Acta 204*, 251–261.
93. Tilvis, R.S., Taskinen, M.R., and Miettinen, T.A. Effect of Insulin Treatment on Fatty Acids of Plasma and Erythrocyte Membrane Lipids in Type 2 Diabetes (1988) *Clin. Chim. Acta 171*, 293–303.
94. Dobrev, D., Terzieva, T., Krustev, I., Svinarov, D., and Petrova, V. Fatty Acids in Diabetes Mellitus (1989) *Vutr. Boles. 28*, 70–74.
95. Salomaa, V., Ahola, I., Tuomilehto, J., Aro, A., Pietinen, P., Korhonen, H.J., and Pentilla, I. Fatty Acid Composition of Serum Cholesterol Esters in Different Degrees of Glucose Intolerance: A Population-Based Study (1990) *Metabolism 39*, 1285–1291.
96. Morita, I., Takahashi, R., Ito, H., Orimo, H., and Murota, S. Increased Arachidonic Acid Content in Platelet Phospholipids from Diabetic Patients (1983) *Prostaglandins Leukotrienes Med. 11*, 33–41.
97. Piper, C.M., Carroll, P.B., and Dunn, F.L. Diet-Induced Essential Fatty Acid Deficiency in Ambulatory Patients with Type I Diabetes Mellitus (1986) *Diabetes Care 9*, 291–293.
98. Howard-Williams, J., Patel, P., Jelfs, R., Carter, R.D., Awdry, P., Bron, A., Mann, J.I., and Hockaday, T.D.R. Polyunsaturated Fatty Acids and Diabetic Retinopathy (1985) *J. Ophthalmol. 69*, 15–18.
99. Kinsell, L.W., Walker, G., Michaels, G.D., and Olson, F.E. Dietary Fats and the Diabetic Patient (1959) *N. Engl. J. Med. 261*, 431–434.
100. King, R.C., Dobree, J.H., Kok, D.A., Foulds, W.S., and Dangerfield, W.G. Exudative Diabetic Retinopathy: Spontaneous Changes and Effect of a Corn Oil Diet (1963) *Br. J. Ophthalmol. 47*, 666–672.

101. Houtsmuller, A.J. Significance of Linoleic Acid in the Metabolism and Therapy of Diabetic Retinopathy (1982) *World Rev. Nutr. Diet. 39,* 85–123.
102. Williams, R., Broughton, M. (1992) in *The Treatment of Diabetic Neuropathy: A New Approach,* Horrobin, D.F., ed., Churchill Livingstone, Edinburgh, pp. 131–135.
103. Monnier, L.H., Colette, C., Chaintreuil, J., and Crastes de Paulet, A. Effects of Dietary Omega 6 Polyunsaturated Fats on Plama Lipids and Platelet Function in Non-Diabetic and Diabetic Subjects (1985) *Diabetes Res. Clin. Pract. (Suppl.) 1,* S390 (abstract).
104. Chaintreuil, J., Monnier, L., Colette, C., and Crastes de Paulet, A. Effects of Dietary Gamma-Linolenate Supplementation on Serum Lipids and Platelet Function in Insulin-Dependent and Diabetic Patients (1984) *Human Nutr. Clin. Nutr. 38C,* 121–130.
105. Van Doormaal, J.J., Idema, I.G., and Muskiet, F.A.J. Effects of Short Term High Dose Intake of Evening Primrose Oil on Plasma and Cellular Fatty Acid Compositions, Alpha-Tocopherol Levels and Erythropoiesin in Normal and Type I (Insulin-Dependent) Diabetic Men (1988) *Diabetologia 31,* 576–584.
106. Uccella, R., Contini, A., and Sartorio, M. Action of Evening Primrose Oil on Cardiovascular Risk Factors in Insulin-Dependent Diabetics (1989) *Clin. Ter. 129,* 381–388.
107. Arisaka, M., Arisaka, O., Yamashiro, Y. Fatty Acid and Prostaglandin Metabolism in Children with Diabetes Mellitus II. The Effect of Evening Primrose Oil Supplementation on Serum Fatty Acid and Plasma Prostaglandin Levels (1991) *Prostaglandins Leukotrienes Med. 43,* 197–201.
108. Jamal, G.A., and Carmichael, H. The Effect of Gamma-Linolenic Acid on Human Diabetic Peripheral Neuropathy: A Double Blind Placebo-Controlled Trial (1990) *Diabetic Med. 7,* 319–323.
109. Keen, H., Payan, J., and Allawi, J. Treatment of Diabetic Neuropathy with Gamma-Linolenic Acid (1993) *Diabetes Care 16,* 8–15.

Chapter 21

Essential Fatty Acids in the Management of Diabetic Neuropathy

David F. Horrobin

Efamol Research Institute, Kentville, Nova Scotia, Canada B4N4H8

Introduction

Holman first reported an abnormality of essential fatty acid (EFA) metabolism in diabetes (1). Diabetic animals required much higher amounts of linoleic acid to counteract EFA deficiency compared with normal animals. The possible explanation for this was provided by Brenner, who observed that the mechanism for conversion of linoleic acid to γ-linolenic acid was defective in diabetic animals (2). Thus, much higher amounts of linoleic acid may be required in the diabetic state to provide the long-chain, highly unsaturated EFAs, dihomo-γ-linolenic acid (DGLA) and arachidonic acid (AA).

Since these original observations, overwhelming evidence has accumulated concerning the defect in conversion of linoleic acid to GLA in insulin-dependent diabetic animals (reviewed in 3, 4, 5). There are no direct studies of linoleic acid desaturation in human diabetes. There are two types of human diabetes mellitus, Type I or insulin-dependent (IDDM), and Type II or noninsulin-dependent (NIDDM) or maturity onset. In Type I diabetes there are several reports of blood EFA abnormalities consistent with impaired conversion of linoleic acid to GLA (reviewed in references 4–6): linoleic acid levels are normal or elevated, whereas levels of DGLA and AA are substantially reduced. There are no equivalent reports in Type II diabetes although all studies reported to date have been small and probably inadequate in size to demonstrate small differences.

Although blood glucose can now be controlled reasonably well with combinations of diet, insulin and other drugs, in both types of diabetes in the long term, all diabetics are at risk for the development of damage to the eyes (retinopathy), kidneys (nephropathy), cardiovascular system, and nerves (neuropathy). The neuropathy is particularly characterized by loss of sensory nerve function, although all nerves, including autonomic nerves may be damaged. Loss of pain sensation and of the normal control of skin circulation required for healing leads to skin damage and ulceration. The ulcers may be difficult to heal, leading eventually to a need for limb amputation. Diabetes is the most common reason for leg amputation in most Western countries. Other common consequences of neuropathy are impotence, muscle weakness, cardiovascular instability and loss of the normal control of the bladder and gastrointestinal tract. After 20 y of diabetes, about half of all patients have clinically detectable symptoms attributable to neuropathy, whereas more than 90% have nerve damage that can be detected by neurophysiological techniques.

DGLA and AA are important in nerve structure and function in several ways. First, they are required for the normal structure of neuronal membranes, without which nerves cannot conduct impulses normally. Second, they are required for the normal regulation of nerve conduction, possibly via the inositol/calcium cycle and also via the release of prostaglandins which are required for normal nerve conduction (5–8). Third, prostaglandin E_1 from DGLA and prostacyclin from AA are required for the normal control of the nerve microcirculation. For these reasons, it has been proposed that the defective conversion of linoleic acid to GLA, with the consequent subnormal levels of DGLA and AA, may be responsible for the long-term nerve damage in diabetes (5–7).

Animal Studies

Animals with streptozotocin-induced diabetes develop a neuropathy which is in many respects similar to the human disorder. Rat diabetic neuropathy is therefore widely used to investigate the pathophysiology of the condition and test possible treatments.

Several groups of investigators have studied the effect of GLA in the form of a selected variety of evening primrose oil (Efamol) on rat diabetic neuropathy. The results have been unusually consistent. All investigations have shown that rat diabetic neuropathy can be both prevented and reversed by the administration of evening primrose oil (9–16).

In the animal model, the neuropathy seems particularly related to reduced nerve blood flow. In the rat, the maintenance of normal nerve blood flow is heavily dependent upon prostacyclin derived from AA. In diabetic animals, nerve blood flow is reduced and can be restored by treatment with GLA (11–13). The reduced nerve blood flow is associated with reduced nerve prostacyclin, and this also can be reversed to normal by the provision of GLA (11–17). GLA also corrects the nerve conduction defects in diabetic animals (11–17). Recent evidence indicates that there is an interaction between prostacyclin and nitric oxide, that both are required for normal regulation of the nerve microcirculation, that production of both is impaired in diabetes, and that both can be normalized by evening primrose oil (17). The effect of GLA on nerve blood flow and on the neuropathy can be blocked by adequate doses of non-steroidal anti-inflammatory drugs which interfere with the synthesis of prostacyclin and prostaglandin E_1 (15).

The animal evidence is therefore highly consistent with Brenner's hypothesis that the complications of diabetes, and in this case the nerve damage, are caused by defective conversion of linoleic acid to GLA. The provision of GLA bypasses this biochemical defect and restores nerve function to normal.

Effects of Different GLA Sources

All of the animal studies reported in the previous section were performed using evening primrose oil (Efamol) which contains about 8% by weight of GLA. Most of this GLA is in the form of a triglyceride which contains two molecules of linoleic acid and one of GLA (18). About one third of the GLA is in the *sn*-2 position with the remainder in the *sn*-1 and *sn*-3 positions (18). The triglyceride can be given the abbreviated name of DLMG (dilinoleoyl-monogammalinolenyl glycerol).

Because 92% by weight of evening primrose oil consists of material other than GLA, much of it linoleic acid (about 73%), Cotter and Cameron conducted a series of experiments to test whether the effects of primrose oil could indeed by attributed to GLA, or might possibly be caused by one of the other components of the oil (19). They did this by developing a precise bioassay in which animals made diabetic for 6 wk were treated with various doses of primrose oil which induced dose-related degrees of restoration of normal nerve conduction.

Using this bioassay, Cameron and Cotter then tested evening primrose oil, pure DLMG isolated from primrose oil by HPLC, and pure tri-GLA prepared by making pure GLA from borage oil followed by enzymatic synthesis of the triglyceride. All three sources of GLA were then tested in the bioassay (19). The three dose/response curves were completely superimposable when plotted on the basis of the GLA content of the various oils, whereas sunflower oil, rich in linoleic acid, had no effect. Artificial primrose oil made by diluting DLMG with sunflower oil to give an 8% final concentration of GLA had exactly the same effect as natural primrose oil. These experiments demonstrate therefore that the effects of primrose oil are attributable to the GLA which is present, primarily, in the form of DLMG (Fig. 21.1).

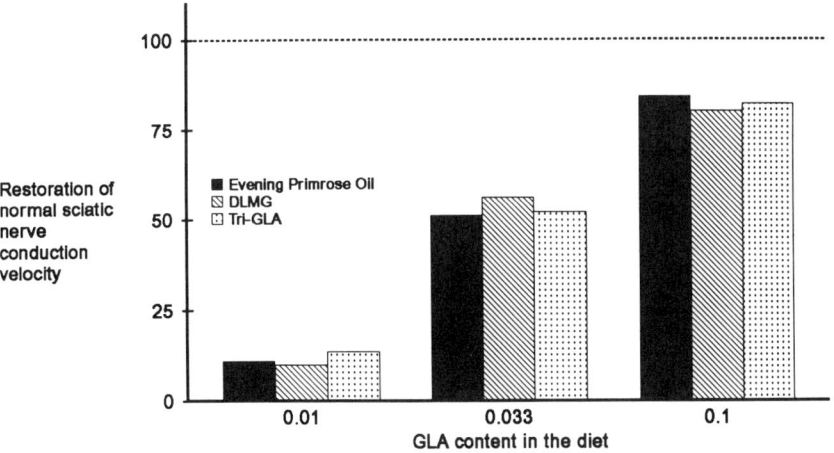

Fig. 21.1. The effects of γ-linolenic acid (GLA) from three different sources on the restoration of normal sciatic nerve conduction velocity (indicated as percentage of normal) in rats with streptozotocin-induced diabetes. The three sources were evening primrose oil, containing approximately 8% GLA by weight, DLMG triglyceride prepared from evening primrose oil, containing about 31% GLA by weight, and tri-GLA prepared by esterification of pure GLA prepared from borage oil and containing about 92% GLA by weight. When expressed as percentage GLA content in the diet, all three GLA sources had virtually identical effects on nerve conduction. *Source:* K.C. Dines *et al.* (19).

Other GLA-containing oils such as borage (22% GLA), black currant (16% GLA), and fungal oil (19% GLA) were then tested in the same system (20,21). Surprisingly, in contrast with primrose oil, DLMG and tri-GLA, there was no clear relationship between the GLA content of the oil and its biological effects. Also surprisingly, the three oils which contained higher levels of GLA than primrose oil were considerably less effective than primrose oil at treating the nerve damage.

Previous studies have reported that the different oils have very different effects on the synthesis of prostaglandins and thromboxanes derived from DGLA and AA (22,23). Thromboxane A_2 is a vasoconstrictor agent, whereas prostaglandin E_1 and prostacyclin are powerful vasodilators. The ratio of prostacyclin to thromboxane synthesis is widely used as an index of vasodilator action. When the ratios of vascular prostacyclin to thromboxane generated by the four oils (22) were plotted against the effectiveness of the oils in restoring nerve function in diabetes, a close linear relationship was observed (Fig. 21.2) (21). The efficacies of borage, black currant and fungal oils, but not of primrose oil, were improved by co-administering them with an inhibitor of thromboxane synthesis. This suggests that the oils contain some unknown factor which stimulates thromboxane synthesis and which counteracts the effects of GLA (21). This strongly suggests that the different efficacies are related to the differing abilities of the oils to modify prostaglandin and thromboxane biosynthesis.

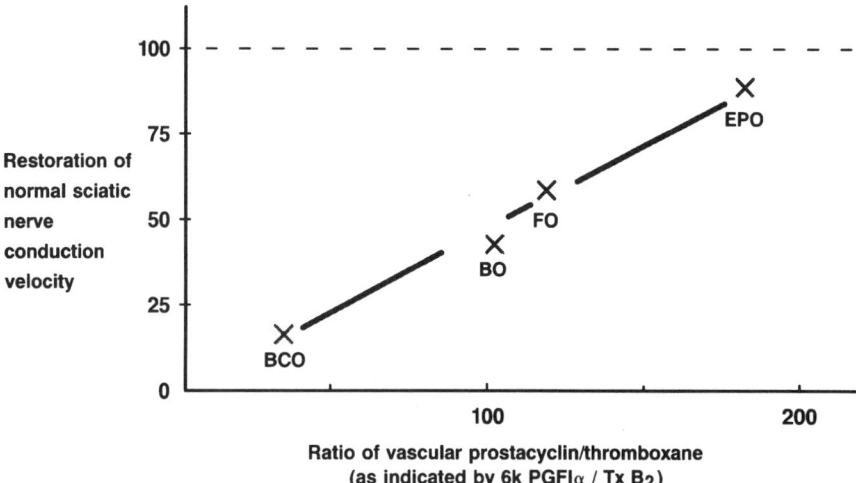

Fig. 21.2. The effects of four different oils which are sources of γ-linolenic acid, added at 1% by weight to the diet, on the restoration of normal sciatic nerve conduction velocity in diabetic animals and on the rate of vascular prostacyclin to thromboxane production. The evening primrose oil (EPO) was most effective in restoring nerve conduction even though it had the lowest content of GLA (8%). Fungal oil (FO) and borage oil (BO) were about equally effective although they contained 19 and 22% GLA, respectively. Blackcurrant oil (BCO) with 17% GLA was the least effective. There was an obvious relationship between the efficacy of an oil and its effects on the prostacyclin/thromboxane ratio in vascular tissue. *Source:* K.C. Dines et al. (21).

The bases for these differences are at present unknown. Clearly, they must be related to components of the oil other than GLA. They may depend on the other triglyceride and fatty acid constituents of the oils which are very different from those of primrose oil, with the other oils having considerably higher levels of saturated and/or monounsaturated and/or n-3 EFAs. They may also depend on minor and as yet unidentified components of the oils which could have inhibitory effects, in particular on the synthesis of prostacyclin. The possibility of such effects on prostacyclin synthesis is indicated by the fact that primrose oil doubles prostacyclin synthesis compared with corn oil, whereas borage oil actually halves the production of prostacyclin compared with corn oil (23). Another indicator of the presence of some inhibitory material in borage oil is the finding of a reversed dose-response curve in neuropathy, with 3% borage oil in the diet being less effective in restoring normal nerve function than 1% borage oil (21). This can be explained reasonably only by the presence in borage oil of some material which adversely affects nerve function, possibly by adversely affecting prostacyclin biosynthesis.

Thus, while the effects of primrose oil in diabetic neuropathy are clearly attributable to GLA, the mere presence of high levels of GLA in an oil does not indicate a desirable effect of that oil. The possibility that natural oils contain toxic materials cannot be ignored (24).

Human Biochemistry

As mentioned earlier, there is good evidence from human studies of a likely defect in conversion of linoleic acid to GLA in type I insulin-dependent diabetes. This is based on normal or elevated levels of linoleic acid and reduced levels of the major metabolites in plasma (4–6, 25–27). There has been no equivalent evidence for type II diabetes for which the results have been variable and based on small numbers.

However, a recent large study compared plasma phospholipid, cholesteryl ester and triglyceride and red cell phospholipid fatty acids in 319 normal controls, 224 type I diabetics and 364 type II diabetics (28). As expected, in all four fractions there was an elevated ratio of linoleic acid to DGLA + AA, consistent with impaired conversion of linoleic acid to GLA, in type I diabetics. In all four fractions the differences from controls were highly significant. In type II diabetics there were similar but smaller elevations of the linoleic to DGLA + AA ratio in three of the four fractions, indicative of a less marked inhibition of desaturation in noninsulin-dependent diabetes. The most striking observation which was present equally in both types of diabetes was a substantial reduction in all of the long-chain essential fatty acids of both n-6 and n-3 types in red cell membranes. DGLA, AA and adrenic acid of the n-6 series, and eicosapentaenoic acid and docosahexaenoic acid of the n-3 series were all highly significantly reduced in the membrane phospholipids of both types of diabetics compared with controls. In compensation, saturated and monounsaturated fatty acids were elevated in the membranes of the diabetic patients (28).

If, as is possible, the red cell membrane composition is indicative of other cell membrane compositions in diabetes, this may suggest that two different biochemical

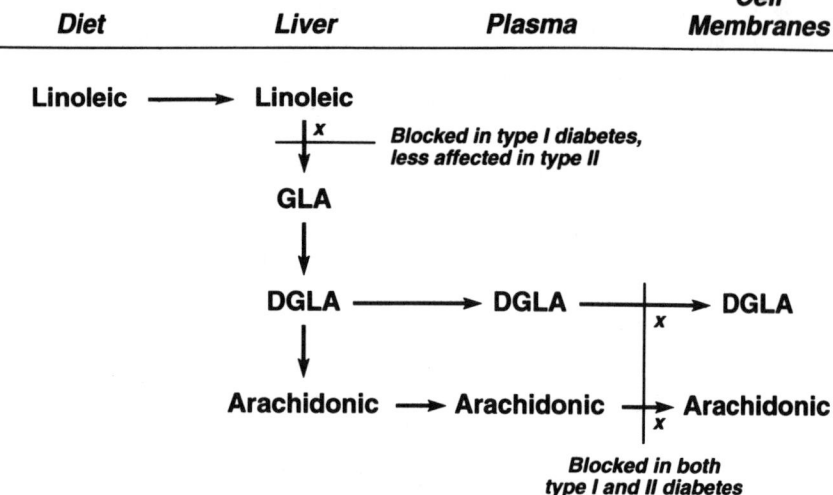

Fig. 21.3. An outline of the metabolism of essential fatty acids in diabetes. Both types of diabetes have some impairment of Δ6-desaturation although this is more marked in insulin-dependent patients. In both types of diabetes, the incorporation of long-chain essential fatty acids from plasma into red cell and possibly other cell membranes is impaired.

abnormalities produce membrane defects in this disease (Fig. 12.3). The first is impaired desaturation of the parent EFAs, present in both types of diabetes, but more evident in insulin-dependent patients. The second is impaired incorporation of the long-chain highly unsaturated EFAs into cell membranes and this applies equally to both types of diabetes. The low levels of the membrane phospholipid EFAs could be attributable to actual reduced incorporation, or to increased loss either because of excessive peroxidation or because of removal by phospholipases or other enzymes. In either situation, there is a case for attempting to correct the situation by treating diabetic patients with EFAs, such as GLA, beyond the first rate-limiting step.

Human Studies in Diabetic Neuropathy

Three randomized, placebo-controlled, human studies of the administration of GLA in patients with human diabetic neuropathy have now been performed. In all three, patients have been randomized to receive a placebo or 480 mg/d GLA provided by 12 × 500 mg capsules of evening primrose oil (Efamol). In all three studies, a range of neurophysiological tests of nerve function involving measurements of conduction velocity and action potential amplitudes, tests of the ability to detect skin temperature changes in the direction of heat or cold, and clinical tests of sensory functions, muscle strength and reflexes have been performed (29–31).

The first pilot study in 22 patients studied for 6 mo was carried out by Jamal and Carmichael (29). They found that all parameters improved in the GLA group, whereas all deteriorated in the placebo group, and that for many of the parameters the differences were statistically significant. The other two trials were multicentered, performed to virtually identical protocols, lasted for 12 mo, and involved measurements of six neurophysiological, six clinical and two thermal parameters in both upper and lower limbs, yielding 28 parameters in all. The first of these multicentered trials involved 111 patients in seven centers (30); the second involved 293 patients in ten centers in the UK, Sweden, Finland, and Germany (unpublished results).

The results in the two multicentered trials were virtually identical: in both trials all 28 parameters were better on active than on placebo. When the two multicentered trials were combined, giving results in 404 patients, all 28 parameters deteriorated over 1 y on placebo, while 26 of 28 improved on GLA. For all 28, GLA was better than placebo, for 25, significantly so, and for 18, the significance of the difference between active and placebo had P values below 0.0001.

These results therefore leave no doubt that GLA is an effective treatment for diabetic nerve damage.

Conclusions

The study of EFAs in diabetes, initiated by the studies by Holman and Brenner and their groups, has followed a classic course. First, abnormalities were demonstrated in animals with the disease. Then, similar abnormalities were demonstrated in humans. Treatment studies in animals, based on biochemical understanding of EFA abnormalities, were successful and led to trials of human treatment. These also have been successful and over the next few years should lead to widespread introduction of this treatment approach. Based on current biochemical understanding, it is unlikely that GLA alone will be the optimum treatment, and it seems probable that other highly unsaturated EFAs will be added to produce even more effective therapeutic regimens.

References

1. Peifer, J.J., and Holman, R.T. Essential Fatty Acids, Diabetes and Cholesterol (1955) *Arch. Biochem. Biophys. 57,* 520–521.
2. Mercuri, O., Peluffo, R.O., and Brenner, R.R. Depression of Microsomal Desaturation of Linoleic to Gamma-Linolenic Acid in the Alloxan Diabetic Rat (1966) *Biochim. Biophys. Acta 116,* 407–411.
3. Brenner, R.R. Nutritional and Hormonal Factors Influencing Desaturation of Essential Fatty Acids (1982) *Prog. Lipid Res. 20,* 41–48.
4. Horrobin, D.F. Nutritional and Medical Importance of Gamma-Linolenic Acid (1992) *Prog. Lipid Res. 31,* 163–194.
5. Horrobin, D.F. The Roles of Essential Fatty Acids in the Development of Diabetic Neuropathy and Other Complications of Diabetes Mellitus (1988) *Prostaglandins, Leukotrienes Essen. Fatty Acids 31,* 181–197.
6. Horrobin, D.F., ed., (1992) *Treatment of Diabetic Neuropathy: A New Approach.* Churchill Livingstone, Edinburgh, 1992.

7. Jamal, G.A. The Use of Gamma Linolenic Acid in the Prevention and Treatment of Diabetic Neuropathy (1994) *Diabetic Med. 11*, 145–149.
8. Horrobin, D.F., Durand, L.G., and Manku, M.S. Prostaglandin E1 Modifies Nerve Conduction and Interferes with Local Anaesthetic Action (1977) *Prostaglandins 14*, 103–110.
9. Julu, P.O.O. Essential Fatty Acids Prevent Slowed Nerve Conduction Velocity in Streptozotocin Diabetes Rats (1988) *J. Diabetic Comp. 2*, 185–188.
10. Julu, P.O.O. Responses of Peripheral Nerve Conduction Velocities to Treatment with Essential Fatty Acids in Diabetic Rats: Possible Mechanisms of Action (1992) in *Treatment of Diabetic Neuropathy: A New Approach*, Horrobin, D.F., ed., pp. 41–62, Churchill Livingstone, Edinburgh, 1992.
11. Tomlinson, D.R., Robinson, J.P., Compton, A.M., and Keen, P. Essential Fatty Acid Treatment—Effects on Nerve Conduction, Polyol Pathway and Axonal Transport in Streptozotocin Diabetic Rats (1989) *Diabetologia 32*, 655–659.
12. Stevens, E.J., Lockett, M.J., Carrington, A.L., and Tomlinson, D.R. Essential Fatty Acids Treatment Prevents Nerve Ischaemia and Associated Conduction Anomalies in Rats with Experimental Diabetes Mellitus (1993) *Diabetologia 36*, 397–401.
13. Stevens, E.J., Carrington, A.L., and Tomlinson, D.R. Prostacyclin Release in Experimental Diabetes: Effects of Evening Primrose Oil (1993) *Prostaglandins Leukotrienes Essen. Fatty Acids 49*, 699–706
14. Cameron, N.E., Cotter, M.A., and Robertson, S. Essential Fatty Acid Diet Supplementation. Effects on Peripheral Nerve and Skeletal Muscle Function and Capillarization in Streptozocin-Induced Diabetic Rats (1991) *Diabetes 40*, 532–539.
15. Dines, K.C., Cotter, M.A., and Cameron, N.E. Contrasting Effects of Treatment with ω-3 and ω-6 Essential Fatty Acids on Peripheral Nerve Function and Capillarization in Streptozotocin-Diabetic Rats (1993) *Diabetologia 36*, 1132–1138.
16. Cameron, N.E., and Cotter, M.A. Potential Therapeutic Approaches to the Treatment or Prevention of Diabetic Neuropathy: Evidence from Experimental Studies (1993) *Diabetic Med. 10*, 593–605.
17. Omawari, N., Mahmood, S., Dewhurst, M., Stevens, E.J., and Tomlinson, D.R. Deficient Nitric Oxide Is Responsible for Reduced Nerve Blood Flow in Diabetic Rats: Prevention by Essential Fatty Acids, *Br. J. Pharmacology*, in press..
18. Redden, P.R., Lin, X.R., Fahey, J., and Horrobin, D.F. Stereospecific Analysis of the Major Triacylglycerol Species Containing Gamma-Linolenic Acid in Evening Primrose Oil and Borage Oil (1995) *J. Chromatogr. 704*, 99–111.
19. Dines, K.C., Cameron, N.E., and Cotter, M.A. Comparison of the Effects of Evening Primrose Oil and Triglycerides Containing γ-Linolenic Acid on Nerve Conduction and Blood Flow in Diabetic Rats (1995) *J. Pharmacol. Exp. Ther. 273*, 49–55.
20. Dines, K.C., Cotter, M.A., and Cameron, N.E. Despite a Greater Gamma-Linolenic Acid Content Borage Oil Is Less Effective than Evening Primrose Oil in Correcting Nerve Conduction Defects in Diabetic Rats: Modulation by a Thromboxane A_2 Antagonist. *British Diabetes Association Annual Meeting*, Lancaster, Sept. 1994.
21. Dines, K.C. (1994) Effects of Oils Containing Gamma-Linolenic Acid on Nerve Function in Diabetic Rats. Ph.D. Thesis, University of Aberdeen, Aberdeen, Scotland.
22. Jenkins, D.K., Mitchell, J.C., Manku, M.S., and Horrobin, D.F. Effects of Different Sources of Gamma-Linolenic Acid on the Formation of Essential Fatty Acid and Prostanoid Metabolites (1988) *Med. Sci. Res. 16*, 525–526

23. Fan, Y.-Y., and Chapkin, R.S. Mouse Peritoneal Macrophage Prostaglandin El Synthesis Is Altered by Dietary Gamma-Linolenic Acid (1992) *J. Nutr. 122,* 1600–1606.
24. Horrobin, D.F. Natural Does Not Equal Safe. *Pharmaceutical Tech. Europe* (1994) December, 14–15.
25. Van Doormaal, J.J., Idema, I.G., Muskiet, F.A.J., Martini, I.A., and Doorenbos, H. Effects of Short-Term High-Dose Intake of Evening Primrose Oil on Plasma and Cellular Fatty Acid Compositions, α-Tocopherol Levels, and Erythropoiesis in Normal and Type I (Insulin-Dependent) Diabetic Men (1988) *Diabetologia 31,* 576–584.
26. Tilvis, R.S., and Miettinen, T.A. Fatty Acid Composition of Serum Lipids Erythrocytes and Platelets in Insulin-Dependent Diabetic Women (1985) *J. Clin. Endocrinol. Metabol. 61,* 741–745.
27. Arisaka, M., Arisaka, O., Fukuda, Y., and Yamashiro, Y. Prostaglandin Metabolism in Children with Diabetes Mellitus. I. Plasma Prostaglandin E_2, $F_{2\alpha}$, TXB_2 and Serum Fatty Acid Levels (1986) *J. Paed. Gastroenterol. Nutr. 5,* 878–882.
28. Horrobin, D.F. Plasma and Red Cell Fatty Acid Abnormalities in Patients with Insulin-Dependent and Non-Insulin-Dependent Diabetes. 2nd International ISSFAL Congress, Bethesda, MD, 8 June, 1995.
29. Jamal, G.A., and Carmichael, H. The Effect of γ-Linolenic Acid on Human Diabetic Peripheral Neuropathy: A Double-Blind Placebo-Controlled Trial (1990) *Diabetic Med. 7,* 319–323.
30. The γ-Linolenic Acid Multicenter Trial Group. Treatment of Diabetic Neuropathy with γ-Linolenic Acid (1993) *Diabetes Care 16,* 8–15.

Chapter 22

Anti-Cancer Actions of γ-Linolenic Acid with Particular Reference to Human Brain Malignant Glioma

U.N. Das

> Department of Medicine, Nizam's Institute of Medical Sciences, Punjagutta, Hyderabad-500 482, India

The major aims of cancer therapy are to kill tumor cells selectively without exerting adverse effects on normal cells, to halt metastasis, and to prevent the development of drug resistance. Current anti-cancer therapeutic modalities have several side effects and are potentially hazardous.

Essential fatty acids (EFAs), the precursors of eicosanoids, are important structural components of cell membranes. They also form substrates for the generation of lipid peroxidation products, which have inhibitory action on cell proliferation. Several studies, which are summarized below, have revealed that essential fatty acids and some of their metabolites have selective tumoricidal action both *in vitro* and *in vivo* and that they can be used in the treatment of human malignant gliomas. Some of the work reported here has already been published, and only a summary of the studies completed to date is reported here.

Metabolism of Essential Fatty Acids

There are two main families of EFAs, the n-6 derived from linoleic acid (LA, 18:2 n-6) and the n-3 from α-linolenic acid (ALA, 18:3n-3). LA and ALA cannot be made by the body and are essential nutrients (1,2). γ-Linolenic acid (GLA, 18:3 n-6), dihomo-γ-linolenic acid (DGLA, 20:3n-6), and arachidonic acid (AA, 20:4n-6) are derived from LA, whereas eicosapentaenoic acid (EPA, 20:5n-3) and docosahexaenoic acid (DHA, 22:6n-3) are derived from ALA by the action of Δ6- and Δ5-desaturases and elongase enzymes (1,2). All of the fatty acids, viz., LA, ALA, GLA, DGLA, AA, EPA, and DHA are known as *cis*-unsaturated fatty acids (*c*-UFAs). DGLA, AA, and EPA form precursors to the 1-, 2-, and 3-series prostaglandins (PGs) and respective thromboxanes (TXs) and leukotrienes (LTs) (Fig. 22.1).

Essential Fatty Acid Metabolism in Tumor Cells

Some prostaglandins (PGs) derived from *c*-UFAs have anti-neoplastic properties (3,4). It is interesting to note that tumor cells such as the human macrophage-like cell line U-937 and human promyelocytic leukemia (HL-60) cells do not constitutively express phospholipase A_2 (PLA_2) activity, but do so when induced to differentiate in vitro (5,6). Because PLA_2 activity is the rate-limiting step in the release of c-UFAs from the cell membrane lipid pool, which form precursors to various PGs, it is likely that their deficiency in tumor cells prevents the formation of anti-neoplastic PGs.

Further, tumor cells are deficient in Δ6-desaturase (7), an enzyme needed for the conversion of LA and ALA to their respective products (Fig. 22.1), and secrete an excess of PGE_2, an immunosuppressive and mutagenic substance (8–10). Such evidence indicates that tumor cells have manipulated the EFA metabolism in such a way that they are able to effectively circumvent the body's defense mechanisms and prevent tumor cell lysis. Our recent observation that chemical hepatocarcinogens block the metabolism of EFAs by inhibiting the activity of the Δ6-desaturase much before the development of hepatoma (11) lends further support to this view. It is likely that other carcinogens also may have similar action on the activity of Δ6-desaturase enzyme. It is also interesting to note that GLA and EPA, the products of Δ6-desaturase action on LA and ALA, respectively, have anti-mutagenic actions (10,12–14).

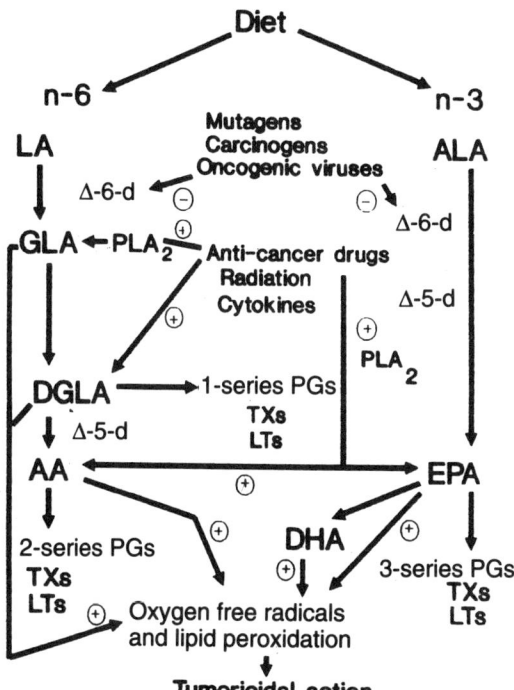

Fig. 22.1. Scheme showing the metabolism of essential fatty acids and its relationship to the cytotoxic action of chemotherapeutic agents. +, release or enhanced action; −, block in release or enzyme activity or inhibition of action.

Tumor Cell Metabolism with Particular Reference to Essential Fatty Acid Metabolism

Metabolic events that are seen in many tumor cells which may have relevance to the present discussion include the following (reviewed in reference 15):

1. excess production of PGE_2 and PGF_{2a}, which have immunosuppressive actions,
2. decrease in free radical generation with a relative increase in anti-oxidative capacity,
3. a decrease in the content of polyunsaturated fatty acids (i.e., c-UFAs),
4. an increase in polyamines, and
5. chromosomal abnormalities that may in part be responsible for the growth of, invasion by, and metastasis of tumor cells and the development of resistance to chemotherapeutic agents due to the overexpression of some oncogenes.

Though this list of metabolic events in the tumor cells is by no means exhaustive, these abnormalities are important to the present discussion.

Both PGE_2 and $PGF_{2\alpha}$ inhibit free radical generation, especially that of superoxide anion, in human neutrophils (16). Polyamines can block lipid peroxidation (15,17). These facts, coupled with the observation that tumor cells have low PUFA (c-UFAs) content (18,19) and relatively more anti-oxidant capacity (20), suggest that tumor cells have evolved a set of metabolic patterns such that there is a decrease in free radical generation. In addition, tumor cells have reduced oxidative and increased glycolytic metabolism (reviewed in reference 15). All of these metabolic events can render the tumor cells extremely sensitive to oxygen- and free radical-dependent cytotoxicity.

Tumoricidal Action of Cytokines and Anti-Cancer Drugs and Their Relationship to c-UFAs and Free Radicals

Several anti-cancer drugs also have the ability to augment free radical generation and enhance lipid peroxidation (reviewed in reference 21). This is supported by the fact that vitamin E, glutathione peroxidase, glutathione, and superoxide dismutase (SOD) can block the action of anti-cancer drugs and reduce toxicity, especially that of adriamycin both *in vitro* and *in vivo* (21). The anti-cancer drugs are able to generate free radicals by enhancing the activity of PLA_2 as indicated by the fact that doxorubicin-induced cardiomyopathy in rats can be inhibited by PLA_2 inhibitors (21). Because c-UFAs can trigger free radical generation (22–25), it is likely that anti-cancer drug-induced free radical generation may at least in part be dependent on the ability of anti-cancer drugs to induce the release of c-UFAs by activating PLA_2. If so, it is possible that a deficiency of c-UFAs and PLA_2 activity in the tumor cells may reduce both free radical generation and the lipid peroxidation process, which may ultimately lead to drug resistance. This relationship between free radical generation, lipid peroxidation, and tumor cell drug resistance has been discussed in detail elsewhere (21).

Similarly, even cytokines can enhance free radical generation and the lipid peroxidation process (26–29) and thus bring about their tumoricidal action. Interferon (IFN) and tumor necrosis factor (TNF) can activate PLA2 (reviewed in Ref. 21). C-UFAs seem to be crucial to the tumoricidal action of IFN and TNF and possibly other cytokines because inhibitors of PLA_2 can block the cytotoxic action of TNF (30), and IFN induces discrete and specific release of c-UFAs (31). Thus, there are many similarities between anti-cancer drugs and cytokines, especially with respect to their action on PLA_2 and c-UFA metabolism (21). If this is correct, the resistance of the tumor cells to the cytotoxic action of IFN and TNF could be secondary to the paucity of c-UFAs in these cells, and this resistance can be overcome by combining cytokines with c-UFAs (21,30). In fact, we observed that TNF-resistant tumor cells can be sensitized to the cytotoxic action of TNF by pretreatment of these cells with suboptimal doses of c-UFAs *in vitro* (Das, U.N., unpublished data). All of these results suggest that if free radical generation is augmented in the tumor cells, cell lysis can be achieved.

Tumoricidal Action of c-UFAs

Several studies (32–42) have shown that c-UFAs such as GLA, AA, EPA, and DHA can selectively kill tumor cells *in vitro*. Jett *et al.* (43) reported that liposomes comprised of plant phosphatidyl inositol (PI) and cholesterol in a 2:1 molar ratio can kill tumor cells in vitro. They noted that free LA and AA are released in significant quantities from PI liposomes after interaction with tumor cells and suggested that the release of free fatty acids (LA and AA) is probably responsible for the cytotoxicity of PI.

In our studies, the cytotoxic action of c-UFAs was found to be dose dependent (32–36,44). Normal MDCK and 41-SK cells (canine normal kidney cells and normal human fibroblasts, respectively) were affected only at AA or EPA doses two to three times the level that is effective in killing the tumor cells (32,33). Further, both virally and chemically transformed mouse fibroblasts but not normal ones can be selectively killed by GLA, AA, and EPA *in vitro* (unpublished data). This is supported by the work of Shimura *et al.* (45) who showed that the viability of rat 3Y1 fibroblasts transformed by adenovirus (AD) type 12 was markedly reduced by the administration of dilinoleoyl glycerol. On that basis, Shimura *et al.* (45) suggested that linoleic acid would be released abundantly in AD 12-transformed cells by PLA_2 or diacylglycerolipase. In an extension of this study, Matsuzaki *et al.* (46) demonstrated that the cytotoxicity of dilinoleonyl glycerol against E1A-transformed 3Y1 cells can be inhibited by the simultaneous administration of anti-oxidants or lipoxygenase inhibitors.

Studies have also suggested that different types of tumor cells show marked variations in their sensitivity to the cytotoxic action of various c-UFAs. For example, lymphoma and leukemia cells are exquisitely sensitive to the cytotoxic action of LA and ALA (unpublished data); human breast cancer cells are sensitive to GLA > AA > EPA and less sensitive to LA and ALA (32,33); human cervical carcinoma cells respond to DHA > EPA > GLA > AA and are almost insensitive to ALA (34); mouse myeloma cells are sensitive to EPA and ALA and are less sensitive to all of the n-6 fatty acids (44); whereas KB-3-1 and KB-8-5 (variants of HeLa) cells are easily killed by EPA, DHA, and GLA (47,48). In general, all types of tumor cells that have been tested were found to be sensitive to the cytotoxic action of at least one type of c-UFA, and the most effective fatty acids seem to be GLA, EPA and DHA. It is also important to note that several studies performed by us and other workers have suggested that GLA, EPA, and DHA can also cause regression of tumor growth *in vivo* (49–53).

Free Radicals as Mediators of the Cytotoxic Action of c-UFAs

Anti-oxidants such as vitamin E, BHA and BHT (butylated hydroxyanisole and butylated hydroxytoluene, respectively), and superoxide dismutase (SOD) can completely block the cytotoxic action of c-UFAs (32–36), indicating a role for free radicals and the lipid peroxidation process. GLA, AA, EPA, and DHA can selectively enhance both superoxide anion and hydrogen peroxide generation and the levels of lipid peroxides in the tumor but not in normal cells (33,35). Further, the uptake of AA and EPA is low in tumor cells compared with normal cells, which is in contrast to the amount of free radicals generated (25), suggesting that the low rates of lipid peroxidation and free radical generation in tumor cells could be due to their low c-UFA content (20) and to decreased activity of NADPH, cytochrome C reductase and cytochrome P-450 (reviewed in reference 21).

There does not seem to be a role for eicosanoids in c-UFA-induced cytotoxicity because both cyclo-oxygenase (CO) and lipoxygenase (LO) inhibitors did not block the cytotoxic action of c-UFAs on human breast, KB-3-1 and KB-8-5 cells (33,47). On the other hand, both CO and LO inhibitors were effective in blocking c-UFA-induced cytotoxicity of human cervical carcinoma cells (34). These results indicate that in some tumor cells free radical generation is dependent on CO and LO enzymes (34,35). In a recent study, we noted that c-UFAs can alter the cellular content of diacyglycerol and protein kinase C which may be responsible for the changes in free radical generation in the tumor cells (Padma, M., and Das, U.N., unpublished data).

Jett and Alving (54) documented a dramatic drop in the uptake of inositol after incubation of tumor cells with plant PI liposomes but not in normal cells or with tumor cells exposed to liposomes of animal PI. This indicates that interference with PI turnover may be an important early event in cytotoxicity for tumor cells. This is particularly interesting because oncogenes and growth factors induce cell growth by the activation of PI turnover, which releases second messengers, diacylglycerol and inositol triphosphate (21,55). It is possible that c-UFAs, free radicals and lipid peroxides may inhibit tumor cell growth by inhibiting the formation of cyclins and cyclin-dependent kinases because lipid peroxides can inhibit mitosis, whereas cyclins trigger cell proliferation. But this suggestion has to be studied and verified.

It is evident from the above discussion that c-UFAs (such as GLA, AA, EPA, and DHA), anti-cancer drugs and cytokines seem to mediate their cytotoxic actions by inducing the generation of free radicals and by enhancing lipid peroxidation. If this is true, is it possible that c-UFAs can be used to eliminate tumor cells in the patient?

γ-Linolenic Acid for the Therapy of Human Gliomas

At present there is no satisfactory treatment for malignant cerebral glioma. Even after aggressive surgery, radiation and chemotherapy, the median survival of patients with human glioma is less than 1 y. The median survival following satisfactory surgery alone is less than 17 wk whereas radiotherapy can prolong the survival to not more than 36 wk. In the majority of patients, treatment failures occur because of local recurrence, suggesting that a more aggressive local therapy of the tumor could be beneficial. It is precisely for these reasons that we have selected human malignant glioma for our clinical study. Further, it is easy to know the effect of the treatment and to follow these patients because the size and progress of the tumor can be conveniently assessed by CT (computerized axial tomography) scan of the brain.

For our preliminary study (56), we selected patients who had (a) histological and radiological (including CT scan) evidence of malignant glioma, (b) clinical and/or radiological evidence of residual tumor after the last course of radiotherapy and/or surgery and (c) a tumor of sufficient size to warrant further therapy. Thus only those patients who had already undergone surgery and radiotherapy with or without chemotherapy and who came to the hospital with recurrence were selected for GLA therapy.

The first six patients recruited for this study (see Ref. 56 for details) demonstrated that injection of GLA from the 8th day after neurosurgical procedure at the rate of 1 mg/d for 10 consecutive days can induce significant necrosis and regression of the tumor. Of the six patients studied, three are still alive and the follow-up period varied from 4 to 5 y. Repeat CT scans have not shown any increase in the size of the residual tumor or recurrence. The most remarkable aspect of this study is that none of the patients showed any neurological, wound or systemic complications following GLA therapy.

In an extension of this study, intratumoral GLA administration was performed in another 15 patients since December 1991. In these patients, unlike in the earlier study, after the neurosurgical procedure and before the closure of the dura, 1 mg of GLA was instilled into the tumor bed and a cerebral catheter was placed in the cavity with the reservoir located on the bone flap under the galea for subsequent injections. These patients with malignant glioma did not undergo any radiotherapy or chemotherapy before entering the study and thus were considered to have undergone GLA therapy for the primary tumor. On the 7th post-operative day, a CT scan of the brain with and without contrast was obtained which was compared with the CT scans obtained following subsequent GLA therapy. One milligram of GLA was instilled every day through the cerebral reservoir for the next 10 d. After GLA therapy, a repeat CT scan was done with and without contrast for post-GLA therapy morphology. After the completion of GLA therapy, all of the patients received standard radiotherapy.

In all of the 15 patients studied, a striking change in the morphology of the tumor was noted in the CT scans. The high density regions (indicating the presence of the tumor) of the gliomas have turned into areas of lesser density (indicating necrosis of the tumor), and an increase in the cystic area was observed. The mass effect and the midline shifts of the brain tissue were also reduced to a significant degree.

These patients have now been followed for more than 2 y (Table 22.1). Twelve patients are still on regular follow-up and are devoid of any significant complications. Three patients (serial no. 6,7, and 14) died after 5 to 6 mo following GLA and radiotherapy due to causes unrelated to GLA therapy. Further details of this study have been submitted for publication.

To determine whether GLA has any effect on normal brain cells, GLA (0.25 mg/d) was injected into the frontal lobe of three normal dogs for six days. On the 7th day, i.e., 24 h after the last GLA injection, CT scan and histopathological examination of their brains did not show any abnormality (unpublished data). This study suggests that GLA is not toxic to normal brain cells.

Conclusions

Cancer therapy aims to eliminate tumor cells selectively without harming the normal cells, a task which is rarely achieved at present. Even adoptive immunotherapy using lypmphokine-activated killer cells and interleukin-2 (IL-2) for human gliomas did not induce regression of the tumor, and in fact, the majority of the patients showed significant side effects (57). In comparison, the results of our studies with GLA in human gliomas suggest that GLA is very effective without producing any side effects (56 and Table 22.1).

In addition, GLA and other c-UFAs can also reverse tumor cell drug resistance (48). In a recent study, we demonstrated that vincristine-resistant KB-8-5 (a variant of HeLa) cells and HeLa cells can be sensitized to the cytotoxic action of vincristine by exposing them to suboptimal doses of GLA, AA, EPA, and DHA (48,58). C-UFAs

TABLE 22.1 Details of Patients Treated with Intratumoral Injection of γ-Linolenic Acid

No.	Age, Sex	Site of tumor	Diagnosis	Date of entry into the study	Present status
1.	60, F	Lt. Temporal	GBM (Gr.IV)	Dec. 91	AUF
2.	55, M	Lt. Parietal	GBM (Gr.IV)	Dec. 91	AUF
3.	46, M	Lt. Parietal	MMG	Dec. 91	AUF
4.	55, F	Bifrontal	MMG	Dec. 91	AUF
5.	55, M	Lt. Parietal	GBM (Gr.IV)	Dec. 91	AUF
6.	74, M	Rt. Parietal	AA (Gr.III)	Dec. 91	Dead
7.	65, M	Lt. Parietooccipital	GBM (Gr.IV)	Dec. 91	Dead
8.	45, M	Lt. FTP	AA (Gr.III)	Jan. 92	AUF
9.	60, M	Rt. Temperoparietal	MA (Gr.III)	Jan. 92	AUF
10.	43, F	Rt. Frontal	MMG	Jan. 92	AUF
11.	40, M	Rt. Temporal	GBM (Gr.IV)	Jan. 92	AUF
12.	60, F	Lt. Temperoparietal	GBM (Gr.IV)	Feb. 92	AUF
13.	45, M	Lt. Frontal	AA (Gr.III)	Feb. 92	AUF
14.	65, F	Lt. Parietal	AA (Gr.III)	July 92	Dead
15.	40, M	Bifrontal	AA (Gr.III)	June 92	AUF

Abbreviations: GBM = Glioblastoma multiforme, AA = Anaplastic astrocytoma, MMG = Malignant mixed glioma, MA = Malignant astrocytoma. AUF = No fresh symptoms and under follow-up. Rt. = Right side, Lt. = Left side, FTP = Frontotemperoparietal.

enhanced the uptake of the anti-cancer drug and inhibited drug efflux, thus augmenting the intracellular concentration of the anti-cancer drugs (48). This could be one, if not the sole, mechanism(s) by which these fatty acids can reverse drug resistance. Further, drug-resistant cells were found to contain low amounts of GLA, AA, and DHA (47). In addition, it was observed that c-UFAs, especially ALA and EPA, can reduce the levels of anti-oxidants such as glutathione, SOD and glutathione peroxidase in mouse myeloma cells in vitro (44). This indicates that c-UFAs are able to tilt the balance between pro-oxidants and anti-oxidants further towards the pro-oxidant system so that the tumor cells are made more vulnerable to the oxidant stress. Because enhanced levels of anti-oxidants could be one of the causes for tumor cell drug resistance, these results suggest that GLA and other c-UFAs will also be effective against drug-resistant tumors.

Because GLA is not toxic to normal cells, it is possible that GLA may be useful in the treatment of other cancers. For example, in hepatoma, GLA can be administered by selective catheterization of the blood vessel feeding the tumor. In a preliminary study, we did observe that GLA is effective against primary hepatoma by this mode of administration (Das, U.N., unpublished data). Similar approaches can be made in the treatment of virtually any tumor by using GLA and other c-UFAs because it is now possible to gain access to any tumor situated anywhere in the body either by selective catheterization of the tumor-feeding blood vessel and/or by using fiber optic instruments (such as endoscopy, colonoscopy, bronchoscopy, etc.). Thus, further studies are required to evaluate the anti-cancer properties of GLA and other c-UFAs in various malignancies, and our studies suggest that, at least for human gliomas, GLA is not only safe but is also an effective agent.

Acknowledgments

Some of the work reported here was supported by grants from the Indian Council of Medical Research, Department of Science and Technology, India, and Scotia Pharmaceuticals Limited, U.K. to Dr. U.N. Das.

References

1. Das, U.N. Essential Fatty Acids: Biology and Their Clinical Implications (1991) *Asia Pacific J. Pharmacol. 6,* 317–330.
2. Das, U.N., Horrobin, D.F., Begin, M.E., Huang, Y.-S., Cunnane, S.C., Manku, M.S., and Nassar, B.A. Clinical Significance of Essential Fatty Acids (1988) *Nutrition. 4,* 337–341.
3. Tanaka, H., Yamamoto, T., Matsumoto, M., Kotoura, Y., and Tanaka, C. The Effect of PGD2 and 9-Deoxy-9-PGD2 on Colony Formation of Murine Osteosarcoma Cells (1985) *Prostaglandins 30,* 167–173.
4. Sakai, T., Yamaguchi, N., Shiroko, Y., Fujii, C., and Nishino, H. Prosaglandin D2 Inhibits the Proliferation of Human Malignant Tumor Cells (1984) *Prostaglandins. 27,* 17–26.
5. Myers, R.F., and Siegel, M.I. The Appearance of Phospholipase Activity in the Human Macrophage-like Cell Line U937 During Dimethyl-Sulfoxide-Induced Differentiation (1984) *Biochem. Biophys. Res. Comun. 30,* 167–174.

6. Bonser, R.W., Siegel, M.I., McConnell, R.T., and Perdrocuatrecasas, P. The Appearance of Phospholipase and Cyclo-Oxygenase Activities in the Human Promyelocytic Leukemia Cell Line HL-60 During Dimethyl-Sulfoxide-Induced Differentiation (1981) *Biochem. Biophys. Res. Commun. 98,* 614–620.
7. Dunbar, L.M., and Bailey, J.M. Enzyme Deletions and Essential Fatty Acid Metabolism in Cultured Cells (1975) *J. Biol. Chem. 250,* 1152–1153.
8. Jaffe, B.M. Prostaglandins and Cancer: An Update (1974) *Prostaglandins 6,* 453–465.
9. Das, U.N. Inhibition of Sensitized Lymphocyte Response to Sperm Antigen(s) by Prostaglandins (1981) *IRCS Med. Sci. 9,* 1087.
10. Devi, G.R., Das, U.N., Rao, K.P., and Rao, M.S. Prostaglandins and Their Precursors Can Modify Genetic Damage Induced by Benzo(a)pyrene and Gamma-Radiation (1985) *Prostaglandins 29,* 911–920.
11. Nassar, B.A., Das, U.N., Huang, Y.-S., Ells, G., and Horrobin, D.F. The Effect of Chemical Hepatocarcinogenesis on Liver Phospholipid Composition in Rats Fed n-6 and n-3 Fatty Acid-supplemented Diets (1992) *Proc. Soc. Exp. Biol. Med. 199,* 365–368.
12. Das, U.N., Devi, G.R., Rao, K.P., and Rao, M.S. Benzo(a)pyrene and Gamma-Radiation-Induced Genetic Damage in Mice Can Be Prevented by Gamma-linolenic Acid but Not by Arachidonic Acid (1985) *Nutr. Res. 5,* 101–106.
13. Das, U.N., Begin, M.E., and Ells, G. Precursors of Prostaglandins and Other n-6 Essential Fatty Acids Can Modify Benzo(a)pyrene-Induced Chromosomal Damage to Human Lymphocytes *in Vitro* (1987) *Nutr. Rep. Int. 36,* 1276–1271.
14. Renner, H.W., and Declincee, H. Different Anti-Mutagenic Actions of Linoleic and Linolenic Acid Derivatives on Busulfan-Induced Genotoxicity in Chinese Hamtser Cells (1988) *Nutr. Res. 8,* 635–642.
15. Das, U.N. Gamma-linolenic Acid, Arachidonic Acid, and Eicosapentaenoic Acid as Potential Anticancer Drugs (1990) *Nutrition 6,* 429–434.
16. Gryglewski, R.J., and Wandzilak, M. The Effect of Six Prostaglandins, Prostacyclin and Iloprost on Generation of Superoxide Anions by Human Polymorphonuclear Leukocytes Stimulated by Zymosan or Formyl-methionyl-leucyl-phenyl-alanine (1987) *Biochem. Pharmacol. 36,* 4209–4212.
17. Tadolini, B. Polyamine Inhibition of Lipoperoxidation (1988) *Biochem. J. 249,* 33–36.
18. Dianzani, M.W. Lipid Peroxidation and Cancer: A Critical Reconsideration (1989) *Tumorigenesis 75,* 351–357.
19. Rossi, M.A., and Cecchini, G. Lipid Peroxidation in Hepatomas of Different Degrees of Deviation (1983) *Cell. Biochem. Funct. 1,* 49–54.
20. Cheeseman, K.H., Collins, M., Proudfoot, K., and Slater, T.F. Studies on Lipid Peroxidation in Normal and Tumor Tissues. The Novikoff Rat Liver Tumor (1989) *Biochem. J. 235,* 507–514.
21. Das, U.N. *Cis*-Unsaturated Fatty Acids as Potential Anti-Mutagenic, Tumoricidal, and Anti-Metastatic Agents (1992) *Asia Pacific. J. Pharmacol. 7,* 305–327.
22. Badway, J.A., Curnutte, J.M., and Karnovsky, M.C. *Cis*-Unsaturated Fatty Acids Induce High Levels of Superoxide Production by Human Neutrophils (1981) *J. Biol. Chem. 265,* 12640–12643.
23. Das, U.N., Begin, M.E., Ells, G., and Horrobin, D.F. Polyunsaturated Fatty Acids Augment Free Radical Generation in Tumor Cells *in Vitro* (1987) *Biochem. Biophys. Res. Commun. 145,* 15–24.

24. Sangeetha, P.S., Das, U.N., and Koratkar, R. Free Radical Generation in Human Leukocytes by *Cis*-Unsaturated Fatty Acids Is a Calmodulin-Dependent Process (1990) *Prostaglandins Leukotrienes Essen. Fatty Acids 39,* 27–30.
25. Das, U.N., Huang, Y.-S., Begin, M.E., Ells, G., and Horrobin, D.F. Uptake and Distribution of *Cis*-Unsaturated Fatty Acids and Their Effect on Free Radical Generation in Normal and Tumor Cells *in Vitro* (1987) *Free Radical Biol. Med. 3,* 9–14.
26. Ghezzi, P., Bianchi, M., Mantovani, A., Spreafici, F., and Salmona, M. Enhanced Xanthine Oxidase Activity in Mice Treated with Interferon and Interferon Inducers (1984) *Biochem. Biophys. Res. Commun. 119,* 144–149.
27. Das, U.N., Ells, G., Begin, M.E., and Horrobin, D.F. Free Radicals as Possible Mediators of the Actions of Interferon (1986) *Free Radical Biol. Med. 2,* 183–188.
28. Berton, G., Zeni, L., Cassatello, M.A., and Rossi, F. Gamma-Interferon Is Able to Enhance the Oxidative Metabolism of Human Neutrophils (1986) *Biochem. Biophys. Res. Commun. 138,* 1276–1282.
29. Tsujimoto, M., Yokota S., Vilcek, J., and Weissman, G. Tumor Necrosis Factor Provokes Superoxide Anion Generation from Neutrophils (1986) *Biochem. Biophys. Res. Commun. 137,* 1094–1100.
30. Hepburn, A., Boeynaems, J.M., Fiers, W., and Dumont, J.E. Modulation of Tumor Necrosis Factor-alpha Cytotoxicity in L929 Cells by Bacterial Toxins, Hydrocortisone, and Inhibitors of Arachidonic Acid Metabolism (1987) *Biochem. Biophys. Res. Commun. 149,* 815–822.
31. Chandrabose, K., Cuatrecasas, P., and Pottathil, R. Changes in Fatty Acyl Chains of Phospholipids by Interferon in Mouse Sarcoma S-180 Cells (1981) *Biochem. Biophys. Res. Commun. 98,* 661–668.
32. Begin, M.E., Das, U.N., Ells, G., and Horrobin, D.F. Selective Killing of Human Cancer Cells by Polyunsaturated Fatty Acids (1985) *Prostaglandins Leukotrienes Med. 19,* 177–186.
33. Das, U.N. Tumoricidal Action of *Cis*-Unsaturated Fatty Acids and its Relationship to Free Radicals and Lipid Peroxidation (1991) *Cancer Lett. 56,* 235–243.
34. Sangeetha, P.S., Das, U.N., Koratkar, R., Ramesh, G., Padma, M., and Sravan Kumar, G. Cytotoxic Action of *Cis*-Unsaturated Fatty Acids on Human Cervical Carcinoma (HeLa) Cells: Relationship to Free Radicals and Lipid Peroxidation and Its Modulation by Calmodulin Antagonists (1992) *Cancer Lett. 63,* 189–198.
35. Das, U.N. (1990) in *Biological Oxidation Systems,* Reddy, C.C., Madyastha, K., and Hamilton, A.K., eds., Academic Press, NY, vol. 2, pp. 607–624.
36. Begin, M.E., Ells, G., Das, U.N., and Horrobin, D.F. Differential Killing of Human Carcinoma Cells Supplemented with n-3 and n-6 Polyunsaturated Fatty Acids (1986) *J. Natl. Cancer Inst. 77,* 1053–1062.
37. Booyens, J., Dippenaar, N., and Fabri, D. The Effect of Prostaglandin Precursor Gamma-Linolenic Acid on the Rate of Proliferation of Human Osteogenic Sarcoma and Oesophageal Carcinoma Cells in Culture (1984) *S. Afr. Med. J. 65,* 240–242.
38. Tolnai, S., and Morgan, J. F. Studies on the in Vitro Anti-tumor Activity of Fatty Acids. V. Unsaturated Fatty Acids. (1962) *Can. J. Biochem. Physiol. 40,* 869–885.
39. Seigel, I., Liu, T.L., Yoghoubzadeh, E., Keskey, T.S., and Gleichner, N. Cytotoxic Effects of Free Acids on Ascites Tumor Cells (1987) *J. Natl. Cancer Inst. 78,* 271–277.
40. Das, U.N. Oxy Radicals and Their Clinical Implications (1993) *Curr. Sci. 65,* 964–968.

41. Leary, W.P., Robinson, K.M., Booyens, J., and Dippenaar, N. Some Effects of Gamma-Linolenic Acid on Cultured Human Oesophageal Carcinoma Cells (1987) *S. Afr. Med. J.* 62, 681–683.
42. Sangeetha, P.S., and Das, U.N. Cytotoxic Action of *Cis*-Unsaturated Fatty Acids on Human Cervical Carcinoma (HeLa) Cells *in Vitro* (1995) Prostaglandins Leukotrienes Essen. Fatty Acids (in press).
43. Jett, M., Chudzik, J., Alving, C.R., and Stanacev, N.Z. Metabolic Fate of Liposomal Phosphotidylinositol in Murine Tumor Cells: Implications for the Mechanism of Tumor Cell Cytotoxicity (1985) *Cancer Res.* 45, 4810–4815.
44. Kumar, S.G., and Das, U.N. Free Radical Dependent Suppression of Growth of Mouse Myeloma Cells by Alpha-linolenic and Eicosapentaenoic Acids in Vitro (1995) *Cancer Lett.* (in press).
45. Shimura, H., Ohtsu, M., Matsuzaki, A., Mitsudoni, T., Onodera, K., and Kimura, G. Selective Cytotoxicity of Phospholipids and Diacylglycerol to Rat 3Y1 Fibroblasts Transformed by Adenovirus Type 12 or Its E1A Genome Gene (1988) *Cancer Res.* 48, 578–583.
46. Matsuzaki, A., Shimura, H., Okuda, A., Ohtsu, M., Sasaki, M., Onodera, K., and Kimura, G. Mechanism of Selective Killing by Dilinoleoylglycerol of Cells Transformed by the E1A Gene of Adenovirus Type 12 (1989) *Cancer Res.* 49, 5702–5707.
47. Madhavi, N., and Das, U.N. Effect of n-6 and n-3 Fatty Acids on the Survival of Vincristine Sensitive and Resistant Human Cervical Carcinoma Cells *in Vitro* (1994) *Cancer Lett.* 84, 31–41.
48. Madhavi, N., and Das, U.N. Reversal of Tumor (KB-3-1 and KB-Ch-8-5) Cell Drug-Resistance by *Cis*-Unsaturated Fatty Acids *in Vitro* (1994) *Med. Sci. Res.* 22, 689–692.
49. Ramesh, G., Das, U.N., Koratkar, R., Padma, M., and Sangeetha, P.S. Effect of Essential Fatty Acids on Tumor Cells (1992) *Nutrition* 8, 343–347.
50. Karmali, R.A., Marsh, J., and Fuchs, C. Effect of Omega-3 Fatty Acids on Growth of a Rat Mammary Tumor (1984) *J. Natl. Cancer Inst.* 73, 457–461.
51. El-Ela, S.H.A., Prasse, K.W., Carroll, R., and Bunce, O.R. Effects of Dietary Primrose Oil on Mammary Tumorigenesis Induced by 7,12-Dimethyl Benz(a)anthracene (1987) *Lipids* 22, 1041–1045.
52. Zhu, Y.P., Su, Z.W., and Li, C.H. Growth Inhibition of Effect of Oleic Acid, Linoleic Acid, and Their Methylesters on Transplanted Tumors in Mice (1989) *J. Natl. Cancer Inst.* 81, 1302–1306.
53. Gabor, H., and Abraham, S. Effect of Dietary Manhadon Oil on Tumor Cell Loss and the Accumulation of Mass of a Transplantable Mammary Adenocarcinoma in BALB/c Mice (1986) *J. Natl. Cancer Inst.* 76, 1223–1229.
54. Jett, M., and Alving, C.R. (1985) in *Inositol and Phosphoinositides*, Bleasdale, J.E., Eichberg, J., and Hauser, G., eds., Humana Press, Clifton, NJ, pp. 91–95.
55. Das, U.N., Huang, Y.-S., Begin, M.E., and Horrobin, D.F. Interferons, Phospholipid Metabolism, Immune Responses and Cancer (1986) *IRCS. J. Med. Sci.* 14, 1069–1072.
56. Naidu, M.R.C., Das, U.N., and Kishan, A. Intra-Tumoral Gamma-Linolenic Acid Therapy of Human Gliomas (1992) *Prostaglandins Leukotrienes Essen. Fatty Acids* 45, 181–184.
57. Barba, D., Saris, S.C., Holder, C., Rosenberg, S.A., and Oldfield, E.H. Intratumoral LAK Cell and Interleukin-2 Therapy of Human Gliomas (1989) *J. Neurosurg.* 70, 175–182.
58. Sangeetha, P., and Das, U.N. Gamma-Linolenic Acid and Eicosapentaenoic Acid Potentiate the Cytotoxicity of Anti-Cancer Drugs on Human Cervical Carcinoma (HeLa) Cells *in Vitro* (1993) *Med. Sci. Res.* 21, 457–459.

Chapter 23

Metabolism of Li-γ-Linolenate (LiGLA) in Human Prostate, Ovarian, and Pancreatic Carcinomas Grown in Nude Mice

R.J. de Antueno, M. Elliot, K. Jenkins, G.W. Ells, and D.F. Horrobin

Efamol Research Institute, P.O. Box 818, Kentville, NS, Canada B4N 4H8

Introduction

There is accumulating evidence that polyunsaturated fatty acids (PUFAs), particularly γ-linolenic acid (GLA, 18:3n-6) and eicosapentaenoic acid (20:5n-3), have anti-tumor and/or anti-proliferative effects (1,2). They may circumvent the Δ6-desaturase deficiency of some malignant cells and/or improve the low levels of PUFAs detected in certain cancer patients (3,4). The altered PUFA pattern may enable the tumor to produce either free radicals, lipid peroxides and/or prostaglandins, many of which have anti-tumor properties (5–7).

Over 30 human cancer cell lines have now been tested in the presence of 18:3n-6 and related essential fatty acids (1). γ-Linolenic acid and its elongation product, dihomo-γ-linolenic acid (20:3n-6), and 20:5n-3 have no harmful effects on normal cells at concentrations which kill malignant cells. In contrast, arachidonic acid (20:4n-6), the Δ5-desaturation product of 20:3n-6, exhibits cytotoxic effects on cancer cells but also frequently harms normal cell lines (7).

Recent reports showed that 18:3n-6 reduced the motility and invasiveness of cancer cells within hours of exposure (8). *In vitro* studies have been followed by nude mouse studies in which 18:3n-6 has been shown to inhibit the growth of transplanted human lung mucoepidermoid carcinoma, breast cancer and malignant melanoma (9,10).

Triglyceride, ester or even free fatty acid forms of 18:3n-6 are appropriate for oral administration, whereas the alkaline salts of fatty acids can be conveniently used for intravenous administration (11,12). Exploration of possible routes of delivering drugs in patients has led to the concept of intravenous administration of a relatively water-soluble lithium salt of 18:3n-6. Potassium salts were discarded because of their potential cardiac effects. The lithium salt has an advantage over the sodium salt in that the rate of infusion could be easily determined by measuring the lithium blood concentrations with analytical techniques routinely available in most hospitals. Lithium-γ-linolenate (LiGLA, Li-18:3n-6) had no important adverse effects and, in particular, none of the serious effects commonly associated with chemotherapy (12). Any toxicity of lithium could be avoided by keeping its blood concentration during infusions below 0.7 mM, which is lower than the concentration used in psychiatric treatments when levels of 0.1–1.0 mM may be maintained for many years. LiGLA has been shown to be a promising experimental compound for the treatment of human cancers. Indeed, LiGLA had a highly significant effect in improving survival of pancreatic cancer patients as assessed by the Cox proportional hazards mode, regression analysis and other statistical techniques (12). However, little is known about the distribution and metabolism of LiGLA among tissues, including the tumor tissue. This information is essential in order to understand the mechanism of action for LiGLA cytotoxicity on cancer cells and for the development of better delivery systems.

In the present study, we examined the uptake, elongation and further desaturation of LiGLA by selected host tissues and three human tumors with different growth rates in athymic mice. Conditions were specifically designed to mimic, as much as possible in this animal model, the infusion protocol followed with cancer patients (11,12).

Materials and Methods

Animals and Tumor Tissue

Seven-week-old athymic CD1BR (nu/nu) mice were obtained from Charles River Canada Inc. (St. Constant, Quebec, Canada) and given free access to γ-irradiated chow diet and sterile water (pH 2.5) in a pathogen-temperature controlled environment ($25 \pm 1°C$) with a 12-h light:dark cycle.

PC-3 and AsPC-1 cells (human prostate and pancreatic carcinomas, respectively) were grown in Dulbecco's modification of Eagle's medium (DMEM; containing 10% fetal bovine serum [FBS], penicillin [50 IU/mL], and streptomycin [50 μg/mL]). OVCAR-3 cells (human ovarian carcinoma) were grown in RPMI 1640 medium supplemented with 20% FBS and antibiotics. Cell culture media and supplements were obtained from ICN Biomedicals Inc., Costa Mesa, CA. All cell lines were suspended in their growth medium and Matrigel (1:1 v/v; Collaborative Research Inc., Bedford, MA). Male mice were injected subcutaneously into the interscapular region with 300 μL of the suspension containing 5×10^6 of either AsPC-1 or PC-3 cells, whereas female mice were injected with the same amount of OVCAR-3 cells.

When tumors became palpable, they were measured twice weekly with slide calipers and the volume was calculated for an ellipsoid using the formula $V = l \times w \times h/2$, where l is the length, w is the width, and h is the height, in millimeters.

LiGLA Infusion and Lipid Analysis

At approximately 300 mm^3 tumor volume, animals were anesthetized with sodium pentobarbital (80 mg/kg; Somnotol, MTC, Ontario, Canada). Mice were then given 125 μL of 0.9% NaCl with 200 IU/kg of heparin and 14 μCi of Li [1-^{14}C]-GLA (radiochemical purity > 98%; specific activity, 52 μCi/μmol; New England Nuclear, Boston, MA) by slow intravenous injection through the tail vein [2.53 mg/(kg·30 min)] using a pediatric 27 G butterfly and infusion pump.

Mice were killed either immediately after the 30-min infusions or left for recovery for either 0.5, 1, 6, 24, 48, 72, or 96 h until exsanguination under Halothane anesthesia.

Organs were perfused and rinsed with cold 0.9% NaCl and blotted dry. Aliquots of each tissue were solubilized with Solvable 0.5 M (New England Nuclear) at 56°C. To reduce chemiluminescence, samples were decolorized with hydrogen peroxide and neutralized with glacial acetic acid before adding the cocktail (Formula 989, New England Nuclear) for scintillation counting.

Lipids from organ and tumor tissues were extracted with chloroform/methanol (2:1, v/v) according to the method of Folch *et al.* (13). The total lipid extract was methylated using BF_3 in methanol at 90°C for 30 min (14). The resultant radiolabeled fatty acid methyl esters (FAMEs) were analyzed as previously described (15). Analyses were carried out on a Waters Associates (Milford, MA) high performance liquid chromatograph equipped with a variable wavelength UV-vis monitor (set at 205 nm), a radioisotope detector (model 171, Beckman, Fullerton, CA) with a solid scintillator cartridge (97% efficiency for ^{14}C-detection) and an ultrasphere ODS column 25 cm × 4.6 mm i.d. (5-μm particle size, Beckman). FAMEs were separated isocratically with acetonitrile:water (95:5 v/v) at a flow rate of 1 mL/min and were identified by comparison with authentic standards.

Results

Tumor Growth

The tumor take (100%) and the time between the injection and a palpable tumor size (latency period, 6–8 d) of AsPC-1, PC-3 and OVCAR-3 cells suspended in Matrigel were all similar (Fig. 23.1). The volume-doubling times (VDT) calculated in the exponential growth phase between 200 and 400 mm^3 (16), were 8 and 16 d for AsPC-1 and PC-3, respectively, whereas the OVCAR-3 carcinoma showed a much longer lag phase with the same VDT as PC-3.

Radiolabeled Fatty Acid Uptake

Figure 23.2 shows the radioactivity recovered in different tissues expressed as a percentage of injected dose per gram of tissue at 0 and 96 h after the slow intravenous infusion of Li [^{14}C]-GLA. To simplify the graph, intermediate time point values were omitted. Because results obtained from PC-3, AsPC-1, and OVCAR-3 were very similar, only PC-3 data are shown as representative of all three tumor tissues. An unidentified radiolabeled compound that may be 22:3n-6, the direct elongation product of 20:3n-6, was included in the figures.

There were considerable variations in the radioactivity per tissue weight among the different organs. At 0.5 h after the infusion, most of the radioactivity was contained in liver, lungs, and urine. The radiolabeled recoveries per gram (or mL) in different tissues ranked as follows: liver, urine, lung, kidneys, heart, spleen, pancreas, plasma, brain, tumor, testes, fat, and red blood cells. In general, the organs showed a maximum uptake of radioactivity within 0.5–1 h after infusion. Thereafter, the percentage of radioactivity declined below 1% at 96 h following infusion. The average

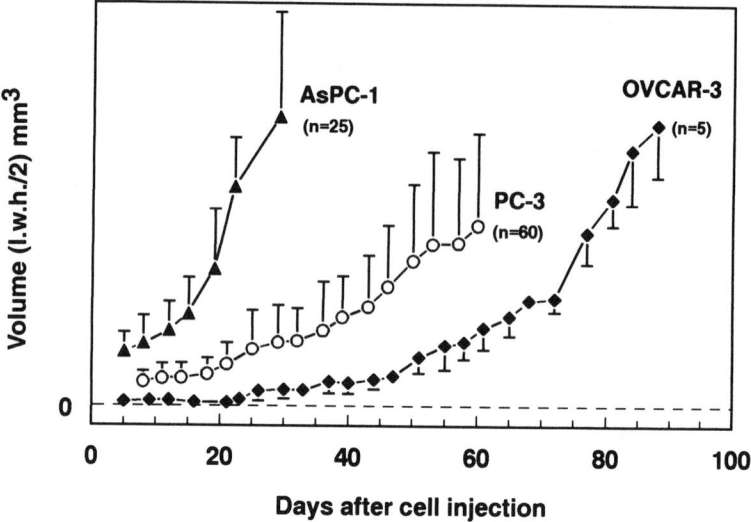

Fig. 23.1. Growth rates of PC-3, AsPC-1, and OVCAR-3 (human prostate, pancreatic, and ovarian carcinomas, respectively) in athymic mice. Animals were injected with malignant cells suspended in a 1:1 (v/v) solution of their growing medium and Matrigel. Tumor volume was measured with slide calipers and calculated for an ellipsoid using the formula $V = l \times w \times h/2$, where l is the length, w is the width, and h the height, in millimeters. Values are the mean ± SD of at least 5 mice.

radioactivity in fat tissue increased by 40% at that time point, whereas kidneys, brain, testes and tumor tissue labeling remained constant throughout the experiment. The differences between the radioactivity in liver and tumor tissue were about 22-fold and 0.45-fold at 0.5 and 96 h after infusion, respectively.

GLA Metabolites

The tissue distribution of specific GLA metabolites was determined for mice bearing the PC-3 tumors. We examined the tissues for the presence of radiolabeled elongation and Δ5-desaturation products of 18:3n-6 (Fig. 23.3). Data from plasma were also included.

All tissues showed a progressive increase in the proportion of radioactivity associated with 20:3n-6 and 20:4n-6 with a concomitant decrease in radiolabeled 18:3n-6 as the time after infusion increased. It is noticeable that 72 h after infusion, 18:3n-6 was detected only in plasma and tumor tissue, whereas 20:3n-6 declined at a much slower rate in brain and tumor tissue.

Figure 23.4 shows the similarities detected in the distribution of radioactivity among 18:3n-6 metabolites of OVCAR-3 and AsPC-1 tumors and selected host tissues to those found with PC-3 carcinoma at 0.5 h (Fig. 23.3). The levels of 20:4n-6 are slightly higher in liver and brain of mice bearing AsPC-1 tumors than in those from mice with PC-3 or OVCAR-3 carcinomas. However, at 96 h after infusion, the

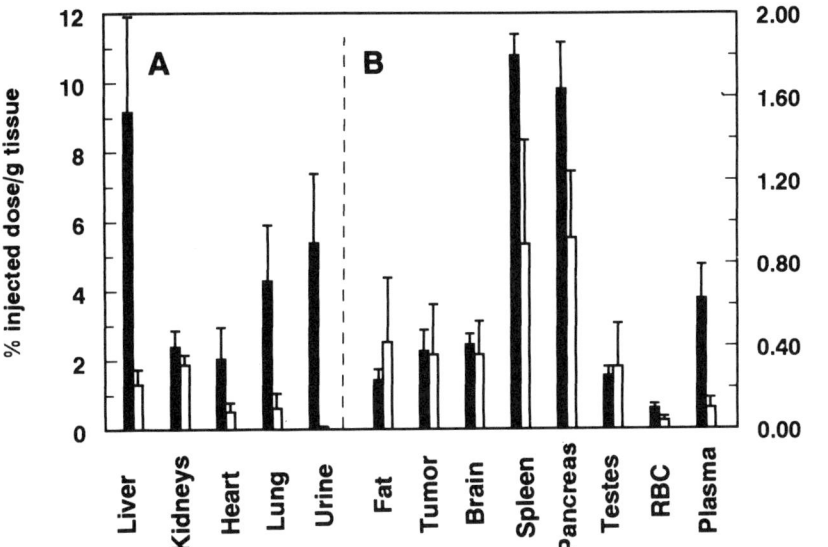

Fig. 23.2. Tissue distribution, as percentage of injected dose/g tissue at 0.5 (■) and 96(□) h post-injection for Li¹⁴C-GLA. Nude mice bearing a human prostate carcinoma (PC-3) received an intravenous infusion of 14 μCi of Li¹⁴C-GLA for 30 min. Data in panels A and B are referred to the left and right y axes, respectively. Abbreviation: RBC, red blood cells. Values are the mean ± SD of at least 4 mice.

radiolabeled fatty acid profiles were almost identical in all three carcinomas and host tissues (data not shown).

When these data were calculated in terms of nmol per gram of tissue, the findings were also consistent with those based on the percentage data. For example, at 72 h, the liver contents of 20:3n-6 and 20:4n-6 were 0.64 and 5.54 nmol/g, respectively, whereas in tumor the levels of 18:3n-6, 20:3n-6 and 20:4n-6 were 0.11, 0.45 and 0.88 nmol/g, respectively. This represents a concentration of about 0.4 μg of total n-6 PUFAs produced from Li [¹⁴C]-GLA per milliliter of tumor tissue, assuming unit density of malignant tissue (17).

When ratios of fatty acid products to substrates are plotted *vs.* time, it is clearly seen that tumor and brain tissues maintained a lower ratio of 20:4n-6/20:3n-6 than plasma and liver tissue (Fig. 23.5A). In tumor tissue, the ratio slowly increased in a similar fashion as in plasma, whereas in liver the ratio reached a plateau at 72 h. The inclusion of 18:3n-6 in this ratio did not substantially change the profiles except for tumor tissue (Fig. 23.5B). In malignant tissue, the ratio 20:3n-6/18:3n-6 reached its maximum at 6 h; thereafter it remained approximately constant throughout the experiment (Fig. 23.5C).

Discussion

Three distinct human carcinomas with different growth rates were grown in male and female nude mice to study the uptake and metabolism of 18:3n-6 administered

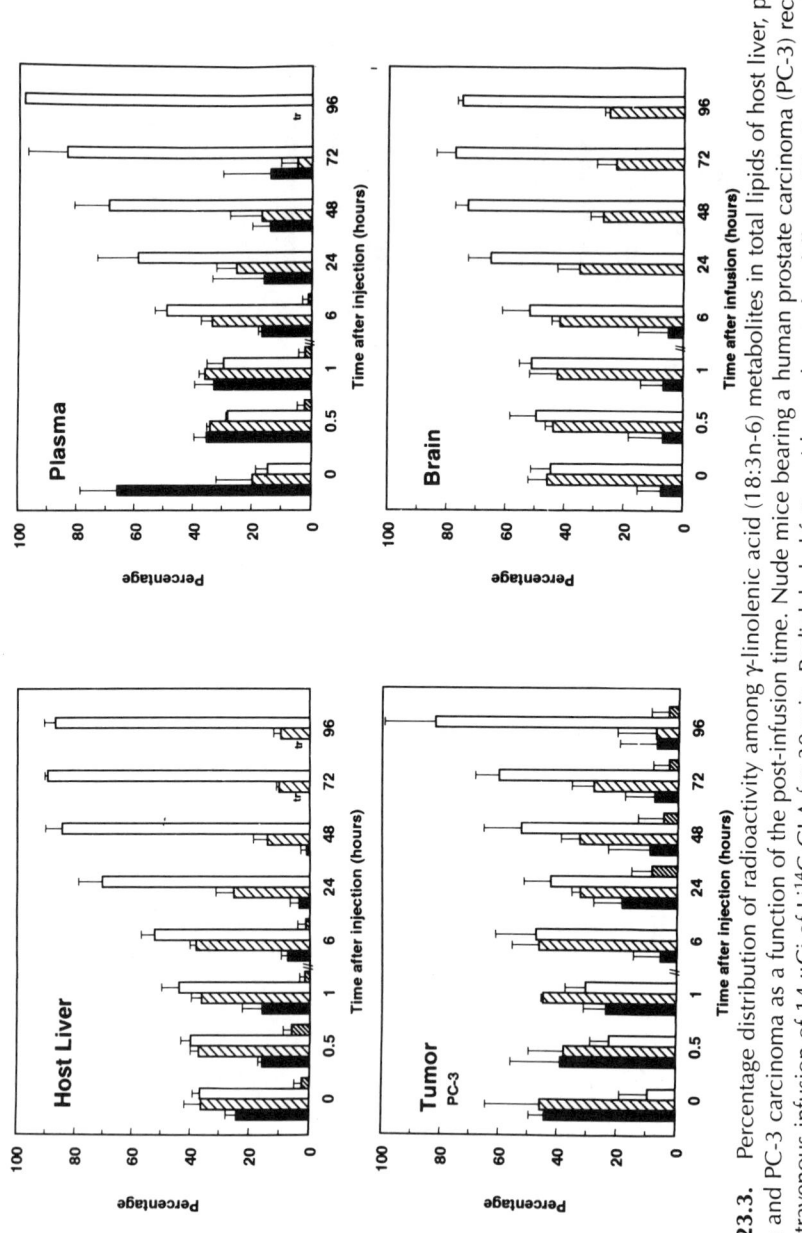

Fig. 23.3. Percentage distribution of radioactivity among γ-linolenic acid (18:3n-6) metabolites in total lipids of host liver, plasma, brain and PC-3 carcinoma as a function of the post-infusion time. Nude mice bearing a human prostate carcinoma (PC-3) received an intravenous infusion of 14 μCi of Li^{14}C-GLA for 30 min. Radiolabeled fatty acids are denoted as follows: ■ γ-linolenic acid (18:3n-6), (heavy diagonal bars) dihomo-γ-linolenic acid (20:3n-6), □ arachidonic acid (20:4n-6), and (lighter diagonal bars) unknown fatty acid (presumably 22:3n-6). Abbreviation: tr, trace amounts. Values are the mean ± SD of at least 4 mice.

intravenously in the form of lithium salt. The differences among tumors were not reflected in differences in their uptake and further metabolism of 18:3n-6. Furthermore, substantial differences were not detected in host liver, plasma and brain except for the liver and brain of mice bearing a pancreatic carcinoma (Figs. 23.2–23.4).

The dose of Li[^{14}C]-GLA (2.5 mg/kg) was scaled down to a 30-min infusion from that used with pancreatic cancer patients (11,12). Under these experimental

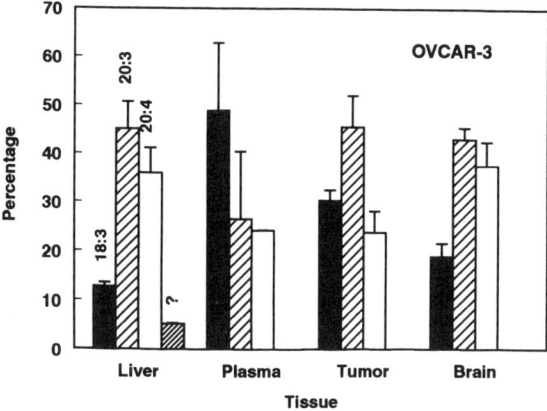

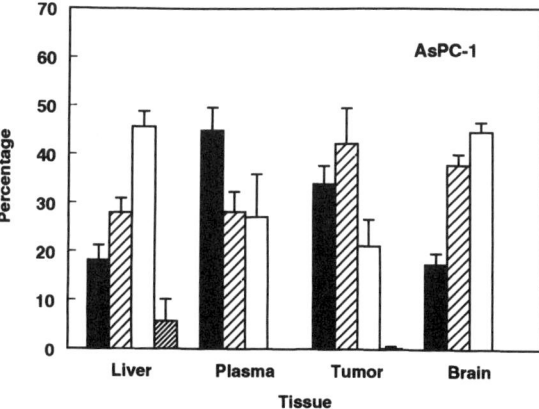

Fig. 23.4. Percentage distribution of radioactivity among γ-linolenic acid (GLA) metabolites in total lipids of host liver, plasma, brain, OVCAR-3, and AsPC-1 carcinomas at 0.5 h after infusion. Nude mice bearing either human ovarian (OVCAR-3) or pancreatic (AsPC-1) carcinomas received an intravenous infusion of 14 μCi of Li^{14}C-GLA for 30 min. Radiolabeled fatty acids are denoted as follows: ■ γ-linolenic acid (18:3n-6), (heavy diagonal bars) dihomo-γ-linolenic acid (20:3n-6), □ arachidonic acid (20:4n-6), and (lighter diagonal bars) unknown fatty acid (presumably 22:3n-6). Values are the mean ± SD of at least 4 mice.

conditions, concentrations of about 0.4 µg/mL of PUFAs derived from radiolabeled 18:3n-6 were reached in tumor tissue at 72 h after infusion. If these values are extrapolated to a dose which would be administrated during a 24-h infusion (120 mg/kg), they could eventually be within the range of cytotoxic concentrations (5–50 µg/mL) for malignant cells according to *in vitro* studies (18). It should be pointed out that total radioactivity per gram of tissue did not vary for at least 96 h in tumor, brain, fat, and testes, whereas in other host tissue, labeling declined substantially.

The higher amount (22-fold) of fatty acids taken up by the liver compared with that recovered in tumors may reflect differences in the vascularization of the liver and subcutaneously transplanted carcinomas as well as differences in liver metabolism of fatty acids (19). In fact, it has already been proposed that subcutaneously transplanted tumors proliferate more rapidly than their blood supply (19). This may partially explain the slower decay of radioactivity in tumor tissue relative to the liver within the 96-h period of the present experiment, although this explanation cannot account for the similar slow decay in brain and testes. Even though the comparisons between human tumor tissue and mouse host liver may not be relevant, similar differences between the malignant and normal tissue uptake after 1 h of intravenous infusion of n-6 PUFAs were reported in early studies using tissues of the same origin, rat hepatoma and host rat liver (20). This suggests that once the PUFAs were taken up and further metabolized by the tumor, they were retained for a longer period of time than in the liver. Our findings with slow infusions of LiGLA are consistent with previous studies (21) in which almost one half of the radioactivity recovered from the liver and plasma lipid fractions 22 h after oral administration of [^{14}C]20:3n-6 was still present as 20:3n-6, probably due to its slower β-oxidation than that showed by 18:3n-6. In this study 18:3n-6, besides being metabolized to 20:4n-6, was also available for incorporation as 18:3n-6 into tissue lipids. Nevertheless, the presence of 18:3n-6 metabolites in tumor tissue did not reflect the ability of the tumors to elongate 18:3n-6 to 20:3n-6 and to Δ5-desaturate 20:3n-6 to 20:4n-6. These metabolites could have been selectively taken by the tumors from the host plasma to establish their particular fatty acid pattern and the observed time-dependent variations of the 20:4n-6/20:3n-6 ratio (Fig. 23.5). Indeed, it has been proposed elsewhere (22) that 20:4n-6 produced in liver can be used for membrane synthesis in cells and tissues that do not have an adequate capacity to make sufficient 20:4n-6 from n-6 precursors. However, it is likely that the altered radiolabeled fatty acid composition mirrors changes in the metabolic pathways of the tumors (19,20).

In summary, intravenous delivery of 18:3n-6 as lithium salt seems to be a promising approach to target malignant cells *in vivo* and thus for cancer treatments because data indicate that LiGLA was well distributed in the host organism and the tumor, with the latter retaining high levels of 18:3-6 and its immediate elongation product (20:3n-6) at 96 h as compared with the liver.

Acknowledgment

We thank I. Pottie for his skillful assistance in the maintenance of nude mice.

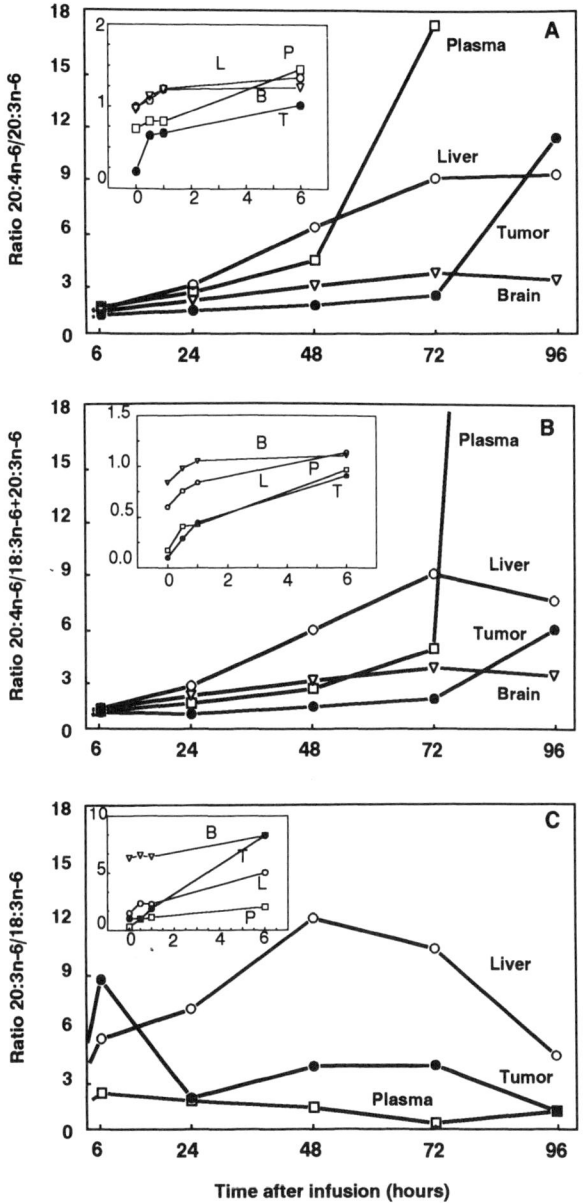

Fig. 23.5. Ratios of radiolabeled fatty acids in total lipids of host liver, plasma, brain and PC-3 carcinoma as a function of the post-infusion time. Nude mice bearing a human prostate carcinoma (PC-3) received an intravenous infusion of 14 µCi of Li-^{14}C-GLA for 30 min. Abbreviations: 18:3n-6, γ-linolenic acid; 20:3n-6, dihomo-γ-linolenic acid; 20:4n-6, arachidonic acid; L, liver; B, brain; P, plasma; and T, tumor. Some brain and plasma ratios are not plotted because 18:3n-6 and 20:3n-6 were found only in trace amounts at certain time points. Values are the mean of at least 4 mice.

References

1. Horrobin, D.F. (1994) in *New Approaches to Cancer Treatment. Unsaturated Lipids and Photodynamic Therapy,* Horrobin, D.F., ed., Churchill Livingstone, London, pp. 1–29.
2. Das. U.N. Gamma-Linolenic Acid, Arachidonic Acid, and Eicosapentaenoic Acid as Potential Anticancer Drugs (1990) *Nutrition 6,* 429–434.
3. Falconer, J.S., Fearon, K.C.H., Ross, J.A., and Carter, D.C. (1994) in *Effects of Fatty Acids and Lipids in Health and Disease. World Rev. Nutr. Diet,* Galli, C., Simopoulos, A.P., and Tremoli, E., eds., Karger, Basel, vol. 76. pp. 74–76.
4. van Hoeven, R.P., and Emmelot, P. (1973) in *Tumor Lipids: Biochemistry and Metabolism,* Wood, R., ed., American Oil Chemists' Society, Champaign, IL, pp. 127–138.
5. Sakai, T., and Yamaguchi, N. Prostaglandin D2 Inhibits the Proliferation of Human Malignant Tumor Cells (1984) *Prostaglandins 27,* 17–26.
6. Takeda, S., Horrobin, D.F., and Manku, M.S. The Effects of Gamma-Linolenic Acid on Human Breast Cancer Cell Killing, Lipid Peroxidation and the Production of Schiff-Reactive Materials (1992) *Med. Sci. Res. 20,* 203–205.
7. Bégin, M.E. Effects of Polyunsaturated Fatty Acids and Their Oxidation Products on Cell Survival (1987) *Chem. Phys. Lipids 45,* 269–313.
8. Jiang, W.G., Hiscox, S., Hallett, M.B., Scott, C., Horrobin, D.F., and Puntis, M.C.A. Inhibition of Hepatocyte Growth Factor-Induced Motility and *in Vitro* Invasion of Human Colon Cancer Cells by Gamma-Linolenic Acid (1995) *Br. J. Cancer 71,* 744–752.
9. Pritchard, G.A., Jones, D.L., and Mansel, R.E. Lipids in Breast Carcinogenesis (1989) *Br. J. Surg. 76,* 1069–1073.
10. de Bravo, M.G., Schinella, G., Tournier, H., and Quintans, C. Effects of Dietary Gamma and Alpha Linolenic Acid on a Human Lung Carcinoma Grown in Nude Mice (1994) *Med. Sci. Res. 22,* 667–668.
11. Reynolds, P.D., Tuffnell, Q., Lee, A., and Hunter, J.O. (1994) in *New Approaches to Cancer Treatment. Unsaturated Lipids and Photodynamic Therapy,* Horrobin, D.F. ed., Churchill Livingstone, London, pp. 79–83.
12. Fearon, K.C.H., Falconer, J.S., Ross, J.A., Carter, D.C., Reynolds, P.D., Tuffnell, Q., and Hunter, J.O. (1994) in *New Appproaches to Cancer Treatment. Unsaturated Lipids and Photodynamic Therapy,* Horrobin, D.F., ed., Churchill Livingstone, London, pp. 84–87.
13. Folch, J., Lees, M. and Sloane-Stanley, G.A. A Simple Method for the Isolation and Purification of Total Lipids from Animal Tissues (1957) *J. Biol. Chem., 226,* 497–509.
14. Morrison, W.R., and Smith, L.M. Preparation of Fatty Acid Methyl Esters and Dimethylacetals from Lipids with Boron Fluoride-Methanol (1964) *J. Lipid Res. 5,* 600–608.
15. de Antueno, R.J., Cantrill, R.C., Huang, Y.-S., Ells, G.W., Elliot, M., and Horrobin, D.F. Metabolism of n-6 Fatty Acids by NIH-3T3 Cells Transfected with the *ras* Oncogene (1994) *Mol. Cell. Biochem. 139,* 71–81.
16. Boven, E. (1991) in *The Nude Mouse in Oncology Research,* Boven, E., and Winograd, B., eds., CRC Press, Boca Raton, FL, pp. 89–101.
17. Houchens, D.P., and Ovejera, A. (1991) in *The Nude Mouse in Oncology Research,* Boven, E., and Winograd, B., eds., CRC Press, Boca Raton, FL, pp. 133–147.
18. Bégin, M.E., Das, U.N., Ells, G., and Horrobin, D.F. Selective Killing of Human Cancer Cells by Polyunsaturated Fatty Acids (1985) *Prostaglandins Leukotrienes Med. 19,* 177–186.

19. Morton, R.E., Waite, M., Lynn King, V., and Morris, H.P. Uptake and Metabolism of Free Fatty Acids by the Morris 7777 Hepatoma and Host Rat Liver (1982) *Lipids 17,* 529–537.
20. De Tomas, M.E., and Mercuri, O. Biosynthesis of Lipids in Tumoral Cells (1977) *Adv. Exp. Med. Biol. 83,* 119–125.
21. Hassam, A.G., and Crawford, M.A. The Incorporation of Orally Administered Radiolabeled Dihomo γ-Linolenic Acid (20:3ω6) into Rat Tissue Lipids and Its Conversion to Arachidonic Acid (1978) *Lipids 13,* 801–803.
22. Voss, A.C., and Sprecher, H. Metabolism of 6,9,12-Octadecatrienoic Acid and 6,9,12,15-Octadecatetraenoic Acid by Rat Hepatocytes (1988) *Biochim. Biophys. Acta 958,* 153–162.

Chapter 24

Global Regulatory Status of γ-Linolenic Acid

F.C. Kulow

Bioriginal Food and Science Corporation, 1-411 Downey Road, Saskatoon, Saskatchewan, Canada

Introduction

Due to a variety of factors, research on the health benefits of γ-linolenic acid (GLA) has recently gained momentum. Demographic changes such as the aging of the "Baby Boomer" generation, economic factors such as the rising cost of health care, and increased nutritional research in areas such as anti-oxidants are behind this momentum. As the link between nutrition and health becomes more clearly established within the Western medical establishment, and the cost savings of nutrition and prevention *vs.* pharmaceutical drugs and curing become better documented, the area of essential fatty acids in general, and GLA in particular, is attracting increasing attention.

The increase in commercial uses of GLA-containing oils reflects this momentum. GLA is the active ingredient in three oilseed crops, borage (starflower), black currant, and evening primrose, as well as in some fungal species; GLA oils are currently used in the health and nutrition industry, the cosmetic industry, the pharmaceutical industry, in functional foods, in pet foods and veterinary applications, and are being assessed for possible use in mass-market foods.

As the interest in GLA grows and its usage increases, so do regulatory implications and scrutiny. This presentation will focus on four areas in the global regulatory status of GLA products:

1. the typical regulatory processes currently used in a number of countries
2. the Swedish regulatory system, which provides the clearest directions in this area
3. the evolution of the regulatory system in the United States and
4. a review of the regulatory situation in Japan, which could serve as a model for the future.

The Typical Regulatory Process

Overall, there is no global regulatory status of GLA. As GLA has increased in prominence, individual regulatory officials around the world have wrestled with the challenge of how to deal with this new area. Government responses have varied, and each country, and sometimes more than one regulatory agency within each country, has developed its own regulations.

Although each country handles these regulations independently, the following generalizations can be made:

1. In most countries GLA products are permitted for use as a food or nutritional supplement, although they may have to be registered.
2. The fewer claims that are made for a product, the less severe the regulation.
3. Once an oil is altered and/or therapeutic or medical claims are made, the product is treated as a pharmaceutical or as a drug.

Involvement in the commercial aspects of GLA importation and sales requires a familiarization with the specific regulatory procedures in the country of interest. Regulations covering the importation of GLA products may differ from those which cover the sale of the product.

Gathering Information

Gathering information on the regulatory processes that govern the import and sale of GLA products can be done by contacting the particular regulatory agency in the country of interest; assistance can often be requested from consulate commercial officers. However, the regulatory process itself is very person specific, and the most valuable information sources are likely to be strategic partners within the country. Such partners are often aware of the best contacts within specific regulatory departments.

Because of the rapidly changing environment for these products, one has to remain in contact with regulatory agencies within each country. In addition, it is important to monitor political changes in the area in which one wishes to do business. For example, the recent institution of the European Union has led to regulations being determined by the Union in some areas and by the individual countries in other areas. Changes in the legal environment also must be monitored. For example, a recent bill passed and signed into law in the United States now makes it easier to import and sell GLA products.

Therapeutic Claims

Understanding what constitutes "therapeutic claims" and how a country determines and defines the term is often more an art than a science. Differences are vast among countries. As an example, in the United States, the proximity of natural health manuals to a GLA product in the retail outlet may be reason enough for the Food and Drug Administration to determine that the retailer, and therefore possibly the distributor and the manufacturer, is making therapeutic claims for the products.

Another interesting example is the regulatory situation in Greece. According to the Greek National Drug Organization (EOF), "GLA is permitted up to a certain quantity and depending on the product in question's composition. In small doses, GLA is considered a food supplement, and in higher doses it is considered a pharmaceutical product. In the event such a product is to be imported into Greece, EOF must be informed of the quantitative and qualitative composition of the product, and it is up to EOF to decide whether the GLA content of the product would classify it as a food supplement, pharmaceutical, or other." Unfortunately, the EOF regulations on exactly what quantities or range of quantities of GLA places a product in each category is information that is not available and EOF does not provide it. In simplistic terms, if a product contains too much GLA, it is classified as a drug, but the definition of what constitutes too much GLA is not available.

Once a product is altered and/or therapeutic or medical claims are made, regulatory agencies will generally require that the product be tested as a pharmaceutical substance or as a drug. The processes involved in the registration of a GLA product as either of the latter are much more stringent, time consuming and expensive than if the product is to be sold as a nutritional supplement.

Country Regulatory Overview

The following overview is not meant to be comprehensive, but only to highlight individual examples of regulatory procedures.

Australia. Australia requires therapeutic goods to be included in the Australian Register of Therapeutic Goods as either "listed" goods or "registered" goods. Listed goods include nutritional supplements and herbal preparations intended only for use in prevention or treatment of minor medical conditions. The listing must include all active ingredients. According to Australian government regulations, "Registered goods are subject to detailed individual evaluation for quality, safety and efficacy. GLA is not permitted as an active ingredient in listed goods, but herbal oils such as evening primrose, black currant, and flax may be included as herbal substance active ingredients and the GLA equivalence may be stated on the product label."

Brazil. Brazilian legislation does not, to date, contain any regulations governing the use of GLA.

Chile. Approval and registration of GLA products for use in drugs, homeopathic medications and cosmetics must be done through the Institute for National Health. A company must be established in Chile or have an arrangement made with an established company for representation. The adminstrative process is quite detailed and lengthy. GLA has to be imported under the regulation for the control of pharmaceutical products. Approval and registration usually require 3 to 6 months.

Czech Republic. In the Czech Republic, GLA is permitted on the market and can be used in health food as well as in cosmetic or pharmaceutical products. No regulations are available in writing. GLA products are subject either to registration as a pharmaceutical by the State Institute for the Control of Pharmaceuticals or to the approval of the State Medical Institute for use as a food or cosmetic product. All products must be tested prior to their introduction into the local market.

Denmark. In Denmark, GLA is permitted for use by the National Food Agency. The use of GLA in food supplements and cosmetics is not as widespread in Denmark as in other European countries.

Egypt. In Egypt, GLA products are not banned from import or use. They do, however, require application to local health authorities for registration of the product. Detailed analytical information and samples must be submitted with an application.

France. The use of GLA as a food ingredient is authorized as a natural component of a vegetable oil. There are strict regulations controlling the nutritional labeling of food products in France. Allegations regarding health are not authorized. If health claims are too explicit, then a GLA product is considered a drug and the manufacturer must obtain official approval based on medical experiments and data.

Germany. GLA may be imported, but its use and sale are subject to a wide range of regulations. The regulatory situation is currently in transition.

Great Britain. No special regulations exist governing the use of GLA-containing oils for food use other than that they must be of high standard food grade.

Hungary. The import and sale of GLA products are under strict control by the National Institute of Food Hygiene and Nutrition. To obtain a permit to import a product, a sample of the GLA product must be tested and specifications provided.

Israel. GLA must be registered as a health food by the Food Directorate or as a drug by the Pharmaceutical Division of the Ministry of Health. The registration of GLA products as drugs is the responsibility of the importer with assistance from local agents.

Korea. In Korea, compounds containing GLA as 100% edible oil are classified as health foods and have to be registered and approved by the National Institute of Health prior to sale.

Malaysia. Dietary and health products containing GLA are required to be registered with the Drug Control Authority prior to being imported and sold. A local agent must be appointed before any registration proceedings can be initiated. This agent must also be responsible for the registration of the product.

Mexico. The use of GLA is practically unknown in Mexico.

Netherlands. There are no special requirements for the importation or sale of GLA products. However, levies are implemented on a sliding scale dependent upon product purity.

New Zealand. Therapeutic claims are not permitted on any dietary supplement label, advertising or promotional material for GLA products sold in New Zealand. If sold for therapeutic purposes, then the product must be classified as a medicine. Regulations are governed by the Therapeutic Section of the Ministry of Health.

Norway. In Norway, there are no special requirements governing GLA products. These products must fulfill the requirements given in the general regulations concerning foodstuffs.

Saudi Arabia. There is no health food industry or cosmetic industry in Saudia Arabia, hence the use of GLA products is practically unknown.

Singapore. GLA is not subject to registration, but GLA products must comply with four specific legislative acts covering medicines and drugs.

South Africa. In South Africa, products are registrable under the Medicines and Related Substances Control Act if a medicinal claim is made. If GLA is a component of other products, specifications, purpose, labeling, and "connected" advertising must be submitted to the Registrar of Medicines.

Spain. In Spain, there are regulations or restrictions on the importation and sale of GLA products.

Switzerland. There are no restrictions for the use of GLA in cosmetic products according to the Cosmetics Division of the Federal Office of Public Health. According to the Food Products Division, regulations vary for use in food products and will depend upon the characteristics of the GLA product and the intended use.

Taiwan. GLA products may be sold in Taiwan, with regulations for some sources being grandfathered and other sources requiring regulatory approval.

Zimbabwe. In Zimbabwe, GLA as a raw material is not controlled as a medicine. However, if GLA is prepared into any pharmaceutical form and any medicinal claims are made for the preparation so produced, the product then becomes subject to registration under the Drugs and Allied Substance Control Act.

The Swedish Regulatory Process

The regulatory process in Sweden is typical of many countries but is unique in that the language used to define "medicinal products" contains a minimum of legal terminology and is quite understandable. The definition of such a product as authorized by the Swedish Medical Product Agency is as follows: "By definition a medicinal product is a product intended to prevent, diagnose, relieve or cure disease or symptoms of disease or to be used for a similar purpose." Therefore, the actual purpose of the product defines its classification. Not only direct claims are taken into consideration when classifying a product. Other factors of importance include ingredient formulations, use in traditional or folk medicine, dosage form, dosage information and the name of the product, which may also provide an idea of claims for the product.

With regard to GLA, the following excerpt is of interest: "Evening primrose oil and borage oil containing GLA are ingredients of several natural remedies which are on the Swedish market for the time being. These products are marketed under indications within the area of self-medication. Some products containing GLA are marketed as cosmetic-hygienic products with no claims allowed but emollient action. We do not regard GLA-containing products as food, as there is not to our knowledge any traditional use of these ingredients as food stuff."

The Swedish Medical Product Agency describes the approval of natural remedies as follows: "The requirements for documentation of the quality of natural remedies are as rigorous as for regular medicinal products. Requirements for safety and efficacy are, on the other hand, usually lower. Applications for approval of natural remedies shall be made by those who wish to sell these products in Sweden. If the applicant is not located within the EEA area, there must be an agent within this area."

The application fee for the registration of GLA products differs between countries and can be a significant consideration for a small company wishing to introduce and market new products. In Sweden, for example, the application fee currently is 23,700 Swedish kronor which is approximately U.S. $3540.00. Once a product has been approved, an annual fee of 4,500 kronor (about U.S. $675.00) must be paid. The time necessary to approve an application is at most 210 days from receipt of the complete application documents as well as the fee. A product can not be marketed until it has received approval. Any modifications which may affect the quality, safety and/or the efficacy of the product may be made only after approval has been given by the Swedish Medical Product Agency. Furthermore, a change in the type or a substantial alteration in the quantity of the active ingredient(s) requires that a new application for marketing authorization be made to the Swedish Medical Product Agency. Even a relatively small company with a short product list may require a full-time compliance manager to monitor regulations.

The Evolution of the Regulatory Status of GLA in the United States

The United States is the only country in the world where the sale of GLA-containing products has been banned. In 1984, because of unsubstantiated medical claims, the importation of evening primrose oil into the United States was halted by the Food and Drug Administration (FDA). The FDA classified GLA-containing oils as "unapproved food additives"; because of this, the burden of proof of product safety shifted to any company selling these products. (In comparison, if a product is classified as a "food," the burden of proof is on the FDA to prove that the product is not safe.) This classification stood until 1992, when Oakmont Investment Co. of Sunapee, NH successfully challenged it in court. In a decision appealed to the United States Supreme Court, the courts ruled that single-ingredient (i.e., nonblended) GLA-containing oils were foods, not food additives. The FDA subsequently lifted its import alert, but maintains an appropriate vigilance regarding product claims made by manufacturers.

Currently, GLA-containing oils can be legally sold in the United States, subject to restrictions. The Dietary Supplement Health and Education Act of 1994 revised the law to allow claims of beneficial attributes without allowing therapeutic and medical claims, with restrictions such as the inclusion of the following disclaimer: "This statement has not been evaluated by the Food and Drug Administration. This product is not intended to diagnose, treat, cure, or prevent any disease."

Japan—A Model for the Future

Looking to the future, there appears to be a global trend toward a new "halfway" industry between the mass market food and pharmaceutical industries. Within this industry, based on rigorous toxicity data and appropriate double-blind, placebo-controlled, peer-reviewed published studies, companies will be able to make limited health claims for products without incurring the years of research and millions of dollars required for pharmaceutical approval. One example of this trend is found in Canada, where claims regarding migraine headaches can be made for the herb, Feverfew.

The most interesting model, however, is evolving in Japan. Here, food products that contain GLA can be registered as "foods with medicinal properties," for which beneficial health claims can be made in the areas of atopic eczema and cholesterol. The parameters for the classification of functional foods in Japan are quite strict; claims must be based on clinical research done on finished products—not just their active ingredients. These "functional foods" in Japan are seen as logical extensions of common foods themselves. Examples in this area include milk with Vitamin D, orange juice with calcium and high fiber waffles. To our knowledge, no GLA-containing products have yet received final approval for classification as a functional food.

Japan is progressive in its approach to nutritional and therapeutic supplements, in part due to the demographic influences associated with an aging population; by the year 2010, more than 25% of the Japanese population will be over 65 years of age. Similar population pressure is being felt by developed countries around the world; it is possible that industry regulations similar to those of Japan will be implemented in these other countries. Because modified regulatory processes could be beneficial from both economic and nutritional standpoints, the growing momentum currently being experienced in GLA research and in the GLA commercial market may signal a concurrent momentum for change in the global regulatory environment.

Index

A

Aceraceae family, 3–4
Acetylcholine, 203
Acetyl-CoA carboxylase, 260
Acute lung injury (ALI), 137–161
Acylation reactions, 15–18, 25, 90–91
  competition with desaturation, 98, 227
Acyl-CoA-dependent desaturation, 14–17, 25, 253, 259
Acyl-lipid-desaturases, membrane-bound, 25, 29
Acylmigration, 55
Adenovirus (AD), 285
Adipose tissue, signal-masking, 70–71, 81
Adult respiratory distress syndrome (ARDS), 137–161
Aging, 109, 184, 258
  and γ-linolenic acid (GLA), 84, 96, 106, 180
Albumin, 44
Alcohol use, 84, 95–96, 184, 228–240
Aldosterone, 214
Algae containing γ-linolenic acid (GLA), 5–6, 248
American Edwards cardiac output computer, 141
Amputation, 273
Angiotensin, 192–193, 202–207, 214, 222
Animal species, variance in essential fatty acid (EFA) metabolism, 87–89, 109, 176–180
Antiatherogenic effect of γ-linolenic acid (GLA), 176
Anti-oxidant studies, 304
Antithrombotic effect of eicosapentaenoic acid (EPA), 208
Apoproteins, 54
Arachidonic acid (AA), 43–46, 66–68, 91–99
  antiinflammatory properties of, 147
  deficiencies in, 200
  desaturated from dihomo-γ-linolenic acid (DGLA), 119–132, 228
  in human milk, 247
  intercellular communication, role in, 246
  γ-linolenic acid (GLA) an indirect source, 246
  in phospholipids, 16–17, 159–160, 262
  preformed, 168, 247–248
  role in reproduction, 87
  sources of, 80–87, 138
  synthesis of, 14–17, 246–247, 257
  tumoricidal properties of, 285, 293
Arachidonic acid (AA)/dihomo-γ-linolenic acid (DGLA) ratio, 92–93, 112, 130, 139–160, 172, 227
Arterial occlusive disease, 221
Arterial oxygen studies, 142–145
Arteriosclerosis, 30
Aspirin, 96–97, 233
Atherogenicity of fatty acids, 9, 55, 89
Atheromatous plaque formation, 222–223
Atherosclerosis, 176, 182–183, 221–223
  effect of γ-linolenic acid (GLA) on, 183, 221–224
Atopy, 112
Autoimmune diseases, 106, 111–112
Autonomic reactivity, 232

B

Bacteremia, 154
Baroreceptor reflex, 215
Basic fibroblast growth factor (bFGF), 222
Binding of fatty acids, 45–49
Bioavailability of γ-linolenic acid (GLA), 7–10, 46, 71–81, 89–90
Black currant oil (BCO), 33–40, 180, 249. See also Seed oils
Bladder control, loss of, 273
Blood pressure (BP) effects of γ-linolenic acid (GLA), 2, 84, 141, 146–154, 189–217, 233
Body temperature regulation, 232, 235

Borage oil (BO), 137–154, 180, 196, 202–213, 219–220, 223, 277. See also Seed oils
Brain cancer, 287–289
Brain membrane phospholipids, 228
  docosahexaenoic acid (DHA) in synaptosomal fraction, 228
  effect on synaptic transmission, 231
Brain studies, 14, 42, 67–81, 93–94, 227–240
  viral infection in, 111
Breath carbon dioxide studies, 67–75, 91
Bronchoalveolar lavage (BAL), 146, 152
Bronchoconstriction, 140–142
B-thromboglobulin (B-TG), 264
  in plasma, 265
Butylated hydroxyanisole (BHA), 286
Butylated hydroxytoluene (BHT), 286

C

Calcium
  effect of prostaglandins (PG) on, 204, 207, 232
  in serum, 204, 207
  transport mechanism, 208
Cancer, 111, 282–303
Canola oil, 193–194
Carbon dioxide in serum, 204
Cardiac myocytes, 44, 70, 90
Cardiopulmonary hemodynamics, 137, 141
Cardiovascular disease, 209, 273
Casein protein, 178, 255–256
Catecholamines, 96, 192, 222
Cerebral glioma, 287–289
Chain elongation, 18–19, 85–99, 106, 209, 218, 228, 246–247, 252–254, 260, 266
  mechanism of, 253
Chemotaxis, 139–140
Chemotherapy, 293
Chloride in serum, 204, 207
Cholesterol, 176–179, 203, 206
  effect of γ-linolenic acid (GLA) on, 30, 54, 84, 175–184
  in plasma, 30, 175–180
  in serum, 204, 265
  supplementation with, 92, 176, 181
Cholesterol 7α-hydroxylase, 181–182
Cholesterol ester (CE), 84–85, 98
  containing essential fatty acids (EFA), 227
  in plasma, 277
Cholesterol ester (CE) hydrolase, 183
Cholesterol ester (CE) synthetase, 183
Chromosomal abnormalities, 284
Chylomicrons (CM), 54–56, 62–64, 99
Circadian running wheel activity, 235–239
Cirrhosis, 98
Coconut oil (CNO), 109, 176
  hydrogenated, 179
Columbinic acid, 175, 184
Commercial potential of γ-linolenic acid (GLA), 304–310
Commercial processing of γ-linolenic acid (GLA), 10, 37–40
Computerized axial tomography (CAT) scan, 287–289
Corn oil, 140–146, 180, 200, 220, 223, 277
Coronary heart disease, 30
Corticosteroids, 110
Cortisol, 106
Cottonseed oil, 132
Cox proportional hazards mode assessment, 294
Cyanobacteria, 22–30
Cyclins, 286
Cyclooxygenase (CO) activity, 109, 112, 118–126, 138–139, 219
  defined, 231
  inhibitors of, 108, 151, 212, 223, 286
  in membrane, 160
Cyclooxygenase (CO) products, macrophage-derived, 223
Cyclosporin, 194–195
Cytokines, 110, 285–286
  proinflammatory properties of, 112

D

Delayed-type hypersensitivity (DTH) skin test, 109, 113
Δ4-desaturase, 107
Δ5-desaturase, 1, 6, 14–15, 43, 84–99, 107, 119, 132, 182, 218, 228, 246, 253
  inhibition of, 141, 159, 183, 264
Δ6-desaturase, 1, 6, 24, 28, 43, 84–99, 107, 118, 218, 246, 253–254. See also Rate-limiting step
  absent in carnivorous animals, 254

acyl-CoA-dependence of, 19
  deficiency in, 111, 118, 139, 282
  desD gene for, 26–29
  inhibition of, 175–184, 200, 229–233, 254–259, 264
Δ8-desaturase, 14–15, 253
Δ9-desaturase, 28, 172
  desC gene for, 26
Δ12-desaturase, 7, 24, 28
  desA gene for, 25–28
Δ15-desaturase, 6–7
ω-3 desaturase (acyl-lipid), 28
  desB gene for, 26
Desaturase cloning, 25–29
Desaturation reactions, 22–25, 90, 106, 179, 227–228, 252–255
  competition with acylation, 98, 227
  zinc as co-factor, 93, 95
Dexamethasone effects, 96–97
Diabetes, 93, 184, 200, 252–266
  effect of γ-linolenic acid (GLA) on, 180, 279
  long-term management of, 263, 273–279
Diabetic
  cataracts, 262
  neuropathy, 2, 84, 93, 95, 261–266, 273–279
  vascular complications, 264–266
Diacylglycerol, 286
Dietary supplementation. See Nutritional supplementation
Dietary Supplement Health and Education Act of 1994, 310
Dihomo-γ-linolenic acid (DGLA), 75, 80, 130–133. See also Arachidonic acid (AA)/dihomo-γ-linolenic acid (DGLA) ratio
  antiinflammatory properties of, 120–123, 130
  deficiencies of, 200
  elongated from γ-linolenic acid (GLA), 1–4, 84–99, 106–112, 143–148, 169–175, 182, 213–214, 219, 228, 231
  metabolism of, 118–125
  in phospholipids, 99, 157–158
  in plasma, 139, 152, 157
Dilinoleoyl glycerol, 285
Dilinoleoyl-monogammalinolenyl glycerol (DLMG), 275
Dipyridamole, 221
DNA, 25–27, 214, 222–223

Docosahexaenoic acid (DHA), 42–43, 68, 71, 93, 107–108, 129
  affected by alcohol, 237
  displacing arachidonic acid (AA), 137
  role in brain and retina function, 237, 248
  tumoricidal action of, 285
Docosapentaenoic acid, 151
Double bonding, 14, 38, 218, 227
  configuration in γ-linolenic acid (GLA), 1, 25, 175, 201
Drug-resistant tumors, 284, 289

E

Ecosatrienoic acid synthesis, 257
Eczema, 30, 111, 139
Efamol, 274–275. See also Evening primrose oil
Eicosanoids, 106–109, 118, 129, 190
  antiinflammatory forms, 218
  antithrombotic properties of, 208, 218
  derived from arachidonic acid (AA), 231
  dienoic, 160
  metabolism of, 140
  monoenoic, 155, 160, 169
  in phospholipids, 157–158
  proinflammatory forms, 137, 146, 151
  secreted by macrophages, 222
  trienoic, 138, 145, 160
  vasodilatory properties of, 208
Eicosapentaenoic acid (EPA), 68, 86, 107–108, 129–132
  antiinflammatory properties of, 137, 154
  decreasing arachidonic acid (AA) levels, 137, 147, 229
  increasing docosahexaenoic acid (DHA) levels, 229
  inhibiting 5-lipoxygenase activity, 147
  tumoricidal properties of, 285, 293
Electrolytes, serum, 203–204, 206
Electroretinogram assessment, 227, 248
Elongase, 1, 6, 86–90, 106–107. See also Chain elongation
Emulsion systems for preparation of fatty acids, 35–36
Endometrium studies, 112
Endoplasmic reticulum, 14–18, 25, 98, 253. See also Microsomes

Endothelium studies, 54, 90, 222
Endotoxemia, 111–112, 140–161
Enterocytes, 54
Enzymatic enrichment of γ-linolenic acid (GLA), 33–40
Epidermal growth factor, heparin-binding (HB-EGF), 222
Epidermis studies, 118–123
Epinephrine, 106
Epoxygenase, 231
Erucic acid, 4
Erythema, 111
Erythrocytes
  lipid composition of, 257, 263–264
  sedimentation rate of, 132
Escherichia coli, 139, 141, 150, 156
Essential fatty acids (EFA), 87–89, 106–111, 129, 279, 282
  in human milk, 247
Esterification, 17, 34–40, 56–57, 90–91, 157
  lipase-catalyzed, 37–40
  and pregnancy outcomes, 42–49
Ethanol. See Alcohol use
Ethanolamine plasmalogen, 258
Ethyl-γ-linoleate, 178
Ethyl-γ-linolenate, 178
Evening primrose oil (EPO), 192–196, 212, 274–277. See also Seed oils
  preferential hypocholesterolemic properties of, 177–179
Excoriation, 111
Exercise, 189

F

Fasting, effects similar to diabetes, 254–255
Fatty acid, 149, 152, 169–170. See also Essential fatty acids; Long-chain polyunsaturated fatty acids (LCPUFA); Monounsaturated fatty acids; Polyunsaturated fatty acids (PUFA); Saturated fatty acids
  absorption of, 6–7, 57–62
  deficiency in, 91–93, 99
  desaturation of, 179
  free (FFA), 44, 91, 157, 227
  higher unsaturated (HUFA), 168–173
  hydroperoxy, 231
  nonesterified, 264
  preferential hydrolysis of, 44, 227
  preparation of, 34–40, 35, 37
  reacylation of, 54–55, 63, 220
  separation of, 39
  synthesis of, 17–19, 44
Fatty acid-binding proteins (FABP), 44–47, 214
Fatty acid methyl esters (FAME), 295
Fetal Alcohol Syndrome, 234
Fetal and neonate development, 42–49, 229–240, 246–250
Fibrinolysis, 17, 86, 90
Fibroblasts, 17, 86, 90
Fish oil, 16, 93–94, 93–97, 112, 129, 137–146, 193–196, 223, 228, 248
  displacing arachidonic acid (AA), 151
Fluid intake problems, 232
Food and Drug Administration (FDA), 309
Food and fluid intake problems, 232
Free radical generation, 108, 284, 293
Freund's adjuvant, 110
Fungi containing γ-linolenic acid (GLA), 4–5, 9–10, 179, 201, 205–207, 212–213, 276

G

Gadoleic acid, 4
Gas chromatography (GC), 35, 66, 142, 149, 156, 169, 208–209, 213
Gas-liquid chromatography (GLC), 55, 120, 229
Gastric lipase, 54
Gender, 96–97
Glomerular sclerosis, 261
Glucagon, 106, 255
Glucocorticoids, 96
Glucose, 203–204
Glutathione, 284, 289
Glutathione peroxidase, 284, 289
Glycerolipids, 22–25
Glycolysis, 256, 259, 284
Gooseberry oil, 201
Growth regulation, 222
  properties of γ-linolenic acid (GLA), 224
Growth retardation, 43, 227, 234

H

HDL-cholesterol, 176–180
Heparin-binding epidermal growth factor (HB-EGF), 222
Hepatic desaturases, 14–15
Hepatic LDL-receptor mRNA, 182
Hepatocarcinogens, 283
15-HETrE, 120–122, 125–127, 152
High-performance liquid chromatography (HPLC), 8, 120, 149, 220, 275, 295
Histadine residues, 27–29
HMG-CoA reductase, 181, 183
Hops, English, 4
Hydrogen peroxide generation, 286
Hydrolysis, lipase-catalyzed, 35–37
15-hydroxy-dihomo-γ-linolenic acid, 130
5-hydroxy-eicosatetraenoic acid (5-HETE), 121–122, 126
12-hydroxy-eicosatetraenoic acid (12-HETE), 121–122
15-hydroxy-eicosatetraenoic acid (15-HETE), 121–122, 126
13-hydroxyoctadecadienoic acid (13-HODE), 126–127
Hypercholesterolemia, 179
Hyperglycemia, 258
Hyperlipidemia, 2, 30, 85
Hypertension, 54, 176, 189–197, 200, 202–208, 214
   environmental factors in, 190
   genetic factors in, 189–197, 200
Hypertriglyceridemia, 85
Hypocholesterolemic properties
   of linoleic acid (LA), 179
   of γ-linolenic acid (GLA), 175–184
   of plant sterols, 176
Hypotension, 154
Hypotriglyceridemic properties of α-linolenic acid (ALA), 175
Hypoxemia, 142

I

Immune-related diseases, 106–113
Immune response-enhancing properties of γ-linolenic acid (GLA), 84, 106–108, 129–131
Impotence, 273
Indomethacin, 222, 233
Inflammatory injury, 54, 96, 106–112, 129–133, 260
   downregulation of, 158
Inflammatory response syndrome, 137
Inositol/calcium cycle, 274
Inositol triphosphate, 286
Insulin, 106, 255
   correction of Δ6-desaturase inhibition, 256
Insulin-like growth factor-1 (IGF-1), 222
Intercellular communication, 246
Interferon (IFN), 285
Interleukins (IL), 108–112, 129–131, 222, 288
Intestinal cell studies, 85–86, 99
Intimal hyperplasia, 222
Intracellular movement in fatty acid synthesis, 17–19, 45
Intrauterine growth retardation, 43
Ischemic heart disease, 182, 184
Isotope ratio mass spectrometry (IRMS), 66–81
Isozymes, 126

J

Jejunal mucosa, 44
Joint injury, 140

K

Keratitis, 110
Kinases, cyclin-dependent, 286

L

Land's equation, 169
LDL-cholesterol, 179, 182
Leukocytes, 110, 183
Leukotrienes (LT), 106, 108–110, 112, 121–130, 222, 232
   cysteinyl, 146
   defined, 231
   noninflammatory forms, 147
   proinflammatory forms, 125–126, 137–141
   suppressed, 139

synthesis of, 246
zymosan-induced, 219
Lichenification, 111
Liliaceae family, 4
Lingual lipase, 54
Linoleic acid (LA), 1, 6–9, 42, 46, 127, 168–169, 202
  conversion to γ-linolenic acid (GLA), 1–2, 84–99, 106–112, 118, 277
  oxidation response to diabetes, 259
  precursor of arachidonic acid (AA), 140
  research needed on Δ6-desaturase desaturation, 266
α-linolenic acid (ALA), 3–9, 42, 46, 86, 110–112, 168–169, 175–176
  precursor of eicosapentaenoic acid (EPA), 132
γ-linolenic acid (GLA), 1, 6, 106–121, 202
  antiinflammatory properties of, 118, 221
  decreasing docosahexaenoic acid (DHA) levels, 229
  different effects from different oils, 276–277
  in human milk, 67, 228
  increasing arachidonic acid (AA) levels, 229
  metabolism of, 66–105
  non-toxicity demonstrated, 288
  in plasma, 209
  purified, 275
  research needed on elongation mechanism, 266
  synthesis of, 6–7, 22–30
  tumoricidal properties of, 285, 293
γ-linolenoyl-CoA, 261
Linolenoyl-CoA-dependent elongation, 260
Linseed oil, 178–181, 196
Lipase-catalyzed hydrolysis, 35–37
Lipase-catalyzed selective esterification, 37–40
Lipid peroxidation, 278, 284–286, 293
Lipoprotein lipase (LPL), 44, 64
5-lipoxygenase, 153
  inhibition of, 147, 223
15-lipoxygenase, 152, 219
Lipoxygenase (LO) activity, 109, 118–126, 130, 138
  defined, 231
  inhibition of, 108, 121, 286
Lithium-γ-linolenic acid (GLA), 293–301
Liver studies, 14–17, 44, 67–81, 90–98, 157, 176, 209, 213–214, 229–230, 259–260

Locomotor problems, 235
Long-chain polyunsaturated fatty acids (LC-PUFA), 42–49, 66–80, 89–96, 218, 228
  synthesis impaired in diabetes, 255–259, 263
  uptake enhanced by γ-linolenic acid (GLA), 265
Loss of water through skin, 227
Low temperature hydrolysis of fatty acids, 34–40
Lung disease, 137–161
Lymphocytes, 90, 106–113, 131
  in mesenteric lymph, 58–62
Lymphokine activation, 111
Lysophosphatidate acyltransferase, 220
Lysophospholipid reacylation, 220
Lysosomal enzymes, 110, 139

M

Macrophage-derived growth factor (MDGF), 222
Macrophages, 86, 231
  alveolar (AM[PHI]), 138, 145, 149, 153
  peritoneal, 148, 218–224
Malonyl-CoA-dependent elongation, 14–19, 119, 253
Malonyl-CoA synthesis, 260
Mania, 233
Marine oil, 231
Maternal long-chain polyunsaturated fatty acid (LCPUFA) metabolism, 49, 229–240
Mechanism of γ-linolenic acid (GLA) effects, 112–113, 182–184, 214–215
  research needed, 266
Medical claims for γ-linolenic acid (GLA), 305–306, 308–310
Membrane
  CoASH-dependent pathway in, 15–16
  defects, 278
  lipid composition of, 227, 231, 252. See also Placental membrane
  transport across, 208, 214, 227, 233, 261
Methylation, 55
Microbial oils containing γ-linolenic acid (GLA), 4, 10
Microsomes, 14–15, 17, 119, 181, 253
Microvascular permeability, 137, 154
Mitachondria, 92, 99

Mold oil containing γ-linolenic acid (GLA), 4–5, 9–10, 177–179, 182
Monocyte-like cells, 85
Monohydroxy fatty acid, 122
Monosodium urate (MSU), 110
Monounsaturated fatty acids, long-chain, 3, 277
Morris-maze, 235
Multiple sclerosis (MS), 111
Muscle weakness, 273
Myelin, 111

N

Natruresis, 214
Neonate studies, 71–81, 92. See also Fetal and neonate development
Neoplastic diseases, 106
Nephropathy, 273
Nephrotoxicity, 194–195
Nerve conduction, 274–275
  effect of γ-linolenic acid (GLA) on, 262
Neuronal membranes, 274
Neuropathy. See Diabetic, neuropathy
Neuropeptides, 222
Neutrophils, 142, 153, 284
Nitric oxide (NO), 222, 274
Non-steroidal antiinflammatory drugs (NSAID), 96, 110, 131–132, 274
Norepinephrine, 192–193, 202207
Nuclear magnetic resonance (NMR) spectroscopy, 66–81
Nucleic acids, 5
Nutritional supplementation, 305
  in critical care settings, 155
  with eicosapentaenoic acid (EPA), 137
  with γ-linolenic acid (GLA), 2–3, 33, 42, 84–98, 109–113, 121–124, 137–161, 168–173, 189–281

O

Octadecatrienoic acids, 175–184
15-OH-20:3, 219
Oleic acid, 5–6, 9, 46, 177, 202, 257
Oligonucleotides, 26
Olive oil, 109, 124–125, 132, 176
  as vehicle, 191–196
Oxidation, 91–92, 99, 118
β-oxidation, 17, 45, 67, 70
Oxygen radicals, 155, 284

P

Pain sensation, loss of, 273
Palmitic acid, 9, 177, 202
Palm oil, 177–178
Pancreatic lipase, 9, 54, 90
Perilla oil, 262
Peripheral blood mononuclear cell (PBMC) studies, 108, 113, 129, 131
Peritoneal macrophage studies, 86, 111, 218
Permeability, microvascular, 137, 154
Peroxidation, lipid, 278, 284–286, 293
Peroxisomes, 17–18, 99
Phosphatidylcholine (PC), 87–88, 91, 94, 98, 229, 247, 258
Phosphatidylethanolamine (PE), 88, 94, 229–230, 257–258
Phosphatidylinositol (PtdIns), 126, 219, 258, 285
Phosphatidylserine (PS), 258
Phospholipase, 220
Phospholipids (PL), 54, 85–92, 95, 98, 143, 172
  membrane, 154, 253
  plasma, 277
  precursors of, 220
  red blood cell, 139, 248, 277
  serum, 168, 172, 247–248
Photoflagellates, 6
Pinolenic acid, 175, 184
Placental membrane
  fatty acid binding on, 45–49
  fatty acid transport across, 42–45
Plaque, 126
Plasma, lipid composition of, 30, 175–180, 257, 264, 277
Plasma renin, 197
Platelet-derived growth factor (PDGF), 222
Platelets, 85, 129, 132
  aggregation enhanced, 138, 142
  aggregation inhibited, 130, 220
  lipid composition of, 208–209
Polyamines, 284
Polymorphonuclear (PMN) cells, 123–125, 130

Polyunsaturated fatty acids (PUFA), 84, 106–109. See also Long-chain polyunsaturated fatty acids (LCPUFA)
 derived from linoleic acid (LA), 253
 displacing arachidonic acid (AA), 18, 138
 displacing eicosapentaenoic acid (EPA), 160
 membrane effects of, 18, 208, 214
 metabolism of, 201, 212–213
 natural, 1
 in phospholipids, 154–161
Porsolt (forced swimming) test, 235, 238–240
Potassium, in serum, 204, 207
Potassium chloride, 203
Pregnancy factor, 42–49, 229–230
Premenstrual syndrome (PMS), 30, 54, 139
Pro-oxidant tumor therapy, 289
Prostacyclins, 222, 262, 274–276
Prostaglandins (PG), 1, 22–25, 84, 106–112, 118–132, 231–232, 293
 autonomic system effects of, 232–233
 defined, 231
 dienoic, 220
 monoenoic, 220
 noninflammatory forms, 139, 147, 151
 proinflammatory forms, 137–141
 short half-life of, 220
 synthesis of, 172, 175, 183–184, 220, 246
 vasodilatory properties of, 143, 212, 215
 vasoregulating properties of, 231
Prostanoids, 262
 mediation of γ-linolenic acid (GLA) effects, 54
Protein, effect on desaturation, 255
Proteinuria, 261
Protozoa containing γ-linolenic acid (GLA), 6
Psychological stress factors, 195–196
Pulmonary disease, 137–161
Pulmonary vascular resistance (PVR), 142–143, 150

R

Radicals, oxygen, 155, 284
Radiochromatogram assessment, 119
Radio-immunoassay (RIA), 142, 149, 220
Radioisotope assessment, 295
Radiotherapy, 287–289
Radio tracer assessment, 67–71

Ranunculaceae family, 4
Rate-limiting step, 1, 15–16, 42, 54, 67, 84, 112, 218, 282
 bypassing, 266
 inhibition of, 92–96, 106, 111
Red blood cell, lipid composition of, 139, 248, 257, 277
Red currant oil, 201
Regression analysis, 169–172, 194
Regulatory procedures, 306–310
Renal studies, 194–195, 258
Reproductive effects, 227, 237
Retinopathy, 264–265, 273
Rheumatoid arthritis (RA), 2, 110–113, 129–133

S

Safflower oil (SFO), 96, 110, 118, 122–126, 176–181, 194, 200
 as vehicle, 234
Salmonella enteritidis, 151
Salt intake stress, 190, 193–194
Saturated fatty acids, 6, 9–10, 106, 277
Scaly dermatitis, 227
Schizophrenia, 85
γ-scintigraphy, 149–150
Scintillation counter assessment, 295
Scrophulareaceae family, 3
Seed oils containing γ-linolenic acid (GLA), 3, 7–10, 33, 38, 54–64, 106–113, 118–132, 139, 177, 200–201, 205–207, 212–213, 228, 231, 276, 304
Septic shock, 137
Serum cholesteryl arachidonate, 249
Serum lipid composition, 168, 172, 204, 207, 247–248, 265
Sesame oil, 203–213
Sesamin, 183
Signal masking, 70–71, 81
Signal/noise ratio, 69
Signal transduction, 126
Skin
 lichenification, 111
 scaly dermatitis, 227
 ulcerations, 273
Sleep-wake cycles, 232, 235
Smoking, 200

Smooth muscle cell (SMC) proliferation, 220–224
Social isolation stress factor, 190–194
Sodium
 in plasma, 207
 reabsorption of, 215
Sodium carbonate, 39–40
Solid phase extraction, 220
Sources of γ-linolenic acid (GLA), 2–10, 54, 130. See also Seed oils
Soybean oil (SBO), 109, 176–179
Soybean protein, 178–179, 262
Spirulina, 22–30
Spleen cell studies, 109
Stearic acid, 202
Stearidonic acid (SDA), 3, 9, 38, 86
Stereospecificity
 of desaturase reactions, 14–15
 of fatty acids, 54–55, 89–90
 of γ-linolenic acid (GLA), 9–10
Steroid excretion, 181–182
Sterol synthesis, 183
Stress, 84, 96, 190–191, 200, 233
Stress management, 189
Stroop color-word conflict task, 194–195, 233
Sunflower oil, 92, 181, 193–196, 275
Superoxide anion generation, 286
Superoxide dismutase (SOD), 108, 284–289
Synovitis, 130, 133

T

Terminal desaturase protein, 256
Therapeutic claims for γ-linolenic acid (GLA), 305–306, 306, 308–310
Thin-layer chromatography (TLC), 35, 55, 156, 229
Thromboxanes (TX), 1, 84, 129, 231
 defined, 231
 in platelets, 262
 suppression of, 143, 153
Thykaloid membranes, 22, 25
Thyroxin, 106
T-lymphocytes, 261
Toxicity of natural oils, possible, 277
Transcapillary fluid flux, 150
Trans fatty acids, 47–48

Transforming growth factor-B (TGF-B), 222
Triacylglycerols (TG), 8–10, 54–57, 85–99
 containing essential fatty acids (EFA), 227, 258
 in serum, 265
Trienoic acids, 14
Tri-γ-linolenic acid (tri-GLA), 275
Triglycerides, 9, 30, 84–85, 203, 206
 in plasma, 30, 277
 in serum, 168, 204, 207
Tumor cells
 access to, 289
 metabolism of, 284, 300
Tumor necrosis factor (TNF), 109, 112, 129, 139, 285
Tumor necrosis factor-α (TNF-α), 222

U

Unsaturated pyrrolidizine alkaloids (UPA), 3

V

Vascular lesions, 264
Vascular lipid studies, 208–215
Vascular reactivity, 138–143, 140, 192, 200–202, 205, 208, 214, 220, 276
Vascular resistivity, 196–197
Verapamil, 205, 207–208
Visual acuity, altered thresholds of, 227
Vitamins, 108, 129, 133, 156, 284, 286
VLDL-cholesterol, 176, 180, 182

Y

Yeast, 25, 26

Z

Zellweger's disease, 17
Zinc
 co-factor in desaturation, 93, 95
 deficiency in, 93–95